Fatigue as a Window to the Brain

Issues in Clinical and Cognitive Neuropsychology
Jordan Grafman, series editor

Fatigue as a Window to the Brain

edited by John DeLuca

A Bradford Book
The MIT Press
Cambridge, Massachusetts
London, England

MIT Press books may be purchased at special quantity discounts for business or sales promotional use. For information, please email special_sales@mitpress.mit.edu or write to Special Sales Department, The MIT Press, 5 Cambridge Center, Cambridge, MA 02142.

This book was set in Stone serif and Stone sans by SNP Best-set Typesetter Ltd., Hong Kong. Printed and bound in the United States of America.

Library of Congress Cataloging-in-Publication Data

Fatigue as a window to the brain / edited by John DeLuca ; foreword by Simon Wessely.
    p. ; cm.—(Issues in clinical and cognitive neuropsychology)
"A Bradford book."
Includes bibliographical references and index.
ISBN 0-262-04227-4 (hc : alk. paper)
1. Fatigue. 2. Neurophysiology. I. DeLuca, John, 1956– II. Series.
[DNLM: 1. Fatigue—physiopathology. 2. Fatigue—etiology. 3. Fatigue—psychology. WB 146 F253 2005]
QP421.F38   2005
612.8′23—dc22
                                                                                        2004062102

Printed on recycled paper.

10 9 8 7 6 5 4 3 2 1

To my children, Jessica, Danielle, and Robbie, who inspire me to achieve and be the best I can be

Contents

Foreword

Fatigue has always been an elusive creature. Poets write about it, newspapers argue about it, patients suffer from it, and scientists occasionally study it. This book represents a substantial, and coherent, attempt to at least partly overcome the neglect, but it is worth spending a moment considering why the subject has never received the serious professional attention it deserves.

There are probably two main reasons for this. First, as several contributors to this book acknowledge, fatigue is difficult to define and measure. While the electrophysiologic fatigue of the myasthenic synapse revealed its secrets to neurophysiologists over a century ago, no such progress was made in measuring the far more common problem of subjective fatigue, although this was not for want of trying (Muscio, 1921). Fatigue, like pain, remains a private experience, which can be measured only at second hand. There will never be an objective fatigue test, in the sense that thyroid function has objective measures, independent of patient experience. There will never be a substitute for the ancient art of talking to patients, either directly as part of the clinical encounter, or indirectly through increasingly impersonal but more reliable questionnaires (Dittner, Brown, & Wessely, 2004). As medicine becomes ever more technological and distanced from the bedside, fatigue has not been a fertile topic for those aiming for the glittering research prizes. Neither I nor the authors of this book share this perspective, but regrettably fatigue studies have so far not figured high on any research funding agenda.

The second reason is that fatigue is unfortunately not a very discriminative symptom for the busy clinician. Doctors afford more attention and respect to symptoms that provide useful diagnostic information, which is arguably their first and most important function—determining what is wrong with the patient. Hence, medical students are taught to pay close attention to symptoms such as hemoptysis, the presence of which indicates a short and usually serious differential diagnosis. Alternatively, the belief that your limbs are controlled by special rays broadcast from your television is equally important for a psychiatric differential diagnosis.

All of this is in marked contrast to the complaint of fatigue. The patient complaining of fatigue could be suffering from nearly any condition listed in a joint edition of the *Oxford Textbooks of Medicine and Psychiatry*. Establishing a complaint of fatigue, thus, barely advances the diagnostic process. More questioning, investigations, and of course, time are needed. This problem is evident even in this book, which includes contributions of a wide range of physical and psychological disorders, though many more could have been included, all strongly associated with fatigue. Human immunodeficiency virus (HIV), cancer, brain injury, lupus, and depression are all appropriately included, but perhaps only limited space prohibited the editor from requesting contributions on pulmonary disease (Breslin, van der Schans, Breukink, et al., 1998), hepatitis C (Wessely & Pariante, 2002) or other hepatic conditions (Kumar, 2002), renal disease (Brunier & Graydon, 1993), and many more. Fatigue is, therefore, the opposite of pathognomic, and hence unlikely to figure largely in medical curricula or multiple choice examinations.

Yet for the patient, fatigue is a vitally important symptom. Not just a source of discomfort in its own right, it can also be associated with sometimes profound disruption of physical and mental function, with the corresponding impact on quality of life.

Psychiatric epidemiologist Bruce Dohrenwend, in his classic midtown Manhattan study, asked professionals and laypeople alike to rate the importance they ascribed to symptoms. Easily the most discrepancy occurred with the complaint of fatigue. "Feeling weak all over for much of the time" was regarded as "very serious" by only 6 percent of psychiatrists and 9 percent of physicians, making it one of the least important of 43 listed symptoms (Dohrenwend & Crandell, 1970). In contrast, the same symptom was listed as one of the most important by nonprofessional samples (Dohrenwend & Crandell, 1970).

Another surprising finding, which does little to increase doctors' interest in fatigue, is that the mechanisms underlying fatigue show considerable overlap between the discrete diagnostic entities. Poor sleep, integral to many disorders, is strongly associated with fatigue across the diagnostic spectrum. Depression, regardless of its cause, is always associated with reduced energy levels. Certain emotional reactions, such as catastrophizing, predict greater fatigue and disability in conditions as diverse as cancer, low back pain, and chronic fatigue syndrome, and probably in other diagnoses as well when someone bothers to look. Lack of exercise is likewise always associated with fatigue.

For this reason, successful treatments are similarly broad based. If lack of exercise is correlated with fatigue in many disorders, it is not surprising that as Lange and colleagues (chapter 18) show, graded exercise effectively alleviates the fatigue found in numerous conditions. Likewise, cognitive behavioral therapy (CBT) is almost always effective.

This information should, and does in the hands of DeLuca and his colleagues, help counter some myths surrounding the treatment of fatigue and fatigue conditions. The book's numerous comparisons between conditions and across the medical/psychiatric divide help demystify interventions that are needlessly stigmatized as "psychiatric" (such as CBT) or considered dangerous or risky (such as graded exercise). Instead, we discuss them as what they are—useful adjunct treatments for disorders of impeccable physical origin (cancer, HIV, rheumatoid, multiple sclerosis) as well as for those whose origins remain obscure, such as chronic fatigue syndrome (CFS) or fibromyalgia (Sharpe, 1997).

Treatment does not necessarily depend on an exact knowledge of the cause of chronic fatigue, only on understanding why it has not gone away. DeLuca, in his final contribution (chapter 19), makes a powerful case to label this chronic condition "secondary fatigue." To date, we have made more progress in treating this "secondary" fatigue than the primary causes. But at least we have made progress.

But what do we now know about the mechanisms of fatigue and fatigability? The central message of this book is, pun intended, that fatigue is predominantly of central origin. Far and away the most promising biological approaches are neurobiological. And we can go further. For me, the most exciting recent developments in our conceptual understanding of fatigue come from the increasing emphasis on the sense of effort. As the editor's own elegant contributions confirm (chapters 3 and 9), patients who suffer from the quintessential fatigue condition, CFS, report greater cognitive effort and more cognitive impairment than is detectable on objective assessment. Put another way, CFS is a disorder of effort perception, both physical and mental. Patients require additional central resources to produce the same amount of mental work (as well as physical work) as neuroimaging is starting to demonstrate (chapter 9). Dedra Buchwald's influential and impressive research group have recently extended these observations to the question of sleep disturbance and CFS as well (Watson et al., 2003). We are at last moving away from fruitless attempts to show structural lesions in the central nervous system to studies of the actual impairment in CFS—the dynamics of physical and mental effort.

Any book on chronic fatigue and its syndromes must sooner or later engage with psychiatry. Actually a few books pointedly do not, while in the United Kingdom an Internet and political campaign is currently underway to promote more research into CFS, a laudable aim, but under the banner of ABP—"anything but psychiatry." Something equally short-sighted is also taking place in one or two quasi-official circles in the United States, among people who ought to know better. Such intolerance will only hamper knowledge and increase the stigma, for psychiatry is like Banquo's ghost at Macbeth's dinner party—an unwelcome guest whose influence is most keenly felt by those who desire it the least. Thankfully, but not surprisingly, DeLuca and colleagues have no truck with such intolerance, preferring to engage with modern psychiatric research and the insights it provides.

Yet, if only the blinkered continue to deny any role for psychiatry in our understanding of chronic fatigue, even the most farsighted have considerable difficulty determining exactly how psychiatry does interact with chronic fatigue. It is also true that those of us who specialize in psychiatry do not make things easier for our colleagues with our own systems of classification. For example, some commentators continue to see somatization as the new harbor for fatigue, but it is a harbor few wish to enter, not just those suffering from the complaint (Mayou, 2003). As Escobar (chapter 11) shows in his contribution, symptom counting alone is certainly simple and reproducible, but replete with difficulties and ambiguities. It is at least better than hysteria, although that is not saying much (Wessely, 2001). "Medically unexplained symptoms" seems a better description; it is intellectually less taxing and carries less baggage but is likely to be only a temporary staging post.

It is left to one of the foremost historians of psychiatry, Edward Shorter (chapter 8), to make perhaps the most subversive contribution to the book. He draws attention to the strange disappearance of fatigue syndromes and synonyms from the psychiatric lexicon in the mid-twentieth century. From its central position in psychiatric thinking, it declined precipitously, and was finally booted out of the new bible of PC (psychiatric correctness), the DSM (*Diagnostic and Statistical Manual of Mental Disorders*).

As Shorter perceptively points out, the ejection of fatigue syndromes from psychiatric classification paradoxically corresponds with its reintroduction into popular culture. Fatigue syndromes such as chronic brucellosis, hypoglycemia, effort syndrome, and most of all, neurasthenia disappeared from professional discourse in the mid-twentieth century. They were replaced by psychologization as fatigue was subsumed under depression and anxiety. Neurasthenia is not found in the new psychiatric bibles, but descriptions of the new depressive disorders emphasize the familiar fatigue and fatigability. This was never likely to find universal favor, however, especially with some sections of the public. Ejected from psychiatry, where were the new fatigue syndromes going to find a home? The sudden interest in chronic Epstein-Barr virus infection in the 1980s, with its high watermark being the 1988 CDC case definition (Holmes, Kaplan, Gantz, et al., 1988) represented an attempt to place fatigue syndromes under infectious diseases or immunology, but after two decades, the commentators, editorialists, and textbook contributors in those disciplines remain to be convinced. At the time of this writing, some vigorous efforts are being made to claim fatigue syndromes for neurology. This would be commendable if it took the broad approach embracing neuropsychiatry and neuropsychology epitomized by this volume. However, as those advancing this cause most often define neurology narrowly as the study of muscle and nerve, this approach is no more likely to be successful than it was in Victorian times (Wessely, Hotopf, & Sharpe, 1998).

So have we progressed in our conceptualization and classification of the fatigue syndromes? Shorter clearly invites us to answer in the negative. And this situation is unlikely to change. The rapid rise of powerful lobby groups and the politics of PC means that fatigue is not likely to return to psychiatry, at least in its old form. The evidence for reintroducing at least one fatigue diagnosis or syndrome into Western psychiatry may be strong, but its chances of happening are remote. Neither the American Psychiatric Association, owners of the DSM, nor the World Health Organization (WHO), creators of the quixotic International Classification of Diseases, show any inclination to enter the bear pit, and who can blame them?

So why then does fatigue continue to pose such problems, albeit fascinating problems, for medical science? To answer that question, we need to return to history. We are probably now in a transition period in conceptualizing fatigue in general and symptoms in particular. We are somewhere between the medicine of symptoms (description), which we have largely left behind, and the medicine of mechanisms (molecular pathology), which we aspire to but have not reached. Until the nineteenth century, chronic fatigue could not be a problem because symptom and disease were synonymous. The diagnosis of a patient with a fever was fever, and likewise for fatigue. Then along came the scientific revolution of the nineteenth century, the great German physiologists and pathologists, and the dawn of genuine understanding of pathological processes. From then on, the symptom was only a guide to the diagnosis. A patient would be fatigued, but the real problem was a dysfunction of the thyroid gland, or a lack of red blood cells. Once that problem was identified, the symptom of fatigue ceased to have much significance; scientific and therapeutic attention would now be focused on understanding and rectifying the pathology, be it endocrine, neoplastic, hematological, or whatever.

This understanding of health and disease is fine for those whose symptoms correspond with a known pathological process. For them, medicine is indeed, as medical historian Roy Porter once put it, "the Greatest Benefit to Mankind," speaking for once without irony. If you are sick with medically explained illness, in the "double plus" box in table F.1, then your relationship with your doctor, and the roles each of your play are fine. The patient is sick and the doctors agree and validate that experience. They have a reasonable understanding of why the patient is sick, even when they cannot do much about it. At the other end of the spectrum, being in the "double negative" box (Health) is also unproblematic—the person feels well and the doctors, if asked, will agree that he or she is free from disease.

Problems arise with those in the disease present but symptoms absent box. These people feel well, but are either about to get sick or carrying a disease of which they

		Symptom	
		Present +	Absent −
Disease as accepted by doctors in 2004	Present +	Medically explained illness	Prodromal, asymptomatic, latent, etc.
	Absent −	Medically unexplained illness	Health

are unaware. These are the targets of screening programs. In this genomic age, more and more people are likely to find themselves in this box, with often profound consequences, but that is another story.

The most serious problems arise among those who have symptoms but contemporary medical opinion believes to be disease free—the current jargon term being "medically unexplained" illness. It is here that we find the fatigue syndromes. Patients in this box pose a real dilemma for doctors and patients alike. Doctors still, despite the increased understanding this book so ably demonstrates, still feel uneasy with this group, while sufferers definitely feel short-changed and stigmatized.

There are many answers to this dilemma. For some, CFS already belongs in the double plus box, as a disease with a known pathology. Medical authorities have simply failed to recognize the evidence that already exists because they are ignorant, stupid, or corrupt. An Internet trawl will reveal examples of all these charges. However, as this book also demonstrates, many professionals are interested in fatigue who are neither stupid, ignorant, nor corrupt but have still to crack the conundrum.

We are not there yet, but what this volume does show is the real progress that has been made in understanding fatigue, even if classification has yet to catch up. DeLuca and his colleagues have produced what is the best multiauthor book yet on the subject of fatigue in medicine and psychiatry. I congratulate all the contributors, and commend their efforts to the reader.

—Simon Wessely

References

Breslin, E., van der Schans, C., Breukink, S., et al. (1998). Perception of fatigue and quality of life in patients with COPD. *Chest, 114,* 958–964.

Brunier, G., & Graydon, J. (1993). The influence of physical activity on fatigue in patients with ESRD on hemodialysis. *ANNAJ, 20,* 457–461.

Dittner, A., Brown, R., & Wessely, S. (2004). The assessment of fatigue: A practical guide to clinicians and researchers. *Journal of Psychosomatic Research, 56,* 157–170.

Dohrenwend, B., & Crandell, D. (1970). Psychiatric symptoms in community, clinic and mental hospital groups. *American Journal of Psychiatry*, *126*, 1611–1621.

Holmes, G., Kaplan, J., Gantz, N., et al. (1988). Chronic fatigue syndrome: A working case definition. *Annals of Internal Medicine*, *108*, 387–389.

Kumar, D. T. R. (2002). Fatigue in cholestatic liver disease—a perplexing symptom. *Postgraduate Medical Journal*, *78*, 404–407.

Mayou, R. (2003). Towards DSM-V: Replacing the somatoform section. *Journal of Psychosomatic Research*, *52*, 363.

Muscio, B. (1921). Is a fatigue test possible? *British Journal of Psychology*, *12*, 31–46.

Sharpe, M. (1997). Cognitive behavior therapy for functional somatic complaints: The example of chronic fatigue syndrome. *Psychosomatics*, *38*, 356–362.

Watson, N. F. J. C., Goldberg, J., Kapur, V., & Buchwald, D. (2003). Comparison of objective and subjective sleepiness in monozygotic twins discordant for chronic fatigue syndrome. *Sleep*, *26*, A359.

Wessely, S. (2001). What are the classifications of hysteria and why don't clinicians use them? In P. Halligan & C. Bass, eds. *Conversion hysteria*, pp. 63–72. Oxford: Oxford University Press.

Wessely, S., Hotopf, M., & Sharpe, M. (1998). *Chronic fatigue and its syndromes*. Oxford: Oxford University Press.

Wessely, S., & Pariante, C. (2002). Fatigue, depression and chronic hepatitis C infection. *Psychological Medicine*, *32*, 1–16.

Preface

After many years of working with issues related to fatigue both clinically and in research, it has became clear how little we have progressed in our theoretical and applied understanding of fatigue and its impact on persons' lives. Even its definition was ubiquitous, unclear, and equivocal. How could we feel we could treat a symptom without a clear understanding of what it is? Some see the presence of fatigue as a major symptom of a psychiatric illness, while others see it as the result of damage to the brain. Still others view fatigue not as a symptom but as an illness. What do we really know about fatigue? Today, we face the same questions first asked after more than 100 years of scientific inquiry.

This book can by no means address the varied and broad questions we need answered regarding the enigma of fatigue. Rather the purpose of this book is specific: to answer the question what does the presence of fatigue tell us about how the brain works? More specifically, what are the neural mechanisms associated with fatigue? Experts from a wide variety of conditions that result in fatigue have shared what they know about fatigue and the brain. We hope that bringing such experts together in a single volume will uncover some pattern(s) to form hypotheses that can drive future research in our quest to understand the underlying causes of fatigue.

This book is divided into six parts. The first part discusses the nature of fatigue. It includes a chapter on the history of fatigue and its epidemiology. A second chapter presents information on assessing and measuring fatigue. The final chapter in this section discusses the issue of cognitive fatigue, its measurement and interpretation.

Part II discusses specific neurological conditions that produce fatigue as a symptom. It includes chapters on multiple sclerosis, stroke, traumatic brain injury, and a more general chapter on other neurological conditions such as Parkinson's disease, dementia, and Lyme's disease.

Part III covers psychiatric conditions in which fatigue is a major symptom. Beginning with a historical overview of fatigue in psychiatry, this section presents chapters on chronic fatigue syndrome, depression, and somatization.

Part IV includes chapters on general medical conditions in which fatigue is a major symptom. These include HIV, sleep disorders, heart disease and cardiovascular dysfunction, autoimmune disorders such as systemic lupus erythematosus, and cancer. A chapter on the emerging field of psychoneuroimmunology and fatigue is also provided.

Part V consists of a single chapter on the treatment of fatigue. While individual chapters in sections III and IV also include information on treatment specific to particular disorders, this chapter provides a broad overview of treatment approaches to fatigue.

Finally, part VI attempts to integrate what has been learned from the previous chapters. The goal of this final chapter is to provide an overall definition of fatigue, explore the brain mechanism that appears to be responsible for "primary" fatigue, and suggest future research and investigation.

I have several people to thank for making this book a reality. I would like to thank George Prigatano, who first suggested that I write a book on the topic of fatigue. I would also like to thank Jordan Grafman, whose initial excitement about this project gave me the impetus to forge ahead. I thank Sara Meirowitz, my associate editor, for her patience and guidance throughout this process. Last, I thank all of the authors whos contributions turned an idea into a reality.

I also wish to recognize and thank the following individuals who served as external reviewers for the manuscripts submitted for this book: Susan Johnson, Wilfred Van Gorp, Carol Armstrong, Nicholas Ponzio, Nancy Chiaravalloti, Gudrun Lange, Anthony Komaroff, and Benjamin Natelson. I am especially grateful to Simon Wessely, for his encouragement, suggestions, chapter reviews, time, and effort in helping me through this project. His attention and thoughtfulness provided the enthusiasm for me to persevere. Finally, I would like to thank Natasha Smith-Dargan and Violeta Gomez for secretarial support throughout the project.

I The Nature of Fatigue

1   What Is Fatigue? History and Epidemiology

Susan Torres-Harding and Leonard A. Jason

Fatigue is a nonspecific symptom because it can be indicative of many causes or conditions including physiological states such as sleep deprivation or excessive muscular activity; medical conditions such as chronic inflammatory conditions, bacterial or viral infections, or autoimmune illnesses; and psychiatric disorders such as major depression, anxiety disorders, and somatoform disorders (Manu, Lane, & Matthews, 1992). Fatigue may be caused by prescription medications such as antihistamines, drugs prescribed for insomnia, or chemotherapy drugs. Fatigue may also result from unhealthy lifestyles, such as frequent disruptions in the wake-sleep cycle, excessive alcohol or caffeine intake, and psychosocial stressors, or from the delayed effects of traumatic events (Manu et al., 1992). Finally, fatigue may be "unexplained," when none of the above causes is present or the causes cannot be determined. Chronic fatigue syndrome has recently received considerable attention, and it is an illness characterized by unexplained severe, persistent, disabling fatigue (Fukuda et al., 1994).

Some describe fatigue in terms of physiological data or "objective" observations of decreasing muscle performance or decrements in work or performance. For example, fatigue has been defined as a failure to maintain a required force or output of power during sustained or repeated muscle contraction (Stokes, Cooper, & Edwards, 1988) or as time-related deterioration in the ability to perform certain mental tasks (Broadbent, 1971). In contrast to physiological fatigue, some have defined fatigue as a subjective self-reported feeling of fatigue. This feeling of fatigue is what people generally report when they seek medical treatment (Berrios, 1990). Fatigue is sometimes defined as "tiredness," feeling tired, being fatigued, feeling weak in part of the body, tired or lacking in energy, or experiencing "everything [as] an effort" (Cope, 1992, p. 273). Physiological definitions are more easily measured, but the subjective feeling of fatigue is not directly observable (Berrios, 1990). Further, this feeling of fatigue does not always correspond directly with physiological manifestations (Berrios, 1990).

In response to its complex nature, most measures of fatigue have moved away from single questions (i.e., "Do you feel tired?") to a more multidimensional approach. These measures assess the effect of fatigue on daily activities, mental and physical aspects of fatigue, and other characteristics and related symptoms (Barofsky & West Legro, 1991; Chalder et al., 1993; Cope, 1992). Fatigue has also been described in terms of level of severity, level of impairment, physiological and psychological characteristics (physical vs. mental), and duration (Barofsky & West Legro, 1991; Cope, 1992). Whereas some researchers have proposed a categorical classification (i.e., absence or presence of fatigue), several research studies suggest that fatigue is best conceptualized on a continuum (Berrios, 1990; Loge et al., 1998; Pawlikowska et al., 1994; Wessely, 1998), with its variability reflecting degrees of severity (Pawlikowska et al., 1994). Despite these more recent attempts to compartmentalize fatigue, the major problem with such measures is their subjectivity.

Historical Perspectives

There has been considerable controversy over both what constitutes and what causes fatigue since the mid-nineteenth century (Wessely, 1991). By the mid-1800s, reports of upper-class women who were too weak to rise from bed were being reported frequently (Shorter, 1993). These women predominantly complained of fatigue and muscle weakness, but pain was often a prominent symptom as well. George Beard, an American neurologist, was one of the first to describe neurasthenia as a distinct clinical entity (Macmillan, 1976). The symptoms of neurasthenia included "general malaise, debility of all function, poor appetite, fugitive neuralgic pains, hysteria, insomnia, hypochondriases, disinclination for consecutive mental labor, severe and weakening attacks of headaches, and other symptoms" (Macmillan, 1976).

By 1900, neurasthenia had become the single most common diagnosis in the domain of neuropathology and psychopathology. Before 1900, however, chronic unexplained fatigue was rarely distinguished from depression (Shorter, 1993). Neurasthenia appeared to be a "wastebasket" category, used alternately as a synonym for general nervousness and evolving psychosis, as the "male" equivalent of hysteria, as a synonym for minor depression, and as a diagnosis of fatigue states in patients who were not depressed (Shorter, 1993). Physicians before 1900 had difficulty distinguishing psychogenic from neurogenic weakness. When they described "exhausted" patients, it is unclear if the problems were due to subjective perceptions of fatigue or an objective dysfunction of the muscles (Shorter, 1993). Further, when persons were described as being too exhausted to rise from bed, it was unclear whether they were simply too tired or suffered from a neurological or medical disorder (Shorter, 1993). These complaints echo contemporary descriptions of unexplained fatigue illness.

The diagnosis of neurasthenia began to fall out of use in the early 1900s, as the conceptualization of this illness shifted from physiological to psychogenic or psychological in origin (Wessely, 1991). Redefined as psychiatric, neurasthenia was less frequently diagnosed because of the stigma of psychiatric labels (Wessely, 1991).

Further, the illness was diagnosed less frequently as more working class people began to suffer from it, and it began to fade from neurological textbooks (Wessely, 1991). Within the psychiatric domain, it was subdivided into various neuroses, including obsessive-compulsive disorders, anxiety neuroses, and hysteria (Wessely, 1991). However, the diagnosis of neurasthenia is still included in the latest revision of the International Classification of Diseases, Tenth Revision (World Health Organization, 1992), and continues to be diagnosed in parts of Europe, the former Soviet Union states, and parts of Asia, where it is considered a physical disorder (Wessely, 1991).

In addition to neurasthenia, other illnesses with unexplained fatigue as a primary symptom were reported in the late nineteenth and early twentieth century. These illnesses were alternately termed effort syndrome, DaCosta's syndrome, irritable heart, disordered action of the heart, soldier's heart, and neurocirculatory asthenia. Irritable heart was noticed in the Crimean war, and later in the American Civil War (Hyams, Wignall, & Roswell, 1996). Its symptoms included diarrhea, rapid pulse, palpitation, shortness of breath, headaches, giddiness, disturbed sleep, itching skin, excessive perspiration, and indigestion. DaCosta attributed the syndrome to fevers, diarrhea, hard field service, wounds, rheumatism, scurvy, and other factors. This illness was seen as organic in origin. DaCosta believed the heart became irritable from overaction and was sustained in this state by disordered innervation (DaCosta, 1871).

During the First World War, Lewis first described effort syndrome. Its symptoms included breathlessness, cyanosis, pain, palpitation, fainting, giddiness, headaches, especially after exertion, and complaints of fatigue. Infection was considered to be a dominant factor in the etiology, as Lewis noted that approximately 32 percent of the cases he studied began with an infectious disease (Bartley & Chute, 1947). In 1918, a group of military doctors termed similar cases "neurocirculatory asthenia" (Ivy & Roth, 1944).

Initially, DaCosta's syndrome or irritable heart, Lewis's effort syndrome, and neurocirculatory asthenia were regarded as arising from anomalies of cardiac function. Over time, however, as efforts to find underlying physiological abnormalities were not successful, these illnesses began to be regarded as primarily psychosomatic or psychogenic. For example, some researchers held that these illness states were due primarily to the emotional reaction of the patient to misinterpretation of symptoms arising from effort (Ivy & Roth, 1944), fundamental nervous instability (Robey & Boas, 1918), or the effects of hyperventilation (Bartley & Chute, 1947). After World War II, a set of influential clinical studies by Paul Wood helped shift the conceptualization of effort syndromes from medical illness to psychoneuroses (Hyams, Wignall, & Roswell, 1996).

Thus, the diagnoses of neurasthenia and such illnesses as neurocirculatory asthenia fell out of favor during the early twentieth century, as they were increasingly seen as psychogenic. However, it is notable that fatigue and chronic fatigue continued to be described as symptoms in the research literature (Bartley & Chute, 1947). Some physicians felt that chronic fatigue was due primarily to psychogenic or psychological factors; for example, Kepler (1942) described chronic fatigue as an outcome of the Western way of life, best thought of as a "psychologic" disease of the "intelligentsia." Alvarez (1941) listed as the most common causes of chronic fatigue overwork neuroses, postinfective neurosis, neurosis associated with arthritis or fibrositis, nervous breakdown, constitutional inadequacy, cerebral thrombosis, equivalents of insanity, and actual insanity.

Other physicians espoused a holistic approach, emphasizing the need to take into account both possible organic or physical factors, such as disease or overwork, and psychogenic or personality factors (Muncie, 1941; Wharton, 1938). For example, Wharton (1938) described patients with fatigue that was not relieved by average rest and whose symptoms appeared to be related to mental or physical depletion or both. He attributed this excessive fatigue primarily to overwork. Muncie (1941) noted that, though fatigue was among the complaints in nearly all important diseases, it was most prominent among endocrine-metabolic disorders, postinfectious states, and emotional and attitudinal states or personality maladjustment. Finally, Allen (1944) analyzed 300 cases in which the chief complaint was weakness or fatigue. Nervous conditions were considered responsible in 80 percent, and physical disorders accounted for 20 percent of the cases. These physical disorders included diabetes, heart disease, chronic infection, nephritis, anemia, and various neurological disorders.

Industrial Fatigue
Another area of research concerned the problem of industrial or occupational fatigue. In the early part of the twentieth century, attention focused on the experience and physiology of fatigue as it affected workers' productivity. To this end, Harvard University's Graduate School of Business set up a Fatigue Laboratory in 1927, where investigators continued research into various aspects of fatigue until 1947 (Chapman, 1990). Because worker fatigue impaired performance, a scientific and systematic study of fatigue was encouraged (Chapman, 1990). Henderson, one of the laboratory's founders, noted that "business leaders, engineers, physiologists, and the general public" all agreed fatigue was important, but found no agreement on its definition (Chapman, 1990). The purpose of the Fatigue Laboratory was therefore to describe the physiological experiences of fatigue in everyday life, and the scope of the studies extended beyond industrial fatigue to encompass exercise physiology and medical applications (Chapman, 1990). Industrial fatigue studies included investigations into muscular exercise and fatigue, resting conditions, and adaptations to physical stress. Some studies indicated that the rest cure, or enforced complete bedrest prescription, was actually contraindicated; physical exercise was considered an important therapeutic measure (Chapman, 1990).

Ward (1941) noted in his study of 600 male and 1200 female workers that 4 percent were chronically fatigued. Many complained of feeling tired, and most also complained of back pain, loss of appetite, and insomnia, and were prone to irritability. Physical findings were increased pulse rate, low blood pressure, pallor, tremor, and weight loss. Ward concluded that anyone who works beyond 100 percent of his capacity is bound to develop fatigue-related symptoms, and overwork was a primary cause of chronic fatigue. Collier (1943) also recognized the hazards of chronic fatigue and noted that fatigue arising from overwork could lead to disease. Interestingly, although overwork was seen as a major contributor to chronic industrial fatigue, researchers such as Collier (1943) also emphasized the importance of psychological factors in industrial or occupational fatigue. Nearly all of the everyday problems of industrial fatigue, Collier noted, were psychological rather than physical (Collier, 1943).

Outbreaks of Fatigue Illnesses

During the twentieth century, several outbreaks of illnesses with fatigue of unknown etiology as a chief or principal symptom were also reported (Wessely, 1991; Levine, 1994). These unexplained fatigue illnesses were variously labeled epidemic neuromyasthenia, myalgic encephalomyelitis, Iceland disease, and atypical poliomyelitis. A major outbreak occurred in 1955 among the nursing and medical staff at the Royal Free Hospital in England (Wessely, 1991). Termed myalgic encephalomyelitis, the illness' symptoms included fatigue and muscle pain as well as other neurological signs (Shorter, 1993). Another outbreak of a severe fatigue illness, atypical poliomyelitis, occurred at the Los Angeles County Hospital in 1934 (Wessely, 1991).

Levine (1994) describes several outbreaks of epidemic neuromyasthenia, another fatigue illness of unknown etiology with fatigue as a principal symptom that often encompassed neurological symptoms and signs. Outbreaks were reported in northern England (1955) among 233 males and females; in a private medical facility near Washington, D.C. (1953); and in Ridgefield, Connecticut (1955–1956), at a small medical research facility and neighboring community. Finally, in Lake Tahoe, Nevada, and the surrounding communities (1984–1986), an outbreak of 184 cases of a severe fatigue illness occurred. The symptoms of the Lake Tahoe outbreak included prolonged fatigue, abrupt onset of symptoms, severe pain, and prominent cognitive disorder (Levine, 1994).

Contemporary Investigations into Fatigue

Interest in fatigue was renewed in the late 1980s with the emergence of chronic Epstein-Barr virus syndrome. This syndrome explained chronic fatigue as a persistent viral illness caused by the same pathogen responsible for acute mononucleosis (Friedberg & Jason, 1998). Later renamed chronic fatigue syndrome, or CFS (Wessely,

1998), the syndrome's criteria were developed in 1988 (Holmes et al., 1988), and later refined in 1994 (Fukuda et al., 1994). The 1994 criteria for CFS include severe, disabling fatigue lasting 6 months or more. The illness also requires four of eight additional symptoms: sore throat, headaches, lymph node tenderness or pain, joint pain, muscle pain, unrefreshing sleep, postexertional malaise, and memory or concentration difficulties. Finally, for a diagnosis of CFS, the fatigue must be "unexplained," that is, not better accounted for by another medical or psychiatric condition (Fukuda et al., 1994).

Unexplained chronic fatigue has also been diagnosed as myalgic encephalomyelitis, ME (Wessely, 1991). The criteria for ME include fatigue after minimal exertion and delayed recovery of muscle power after exertion; symptoms of circulatory impairment; and central nervous system involvement (cerebral problems). These symptoms often have a chronic, fluctuating course (Ramsay, 1988).

Fatigue has been a frequent reason for visits to physicians (Nelson et al., 1987), and the chief complaint in 4 to 9 percent of all visits to a family practitioner or internist (Manu, Lane, & Matthews, 1992). Studies of people presenting with fatigue in primary care settings show an estimated 7.6 to 32 percent of these patients have fatigue as either a symptom or chief complaint (Cathebras et al., 1992; Fuhrer & Wessely, 1995; Kroenke, Wood, Mangelsdorff, Meier, & Powell, 1988). Further, excessive fatigue affects a significant proportion of the general population. It has been noted to be a common symptom in both community-based studies (Cope, 1992; Pawlikowska et al., 1994) and primary care and hospital-based studies of fatigue prevalence (Fuhrer & Wessely, 1995; Cope, 1992). Fatigue can also have a powerful, adverse effect on quality of life (Nelson et al., 1987).

The problem of chronic fatigue has also received considerable attention. Typically defined as excessive fatigue lasting more than 6 months (Fukuda et al., 1994), chronic fatigue is considered more severe and disabling then acute fatigue because of its persistent, chronic course (Fukuda et al., 1994). Chronic fatigue is estimated to occur in approximately 4 to 5 percent of the general population (Jason, Jordan et al., 1999).

Gender and Fatigue

Many studies have examined the role of gender in fatigue. Some studies have found gender differences in fatigue, with women more likely to report having both fatigue and chronic fatigue (Chen, 1986; Nelson et al., 1987; Loge et al., 1998; Nisenbaum et al., 1998; Jason, Jordan et al., 1988). Some researchers have also found that women tend to report more severe fatigue (Chen, 1986; Kroenke et al., 1988; Loge et al., 1998; Jason, Jordan et al., 1998; Nisenbaum et al., 1998; Pawlikowska et al., 1994). Further, women are also more than twice as likely to seek medical help for their fatigue (Cope, 1992). For example, two-thirds of the people in one study who presented with fatigue in a primary care practice were women (Nelson et al., 1987). However, some primary care and hospital studies have found no statistically significant gender differences in fatigue (Cathebras et al., 1995; Kirk, Douglas, Nelson, Jaffee, & Lopez, 1990).

Ethnicity and Fatigue
Relatively few studies have examined fatigue levels among different ethnic groups (Richman, Flaherty, & Rospenda, 1994). Cathebras and associates (1995), in examining English-speaking and French-speaking Canadians, found an ethnic difference in reported rates of fatigue, with French-speaking Canadians reporting more fatigue. Buchwald and others (1996), however, found no ethnic differences in their study of white and "nonwhite" (African American, Asian American, American Indian, and Latino) people attending a university health center. Similarly, Nisenbaum and coworkers (1998), in a representative sample of people living within the San Francisco urban area, failed to find any ethnic differences in reported levels of fatigue. However, Steele and associates (1998) reported higher levels of fatigue among Native Americans. Finally, Song, Jason, and Taylor (1999) found that the mean fatigue severity scores were significantly higher for African Americans and Latinos than for Caucasians.

Although these community-based studies seem to point to some ethnic group differences, the problem of fatigue in multiethnic populations continues to be understudied. Selection bias may play a part in the lack of ethnic minority studies, as many primary care or hospital-based studies report few ethnic minority group members among their sample. People of color may have poorer access to quality health care, because of their disproportionate representation in lower socioeconomic populations (Richman, Flaherty, & Rospenda, 1994). This relative absence of people of color in research is especially disconcerting since some studies suggest they may be at higher risk for severe fatigue (Song, Jason, & Taylor, 1999), and inappropriate conclusions about the etiology of this illness may be drawn from a highly select, ethnically homogenous population. Community-based studies hold more promise of representing persons of color, and sampling from ethnically diverse populations may help to elucidate the prevalence and experience of fatigue in these traditionally understudied groups.

Physical versus Psychological Causes of Fatigue
The debate as to whether fatigue has primarily a physical or psychological etiology continues in contemporary investigations. Some researchers have distinguished between central and peripheral fatigue. Peripheral fatigue is defined as failure to sustain force or power output because of "failure in neuromuscular transmission, sarcolemmal excitation, or excitation-contraction coupling," implying neuromuscular dysfunction outside of the central nervous system, or CNS (Edwards, Newham, & Peters, 1991; Swain, 2000). In contrast, central fatigue is defined as resulting from failure to achieve and maintain the recruitment of high-threshold motor

units (Edwards, Newham, & Peters, 1991), implicating dysfunction in CNS neuro-transmitter pathways (Swain, 2000). However, the contributions of neither peripheral fatigue nor central fatigue to overall subjective reports of fatigue is well understood.

Clinical studies tend to focus on self-reported feeling of fatigue (Swain, 2000). Such studies often find a mixed presentation of both physical and psychological factors in unexplained chronic fatigue (Hall et al., 1994). Elevated rates of psychiatric comorbidity or indicators of psychological disorder have been found among chronic fatigue patients in primary care settings (Cathebras et al., 1995; Manu et al., 1989; McDonald, David, Pelosi, & Mann, 1993). Community-based studies have also found that persons suffering from chronic fatigue were more likely to have psychiatric symptoms or be diagnosed with psychiatric disorders (Lawrie et al., 1997; Pawlikowska et al., 1994). Somatic symptoms often occur together with self-reported fatigue as well. Manu and associates (1989) found that the most frequent somatic symptoms in fatigue patients were pain in extremities, joints, chest, and other parts of the body; shortness of breath; blurred vision; muscle weakness; and sexual indifference (Manu et al., 1989). Hartz and coworkers (1998) noted that the number of symptoms was strongly associated with the severity of fatigue, the response of fatigue to mental and physical activity, and the following participant characteristics: a greater frequency of sinus and respiratory infections, a higher frequency of migraines, a greater number of somatoform symptoms not included as criteria for CFS, and abstinence from alcohol (Hartz et al., 1998). Nisenbaum and associates (1998) found the most common symptoms experienced by fatigued persons were sleep problems, general weakness, muscle aches and pain, difficulty thinking or concentrating, depression, and unusual fatigue after exertion. These findings suggest that other somatic symptoms are likely to arise as unexplained severe fatigue persists (Nisenbaum et al., 1998).

Factor analytic studies tend to find multiple factors or clusters of fatigue-related symptoms. Ray, Weir, Cullen, and Phillips (1992) analyzed a list of symptoms in 208 patients with postviral fatigue and found four factors: emotional distress, fatigue, somatic symptoms, and cognitive difficulty. Hall, Sanders, and Replogle (1998), in a sample of 197 primary care patients, performed a factor analysis using 34 reported symptoms. In this investigation, four clusters of symptoms emerged: organic symptoms, anxiety, depression, and mixed-anxiety depression. Nisenbaum and associates (1998) also conducted a factor analysis of 30 symptoms experienced by people who were fatigued for 6 months or more, finding fatigue/mood/cognition, flu-type, and visual problem factors (Nisenbaum et al., 1998). Finally, Jason and coworkers (2002) factor analyzed fatigue-related symptoms reported by 780 persons with chronic fatigue and found four factors: lack of energy, physical exertion, cognitive problems, and fatigue and rest.

As Berrios (1990) noted, it is unclear whether the feeling of fatigue represents a primary state or a composite of symptoms that may vary depending on the etiology of the medical condition. These studies suggest that subjective unexplained fatigue may not always represent strictly "psychological" or "physical" etiologies; there may be separate physiological and psychological contributions to the experience of fatigue. This echos Bartley and Chute's recommendation in 1947, that fatigue and chronic fatigue research should examine the relative importance of multiple physical and psychological contributions (Bartley & Chute, 1947) to the experience of overall fatigue.

Unexplained Fatigue in Chronic Fatigue Syndrome

Only a small minority of patients presenting with chronic or severe fatigue are actually diagnosed with chronic fatigue syndrome. The prevalence of this disorder has been estimated at 0.24 percent (Reeves, 1999) to 0.4 percent (Jason et al., 1999) in community-based studies, and 2.6 percent of patients in primary care (Wessely, Chalder et al., 1997). As fatigue is the defining symptom of this illness, all persons diagnosed with chronic fatigue syndrome have experienced severe and disabling fatigue for 6 months or more (Fukuda et al., 1994). The effects of this chronic, unexplained fatigue appear to differ from individual to individual, with some persons experiencing only mild impairment, while others experience severe or very severe limitations (Carrico, Jason, Torres-Harding, & Witter, 2004; Cox & Findley, 2000). The fatigue in CFS can lead to a markedly higher degree of impairment than is found other chronically ill populations (Anderson & Ferrans, 1997).

As an illness of unexplained fatigue, CFS is diagnosed only when other fatigue-causing conditions are ruled out as the primary source of the fatigue. Because the fatigue is designated as "unexplained," some have proposed psychiatric explanations for the illness, while others propose several physiological hypotheses to explain the illness process and its resulting symptomatology. Regarding physiological findings, Clauw and Chrousos (1997) suggest that individuals who develop CFS might be genetically predisposed to develop this condition. In support of this, Torres-Harding and Jason (2003) found that persons with CFS were significantly more likely to report a family history of metabolic disorders than a control group. Recent twin studies of complex genetic and environmental relationships between psychological distress, fatigue, and immune system functioning suggest the need to acknowledge the increasing importance of the individual's genotype (Hickie, Bennett, Lloyd, Heath, & Martin, 1999). Clauw and Chrousos further posit that susceptible individuals might evidence a number of organ-specific illnesses before progressing to CFS. Supportive data support this thesis, showing CFS patients have had significantly more upper respiratory tract infections, lethargy, and vertigo than controls (Hamilton et al., 2001).

Clauw and Chrousos also suggest that once CFS develops, either abruptly or slowly through viral infections or emotional stressors, the human stress response is blunted, along with blunting of the hypothalamic-pituitary axis and autonomic nervous system instability. Symptom heterogeneity might be due to different axes of the stress response, either independently or concurrently functioning in aberrantly. Patients with CFS experience blunted biological stress response, and a low corticotrophin-releasing hormone (CRH) state is exacerbated if exercise further reduces cortisol levels; this postexercise adrenal insufficiency could be responsible for the patients' severe postexertional fatigue. One strength of such a biopsychosocial understanding of CFS is that it may bridge the theoretical gap between mind versus body explanations of these illnesses.

Fatigue in Chronic Disease

In addition to unexplained fatigue, the occurrence of fatigue in specific medical diseases has also been investigated. Fatigue has come be recognized as a serious symptom of many illnesses that can significantly impair a person's functioning and have a negative impact on quality of life in many chronic illnesses, including after cancer treatment (Bartsch, Weis, & Moser, 2003; Irvine, Vincent, Graydon, Bubela, & Thompson, 1994; Smets et al., 1993), systemic lupus erythematosus (SLE) (Jacobson, Gange, Rose, & Graham, 1997), multiple sclerosis (Schwid, Covington, Segal, & Goodman, 2002), human immunodeficiency virus (HIV) infection, viral and cholestatic liver diseases, and rheumatoid arthritis (Swain, 2000).

However, understanding fatigue in chronic medical disease continues to prove difficult. Even when fatigue is considered a primary or a common symptom, such as in multiple sclerosis or SLE, fatigue often does not correlate with disease status or physiological findings (Schwid, Covington, Segal, & Goodman, 2002; Krupp et al., 1990; Wang et al., 1998; Omdal et al., 2003). Despite the recognition that fatigue is an integral component of chronic disease, its etiology in many chronic illnesses is not well understood, although some have proposed it is mainly of central origin (Swain, 2000). Swain (2000) proposes that corticotropin-releasing hormone and chronic stress, cytokines and immune activation, central neurotransmitter pathways, and mood disorders such as depression are possible factors contributing to fatigue in chronic diseases. Further, different chronic illnesses may vary in the relative contributions of peripheral and central fatigue to the overall experience of fatigue (Swain, 2000). Finally, other factors such as stress, sleep disturbance, distress of other somatic symptoms, and personality traits have been reported to contribute to the subjective experience of fatigue in chronic disease (Berger, 2003; Irvine et al., 1994; Schwid, Covington, Segal, & Goodman, 2002).

Summary

The problem of excessive or unexplained fatigue has been common from the middle of the nineteenth century to the present day. Today, both unexplained fatigue and fatigue occurring as a symptom of illness are recognized as serious symptoms that can severely limit physical functioning and have a negative impact on quality of life. Research supports the involvement of multiple dimensions, with physiological, psychological, and psychosocial factors contributing to the experience of fatigue. Fatigue often occurs in conjunction with other somatic and psychiatric symptoms.

The relationship between physiological fatigue or disease states and the feeling of fatigue remains poorly understood, partly because fatigue is difficult to define and measure. Unfortunately, theories on the nature of fatigue from the last century are closely echoed by contemporary views, with little progress made in understanding this symptom. A recurring theme in research, however, is the need for a biopsychosocial approach, incorporating physiological, psychological, and psychosocial factors, in understanding the experience of fatigue. Continued research into the factors contributing to fatigue may help elucidate this complex symptom.

Acknowledgment

The authors appreciate the financial support of NIAID and grant number AI49720.

References

Anderson, J. S., & Ferrans, C. E. (1997). The quality of life of persons with chronic fatigue syndrome. *Journal of Nervous and Mental Disease, 185*, 359–367.

Allen, F. N. (1944). The differential diagnosis of weakness and fatigue. *New England Journal of Medicine, 231*, 414–418.

Alvarez, W. C. (1941). What is the matter with the patient who is chronically tired? *Journal of Missouri Medical Association, 38*, 365–368.

Barofsky, I., & West Legro, M. (1991). Definition and measurement of fatigue. *Reviews of Infectious Diseases, 13*, S94–S97.

Bartley, S. H., & Chute, E. (1947). *Fatigue and Impairment in Man.* New York: McGraw-Hill.

Bartsch, H. H., Weis, J., & Moser, M. T. (2003). Cancer-related fatigue in patients attending oncological rehabilitation programs: prevalence, patterns, and predictors. *Onkologie, 26(1)*, 51–57.

Berger, A. (2003). Treating fatigue in cancer patients. *Oncologist, 8(Suppl 1)*, 10–14.

Berrios, G. E. (1990). Feelings of fatigue and psychopathology: a conceptual history. *Comprehensive Psychiatry, 31(2)*, 140–151.

Broadbent, D. (1971). *Decision and Stress.* London: Academic Press.

Buchwald, D., Manson, S. M., Pearlman, T., Umali, J., & Kith, P. (1996). Race and ethnicity in patients with chronic fatigue. *Journal of Chronic Fatigue Syndrome, 2(1)*, 1996.

Carrico, A. W., Jason, L. A., Torres-Harding, S. R., & Witter, E. A. (2004). Disability in chronic fatigue syndrome and idiopathic chronic fatigue. *Review of Disability Studies: An International Journal, 1*, 79–88.

Cathebras, P. J., Robbins, J. M., Kirmayer, L. J., & Hayton, B. C. (1992). Fatigue in primary care: prevalence, psychiatric comorbidity, illness behavior, and outcome. *Journal of General Internal Medicine, 7*, 276–286.

Chalder, T., Berelowitz, G., Pawlikowska, T., Watts, L., Wessely, S., Wright, D., & Wallace, E. P. (1993). Development of a fatigue scale. *Journal of Psychosomatic Research, 37(2)*, 147–153.

Chapman, C. B. (1990). The long reach of Harvard's Fatigue Laboratory, 1926–1947. *Perspectives in Biology and Medicine, 34(1)*, 17–33.

Chen, M. (1986). The epidemiology of self-perceived fatigue among adults. *Preventive Medicine, 15*, 74–81.

Clauw, D. J., & Chrousos, G. P. (1997). Chronic pain and fatigue syndromes: overlapping clinical and neuroendocrine features and potential pathogenic mechanisms. *Neuroimmunomodulation, 4*, 134–153.

Collier, H. E. (1943). *Outlines of Industrial Medical Practice*. Baltimore: Williams & Wilkins Company.

Cope, H. (1992). Fatigue: a non-specific complaint? *International Review of Psychiatry, 4*, 273–280.

Cox, D. L., & Findley, L. J. (2000). Severe and very severe patients with chronic fatigue syndrome: perceived outcome following an inpatient program. *Journal of Chronic Fatigue Syndrome, 7(3)*, 33–47.

DaCosta, J. M. (1871). On irritable heart: a clinical study of a form of functional cardiac disorder and its consequences. *American Journal of Medical Science, 61*, 17–52.

Edwards, R. H. T., Newham, D. J., & Peters, T. J. (1991). Muscle biochemistry and pathophysiology in postviral fatigue syndrome. *British Medical Bulletin, 47(4)*, 826–837.

Friedberg, F., & Jason, L. A. (1998). *Understanding Chronic Fatigue Syndrome*. Washington, DC: American Psychological Association.

Fuhrer, R., & Wessely, S. (1995). The epidemiology of fatigue and depression: a French primary care study. *Psychological Medicine, 25*, 895–905.

Fukuda, K., Straus, S., Hickie, I., Sharpe, M. C., Dobbins, J. G., & Komaroff, A., & The International Chronic Fatigue Syndrome Study Group (1994). The chronic fatigue syndrome: a comprehensive approach to its definition and study. *Annals of Internal Medicine, 121*, 953–959.

Hall, D. G., Sanders, S. D., & Replogle, W. H. (1994). Fatigue: a new approach to an old problem. *Journal of the Mississippi State Medical Association, 35*, 155–160.

Hamilton, W. T., Hall, G. H., & Pound, A. P. (2001). Frequency of attendance in general practice and symptoms before development of chronic fatigue syndrome: a case-control study. *British Journal of General Practice, 51*, 553–558.

Hartz, A. J., Kuhn, E. M., & Levine, P. (1998). Characteristics of fatigued persons associated with features of chronic fatigue syndrome. *Journal of Chronic Fatigue Syndrome, 4(3),* 71–97.

Hickie, I., Bennett, B., Lloyd, A., Heath, A., & Martin, N. (1999). Complex genetic and environmental relationships between psychological distress, fatigue and immune functioning: a twin study. *Psychological Medicine, 29,* 267–277.

Holmes, G. P., Kaplan, J. E., Gantz, N. M., et al. (1988). Chronic fatigue syndrome: a working case definition. *Annals of Internal Medicine, 108,* 387–389.

Hyams, K. C., Wignall, F. S., & Roswell, R. (1996). War syndromes and their evaluation: from the US Civil War to the Persian Gulf War. *Annals of Internal Medicine, 125,* 398–405.

Irvine, D., Vincent, L., Graydon, J. E., Bubela, N., & Thompson, L. (1994). The prevalence and correlates of fatigue in patients receiving treatment with chemotherapy and radiotherapy. A comparison with the fatigue experienced by healthy individuals. *Cancer Nursing, 17(5),* 367–378.

Ivy, A. C., & Roth, J. A. (1944). A review of neurocirculatory asthenia, cardiovascular neurosis, effort syndrome, or DaCosta's syndrome. *Quarterly Bulletin of Northwestern University, 18,* 112–124.

Jacobson, D. L., Gange, S. J., Rose, N. R., & Graham, N. M. (1997). Epidemiology and estimated population burden of selected autoimmune diseases in the United States. *Clinical Immunology and Immunopathology, 84(3),* 223–243.

Jason, L. A., Jordan, K. M., Richman, J. A., Rademaker, A. W., Huang, C., McCready, W., Shlaes, J., King, C. P., Landis, D., Torres, S., Haney-Davis, T., & Frankenberry, E. L. (1999). A community-based study of prolonged and chronic fatigue. *Journal of Health Psychology, 4,* 9–26.

Jason, L. A., Richman, J. A., Rademaker, A. W., Jordan, K. M., Plioplys, A. V., Taylor, R. R., McCready, W., Huang, C. F., & Plioplys, S. (1999). A community-based study of chronic fatigue syndrome. *Archives of Internal Medicine, 159(18),* 2129–2137.

Jason, L. A., Taylor, R. R., Kennedy, C. L., Jordan, K., Huang, C. F., Torres-Harding, S., Song, S., & Johnson, D. (2002). A factor analysis of chronic fatigue symptoms in a community-based sample. *Social Psychiatry and Psychiatric Epidemiology, 37,* 183–189.

Kepler, E. J. (1942). Chronic fatigue. *Proceedings of the Staff Meetings, Mayo Clinic, 17,* 340–344.

Kirk, J., Douglass, R., Nelson, E., Jaffee, J., & Lopez, A. (1990). Chief complaint of chronic fatigue: a prospective study. *Journal of Family Practice, 30(1),* 33–41.

Kroenke, K., & Mangelsdorff, A. D. (1989). Common symptoms in ambulatory care: incidence, evaluation, therapy, and outcome. *The American Journal of Medicine, 86,* 262–266.

Kroenke, K., Wood, D. R., Mangelsdroff, A. D., Meier, N. J., & Powell, J. B. (1988). Chronic fatigue in primary care: prevalence, patient characteristics, and outcome. *Journal of the American Medical Association, 260(7),* 929–934.

Krupp, L. B., & Christodoulou, C. (2001). Fatigue in multiple sclerosis. *Current Neurology and Neuroscience Reports, 1(3),* 294–298.

Lawrie, S. M., Manders, D. N., Geddes, J. R., & Pelosi, A. J. (1997). A population-based incidence study of chronic fatigue. *Psychological Medicine, 27*, 343–353.

Levine, P. H. (1994). Epidemic neuromyasthenia and chronic fatigue syndrome: epidemiological importance of a cluster definition. *Clinical Infectious Diseases, 18(Suppl 1)*, S16–S20.

Loge, J. H., Ekeberg, O., & Kaasa, S. (1998). Fatigue in the general Norwegian population: normative data and associations. *Journal of Psychosomatic Research, 45(1)*, 53–65.

Macmillan, M. B. (1976). Beard's concept of neurasthenia and Freud's concept of the actual neuroses. *Journal of the History of the Behavioral Sciences, 12(4)*, 376–390.

Manu, P., Lane, T. J., & Matthews, D. A. (1992). Chronic fatigue syndromes in clinical practice. *Psychotherapy and Psychosomatics, 58*, 60–68.

Manu, P., Matthews, D. A., Lane, T. J., Tennen, H., Hesselbrock, V., Mendola, R., & Affleck, G. (1989). Depression among patients with a chief complaint of chronic fatigue. *Journal of Affective Disorders, 17*, 165–172.

McDonald, E., David, A. S., Pelosi, A. J, & Mann, A. H. (1993). Chronic fatigue in primary care attenders. *Psychological Medicine, 23(4)*, 987–998.

Muncie, W. (1941). Chronic fatigue. *Psychosomatic Medicine, 3*, 277–285.

Nelson, E., Kirk, J., McHugo, G., Douglass, R., Ohler, J., Wasson, J., & Zubkoff, M. (1987). Chief complaint fatigue: a longitudinal study from the patient's perspective. *Family Practice Research Journal, 6(4)*, 175–188.

Nisenbaum, R., Reyes, M., Mawle, A. C., & Reeves, W. (1998). Factor analysis of unexplained severe fatigue and interrelated symptoms. *American Journal of Epidemiology, 148(1)*, 72–77.

Omdal, R., Waterloo, K., Koldingsnes, W., Husby, G., & Mellgren, S. I. (2003). Fatigue in patients with systemic lupus erythematosus: the psychosocial aspects. *The Journal of Rheumatology, 30(2)*, 283–287.

Pawlikowska, T., Chalder, T., Hirsch, S. R., Wallace, P., Wright, D. J. M., & Wessely, S. C. (1994). Population based study of fatigue and psychological distress. *British Medical Journal, 308*, 763–766.

Ramsay M. A. (1988). *Myalgic encephalomyelitis and postviral fatigue states: the saga of Royal Free Disease*, 2nd ed. Aldershot, Hampshire, UK: Gower.

Ray, C., Weir, R. C., Cullen, S., & Phillips, S. (1992). Illness perception and symptom components in chronic fatigue syndrome. *Journal of Psychosomatic Research, 36(3)*, 243–256.

Reeves, W. C. (1999). Transcript of U.S. Chronic Fatigue Syndrome Coordinating Committee of April 21–22, 1999, Bethesda, MD. Available at http://www.cais.net/cfs-news/cfscc-9904.txt. Accessed August 10, 1999.

Richman, J. A., Flaherty, J. A., & Rospenda, K. M. (1994). Chronic fatigue syndrome: Have flawed assumptions been derived from treatment-based studies? *American Journal of Public Health, 84(2)*, 282–284.

Robey, W. H., & Boas, E. P. (1918). Neurocirculatory asthenia. *Journal of the American Medical Association, 71*, 525–529.

Schwid, S. R., Covington, M., Segal, B. M., & Goodman, A. D. (2002). Fatigue in multiple sclerosis: current understanding and future directions. *Journal of Rehabilitation Research and Development, 39(2)*, 211–224.

Shorter, E. (1993). Chronic fatigue in historical perspective. In *Chronic Fatigue Syndrome: CIBA Foundation Symposium*. G. R. Bock & J. Whelan, eds. Pp. 6–22. Chichester, Engl.: John Wiley & Sons.

Smets, E. M. A., Garssen, B., Schuster-Uitterhoeve, A. L. J., & de Haes, J. C. J. M. (1993). Fatigue in cancer patients. *British Journal of Cancer, 68(2)*, 220–224.

Song, S., Jason, L. A., & Taylor, R. R. (1999). The relationship between ethnicity and fatigue in a community-based sample. *Journal of Gender, Culture, and Health, 4(4)*, 255–268.

Steele, L., Dobbins, J. G., Fukuda, K., Reyes, M., Randall, B., Koppelman, M., & Reeves, W. C. (1998). The epidemiology of chronic fatigue in San Francisco. *American Journal of Medicine, 105*, 835–905.

Stokes, M. J., Cooper, R. G., & Edwards, R. H. T. (1988). Normal muscle strength and fatigability in patients with effort syndromes. *British Medical Journal, 297*, 1014–1016.

Swain, M. G. (2000). Fatigue in chronic disease. *Clinical Science, 99*, 1–8.

Torres-Harding, S. R., & Jason, L. A. (2003). "Family medical history of persons with chronic fatigue syndrome." Paper presented at the meeting of the American Association of Chronic Fatigue Syndrome. Chantilly, Virginia.

Wang, B., Gladman, D. D., & Urowitz, M. B. (1998). Fatigue in lupus is not correlated with disease activity. *The Journal of Rheumatology, 25*, 892–895.

Ward, R. V. (1941). Chronic fatigue symptoms among industrial workers. *Canadian Public Health Journal, 32*, 464–467.

Wessely, S. (1991). History of postviral fatigue syndrome. *British Medical Bulletin, 47(4)*, 919–941.

Wessely, S. (1998). The epidemiology of chronic fatigue syndrome. *Epidemiologia e Psychiatria Sociale, 7(1)*, 10–24.

Wessely, S., Chalder, T., Hirsch, S., Wallace, P., & Wright, D. (1997). The prevalence and morbidity of chronic fatigue and chronic fatigue syndrome: a prospective primary care study. *American Journal of Public Health, 87*, 1449–1455.

Wharton, G. K. (1938). The fatigue syndrome. *Canadian Medical Association Journal, 38*, 339–342.

World Health Organization (1992). *International Classification of Diseases and Related Health Problems*, Tenth Revision. Albany, NY: WHO Publications Center USA.

2 The Assessment and Measurement of Fatigue

Christopher Christodoulou

The Multifaceted Nature of Fatigue

The quest to clarify the meaning and measurement of fatigue has challenged researchers and clinicians for many years. Despite its broad use in casual conversation and scientific discourse, or perhaps partly because of it, the term "fatigue" has defied efforts to provide a single, broadly acceptable definition. Instead, its meaning and measurement tend to vary with the circumstances in which it is used. In their classic text, Bartley and Chute (Bartley & Chute, 1947) reviewed dozens of definitions and views of fatigue presented in psychological and physiological texts, as well as articles, monographs, periodicals, and conferences.

Broadly speaking, fatigue can be conceptualized as either a *subjective feeling* or a *performance decrement* (Wessely, Hotopf, & Sharpe, 1998). Bartley and Chute (Bartley & Chute, 1947) advocated a primary focus on the individual's feelings of fatigue. For example, among patients suffering from excessive fatigue the most salient feature might be the uncharacteristic feelings of exhaustion accompanying their pathological condition. This emphasis on subjective experience is also evident in a consensus definition of fatigue in persons with multiple sclerosis (MS) as "a subjective lack of physical and/or mental energy that is perceived by the individual or caregiver to interfere with usual or desired activities" (Multiple Sclerosis Council for Clinical Practice Guidelines, 1998). In contrast, athletic trainers, muscle physiologists, business leaders, and other results-oriented individuals tend to use measures that directly assess performance-based decrements associated with fatigue, such as reduced muscle strength after a period of exertion or increased error rate over time on tasks requiring vigilance. Consistent with an interest in measuring changes in objective performance, muscle fatigue has been defined as "any exercise-induced reduction in the maximal capacity to generate force or power output." (Vollestad, 1997, p. 220).

The two conceptualizations of fatigue (as a feeling state versus performance decrement) are partly reflected in the two basic approaches to measuring fatigue through self-report questionnaires or direct observation of behavior. Self-report measures are uniquely able to assess the feelings associated with fatigue, but can only indirectly assess changes in performance from the respondent's perspective. Direct observation of behavior provides objective measurement of behavioral performance changes associated with fatigue, but lacks the ability to assess underlying feelings. The different focuses on subjective feelings or performance decrements would not be so consequential if empirical studies did not often fail to find an association between these two approaches (Krupp & Elkins, 2000; Sharma, Kent-Braun, Mynhier, Weiner, & Miller, 1995). This chapter reviews and compares the two approaches to the measurement of fatigue.

Pathological versus Normal Fatigue

Fatigue measures have been designed for a variety of purposes. Some were designed to study individuals with medical disorders and others for healthy persons. Fatigue is a pathological feature of a variety of medical conditions, but it is obvious that otherwise healthy individuals also experience periods of fatigue. Pathological fatigue can be distinguished from nonpathological fatigue by a combination of features including greater intensity, longer duration, and more disabling effects on functional activities. Fatigue in healthy persons is generally a time-limited phenomenon that follows a period of exertion or sleep deprivation and is reduced if not eliminated by rest or sleep. Pathological fatigue, in contrast, remains after rest as a severe chronic condition, disrupting an individual's ability to carry out important daily social and occupational activities and obligations.

As detailed in later chapters, pathological fatigue is one of the most common features identified in a broad range of medical conditions, including chronic heart disease, cancer, MS, chronic insomnia, and depression. In addition, fatigue can manifest as chronic fatigue syndrome (CFS) following the onset of persistent debilitating fatigue lasting 6 months or more and the exclusion of other known causes of the condition (Fukuda et al., 1994).

Wherever possible, it is important to identify other causes of fatigue and existing comorbid medical disorders, in part because their treatment might reduce fatigue as well. For example, a recent study found that successful treatment of depression in MS patients also reduced their fatigue (Mohr, Hart, & Goldberg, 2003), although a similar study in oncology patients found no improvement in fatigue (Morrow, Hickok, Roscoe, et al., 2003). The development of fatigue in any situation is clearly a complex process, and a more comprehensive understanding of this multifaceted phenomenon will require a broad approach integrating information gathered from physiological, affective, cognitive, behavioral, and psychosocial factors (Wessely, Hotopf, & Sharpe, 1998).

Questionnaires

A remarkable number of fatigue questionnaires have been developed over the years. Scales have been developed for use in a variety of clinical populations, including cancer (Hann, Denniston, & Baker, 2000; Piper et al., 1998; Stein, Martin, Hann, & Jacobsen, 1998), MS (Iriarte, Katsamakis, & de Castro, 1999; Krupp, LaRocca, Muir-Nash, & Steinberg, 1989; Multiple Sclerosis Council for Clinical Practice Guidelines, 1998), rheumatoid arthritis (Belza, 1995), CFS (Vercoulen et al., 1994), and myasthenia gravis (Grohar-Murray, Sears, Hubsky, & Becker, 1994; Kittiwatanapaisan, Gauthier, Williams, & Oh, 2003), as well as for healthy individuals engaged in work and sports (Ahsberg, Gamberale, & Kjellberg, 1997; Borg, 1970; Borg, 1982a; Borg, 1982b; Haylock & Hart, 1979; Kogi, Saito, & Mitsuhashi, 1970). While item content does vary to some extent with the targeted audience (e.g., questions regarding the particular vulnerability of MS patients to heat-related fatigue) (Schwartz, Jandorf, & Krupp, 1993), there is also a good deal of item similarity across scales. The questionnaires range in length from single stem scales (Borg, 1970; Borg, 1982b; Krupp et al., 1989; Lee, Hicks, & Nino-Murcia, 1991) to longer, multidimensional assessments (Schwartz et al., 1993; Smets, Garssen, Bonke, & De Haes, 1995; Stein et al., 1998). The authors of some multidimensional scales argue that including many factors is necessary to assess the complex pattern of fatigue patients experience (Stein et al., 1998). Those favoring more focused scales, however, might argue that pure measures of fatigue should be more homogeneous, perhaps measuring only the core feelings of fatigue and excluding such aspects as affective feelings, which might be better assessed by separate instruments.

Item Scaling

Some of the earliest scales included items requiring a binary response to indicate the presence or absence of a fatigue symptom (Kogi et al., 1970). The most common approach, however, is a Likert scale format, which gauges a fatigue symptom's severity/intensity by asking subjects to report the degree to which they endorse a particular item (e.g., "feeling exhausted") on an ordered scale (e.g., ranging from 0 = not at all to 5 = completely) (table 2.1). Alternatively, subjects can be asked to bisect the line of a visual analogue scale (VAS) for the same purpose. Fatigue researchers comparing the two formats have generally found they provide relatively equivalent data, but Likert scales are preferred because they are easier for subjects to understand and for the researchers to score (Hartz, Bentler, & Watson, 2003; Piper et al., 1998).

Borg (Borg, 1970; 1982a; 1982b) has developed an interesting approach to measuring fatigue intensity that has been quite influential in the work of physiologists and those interested in measuring physical work capacity (Noble, 1982). His first scale measures ratings of perceived exertion (RPE), based on a series of verbal descriptors

Table 2.1
Fatigue scales

Name of Scale	Author, Year	Initial Population	Specified Fatigue Subscales	Item Length	Item Scoring	Time Frame
Fatigue Symptom Checklist	Japanese (Kogi et al., 1970) English (Haylock et al., 1979)	Healthy (Koji), cancer (Haylock & Hart)	Drowsiness and dullness, projection of physical disintegration, difficulty in concentration,	30	Yes/no	Now
Borg Rating of Perceived Exertion (RPE) scale	(Borg, 1970)	Healthy	Rating of perceived exertion	Single item	6–20*	Now
Borg Category Ratio scale (CR-10)	(Borg, 1982a; Borg, 1982b)	Healthy	Rating of perceived exertion	Single item	0–10**	Now
Piper Fatigue Scale (PFS)	(Piper et al., 1989), Revised in (Piper et al., 1998)	Cancer	Behavioral/severity, affective meaning, sensory, Cognitive/mood	22 items (+5 short answer)	0–10	One item asks for duration
Fatigue Severity Scale (FSS)	(Krupp et al., 1989)	MS, lupus, healthy	None	9	1–7	Not stated, past 2 weeks appropriate***
Single Item Visual Analogue Scale (VAS) of Fatigue	(Krupp et al., 1989)	MS, lupus, healthy	None	1	Visual analogue scale	Not stated
Visual Analogue Scale for Fatigue (VAS-F)	(Lee et al., 1991)	Sleep disordered and healthy	Energy, fatigue	18	Visual analogue scale	Not stated
Fatigue Assessment Instrument (FAI)	(Schwartz et al., 1993)	Lyme, CFS, lupus, MS, dysthymia, healthy	Fatigue severity, situation-specificity, consequences of fatigue, responds to rest/sleep	29	1–7	Past 2 weeks

Scale	Reference	Population	Dimensions	Items	Response scale	Time frame
Fatigue Scale (FS)	(Chalder et al., 1993)	Primary care patients	Physical, mental	14	Yes/No	Not stated
Checklist Individual Strength (CIS)	(Vercoulen et al., 1994)	CFS	Subjective experience of fatigue, concentration, motivation, physical activity	24	7-point scale	Not stated
Fatigue Impact Scale (FIS)	(Fisk et al., 1994), Modified by (Multiple Sclerosis Council for Clinical Practice Guidelines, 1998)	MS	Physical, cognitive, psychosocial	21 (short form: 5 items)	0–4	Past 4 weeks
Myasthenia Gravis Fatigue Scale (MGFS)	(Grohar-Murray et al., 1994; Kittiwatanapaisan et al., 2003)	Myasthenia gravis	Perception of fatigue, task avoidance, observable motor signs or symptoms	26	1–5	In general since illness onset
Multidimensional Assessment of Fatigue (MAF)	(Belza, 1995)	Rheumatoid arthritis	Degree, severity, distress, impact on activities of daily living	15	1–10	One item asks for duration
Mulitidimensional Fatigue Inventory (MFI)	(Smets et al., 1995)	Students, physicians, cancer, CFS, soldiers	General fatigue, physical fatigue, mental fatigue, reduced motivation, reduced activity	20	1–7	Not stated
Swedish Occupational Fatigue Inventory (SOFI)****	(Ahsberg et al., 1997)	Healthy persons in 16 different occupations	Lack of energy, physical exertion, physical discomfort, lack of motivation, sleepiness	25	0–10	At present
Multicomponent Fatigue Scale	(Paul et al., 1998)*****	MS, myasthenia gravis	Mental, physical	15	0–5	At present, & compared to recent past

Table 2.1
(continued)

Name of Scale	Author, Year	Initial Population	Specified Fatigue Subscales	Item Length	Item Scoring	Time Frame
Multidimensional Fatigue Symptom Inventory (MFSI)	(Stein et al., 1998)	Cancer	Global, somatic, affective, behavioral, cognitive symptoms of fatigue	83, (short form: 30 items)	0–4	Last week
Fatigue Descriptive Scale (FDS)	(Iriarte et al., 1999)	MS	Spontaneous mention of fatigue, antecedent conditions, frequency, impact on life	5	0–3	Not stated
Fatigue Symptom Inventory (FSI)	(Hann et al., 2000)	Cancer	Intensity, duration, impact on quality of life	13	0–10	Past week
Rochester Fatigue Diary (RFD)	(Schwid, Covington, Segal, & Goodman, 2002)	MS	Lassitude (reduced energy)	12 (1 item, 12× over 24 hrs)	Visual analogue scale	Past 2 hours
IOWA Fatigue Scale (IFS)	(Hartz et al., 2003)	Primary care patients	Cognitive, fatigue, energy, productivity	11	5-point scale	
Child Fatigue Scale (CFS)	(Hockenberry et al., 2003)	Children with cancer (also versions for parents & staff)	Lack of energy, not able to function, altered mood	14	Frequency (yes/no), Intensity (1–5)	Past week

* Designed to increase linearly with workload & heart rate. Some items anchored with verbal expressions (e.g., very light = 9, very hard = 17).

** Borg designed this category scale to display ratio properties. Some items are again anchored with verbal expression.

*** Krupp, personal communication.

**** In Swedish. English translations of each item provided, but not validated.

***** A variation on the Chalder Fatigue Scale.

(e.g., "very, very light" to "very, very hard") tied to a scale from 6 to 20. The RPE scale was designed to increase linearly with heart rates ranging from 60 to 200 beats per minute while subjects pedal a cycle ergometer, and, indeed, it correlates strongly with heart rate ($r = 0.80 - 0.90$) as well as other physiological variables (Borg, 1982b). Borg also developed a newer scale to provide a ratio level of measurement of verbal descriptors, on a scale from 0 to 10 (Category Ratio Scale, or CR-10) (Borg, 1982a; 1982b). This new scale has also displayed strong correlations with physiological measures (Borg, 1982b). One of the few studies to compare Borg's approach to traditional Likert and VAS scales found that the VAS was most reproducible, but the CR-10 was most sensitive to pharmacologically induced changes in general fatigue in healthy subjects (Grant et al., 1999).

Characteristics Commonly Assessed by Fatigue Questionnaires

Most scales, particularly the multidimensional ones, include items to assess both the feelings of fatigue and the perceived impact of fatigue on the lives of respondents (see Table 2.1). The subjective feelings measured include not only the *core feelings of fatigue* (e.g., tiredness), but also *motivational* (e.g., reduced motivation) and *affective* (e.g., negative affective feelings) feelings accompanying fatigue. To assess the impact of fatigue, some scales ask about the degree of *interference with daily activities* (e.g., occupational activities). Scales commonly distinguish between the impact of fatigue on *mental/cognitive* (e.g., impaired concentration) and *physical/muscular* (e.g., reduction in sustained physical activity) activities. It is important to note that, though subjective feelings and fatigue impact are separate categories of items, both types of items are measured on the basis of the subject's self-report rather than direct performance assessment. As stated earlier, directly measuring performance decrement (e.g., a decline in cognitive performance over time) is a separate approach to fatigue measurement.

Feelings of Fatigue

To measure the *core feelings of fatigue*, questionnaires generally ask respondents to report on the degree to which they feel tired, fatigued, sluggish, pooped, or worn out. The questionnaires that most emphasize the measurement of such feelings include the Piper Fatigue Scale (PFS) (Piper et al., 1998) and the Multidimensional Fatigue Symptom Inventory (MFSI) (Stein et al., 1998), which both include many fatigue synonyms. The Profile of Mood States (POMS), a more general self-report measure, also includes a fatigue subscale with a number of items examining core feelings of fatigue (McNair, Lorr, & Droppleman, 1992). A few fatigue-specific questionnaires measure *affective* feelings that commonly accompany fatigue (e.g., PFS and MFSI) (Hartz et al., 2003; Piper et al., 1998).

Although the feelings assessed are generally negative (e.g., depressed, tense, distressed), it is important to note that not all fatigue is associated with negative affect.

For example, people often report a pleasant sense of fatigue after exercise. Piper's PFS scale measures this less common positive affect (Piper et al., 1998). Some question-naires include items of a *motivational* nature, asking if persons feel unmotivated, indif-ferent, or apathetic. Among the scales emphasizing motivational items are the Multidimensional Fatigue Inventory (MFI) (Smets et al., 1995), the Checklist of Indi-vidual Strength (CIS) (Vercoulen et al., 1994), and the Swedish Occupational Fatigue Inventory (SOFI) (Ahsberg et al., 1997).

Impact of Fatigue

The degree to which fatigue interferes with daily activities can indicate pathology. The more fatigue negatively affects occupational, social, and basic activities of daily living (e.g., bathing, dressing), the greater its pathology. Among the self-report measures including items emphasizing interference with daily activities are the Fatigue Severity Scale (FSS) (Krupp et al., 1989), the Modified Fatigue Impact Scale (MFIS) (Multiple Sclerosis Council for Clinical Practice Guidelines, 1998), and the Fatigue Symptom Inventory (FSI) (Hann et al., 2000).

Mental versus Physical Fatigue

Fatigue scales commonly distinguish between fatigue's impact on *mental/cognitive* (e.g., impaired concentration) versus *physical/muscular* (e.g., reduction in sustained physical activity) activities (Ahsberg et al., 1997; Chalder et al., 1993; Multiple Sclerosis Council for Clinical Practice Guidelines, 1998; Paul, Beatty, Schneider, Blanco, & Hames, 1998; Piper et al., 1998; Smets et al., 1995; Stein et al., 1998; Vercoulen et al., 1994)). Scales measuring fatigue that interferes with physical/muscular activities include items such as "physically I feel only able to do a little" (Smets et al., 1995), or items referring to reduced sustained physical functioning (Krupp et al., 1989), weakness (Chalder et al., 1993), or a heavy feeling (Stein et al., 1998). Mental/cognitive impairment is assessed through items focusing on difficulties with vigilance/concentration (Chalder et al., 1993; Multiple Sclerosis Council for Clinical Practice Guidelines, 1998; Smets et al., 1995), confused thinking (Chalder et al., 1993; Multiple Sclerosis Council for Clinical Practice Guidelines, 1998), and decision-making problems (Multiple Sclerosis Council for Clinical Practice Guidelines, 1998).

Factor analyses of a number of scales support a general differentiation between phys-ical and mental self-reported fatigue (Ahsberg et al., 1997; Smets et al., 1995; Stein et al., 1998). Work by Ahsberg and colleagues (Ahsberg & Gamberale, 1998; Ahsberg, Gamberale, & Gustafsson, 2000; Ahsberg et al., 1997) on fatigue in occupational set-tings (i.e., SOFI) further supports this distinction. They found that persons employed in jobs that are physically highly demanding (e.g., firefighters and factory workers) experience greater physical fatigue, while those with monotonous, mentally demand-ing occupations (e.g., nightshift operators at a nuclear power plant) experience more mental fatigue (Ahsberg et al., 1997). They also found that strenuous physical activity increases the scores of physical fatigue subscales (Ahsberg & Gamberale 1998), and demanding mental activity increases scores on mental fatigue subscales (Ahsberg et al., 2000). It should be noted, however, that neurophysiological differences between fatigue subtypes, which would lend additional support to such distinctions, have not been well established.

Duration of Fatigue

Many questionnaires neglect the important issue of fatigue duration (see Table 2.1), failing to ask subjects how long they have experienced fatigue symptoms. This omission is unfortunate because longer-lasting fatigue can signal greater pathology (Piper, 1989; Wessely et al., 1998). Many scales fail to specify the time frame in which respondents should focus when answering items (e.g., right now, over the past week, in general), reducing the measure's reliability and limiting its utility in assessing changes in fatigue over time or in response to experimental manipulation (though researchers could add a time specification to the scale's instructions).

The most appropriate time frame depends in part on the clinical or research objective at hand. In examining the effects of physically demanding work on otherwise healthy individuals, present fatigue might be the appropriate focus. However, in examining pathological fatigue associated with a medical disorder, a longer duration may be more appropriate. A specific time frame can be helpful in monitoring changes in fatigue associated with disease course or treatment approach. Another temporal aspect of fatigue is its diurnal pattern, involving assessment of whether symptoms are worse at particular times of the day (Schwartz et al., 1993).

Measurement of Performance Decrement

Aside from questionnaires, the other major approach to assessing fatigue is the direct measurement of performance decrement. Almost any behavioral or cognitive performance could conceivably be assessed, including muscular contractions, eye blinking, overall motoric activity, and various cognitive tasks.

Behavioral Measures of Performance Decrement

One of the most common and useful behavioral measure of fatigue involves assessing of muscle fatigue. For example, muscle fatigue has been found to be higher in MS patients who report fatigue than in healthy controls (Sheean, Murray, Rothwell, Miller, & Thompson, 1997). The process of measuring muscle fatigue is not quite as straightforward as one might expect. If muscle fatigue is defined as "any exercise-induced reduction in the maximal capacity to generate force or power output" (Vollestad, 1997, p. 220), a key problem is in determining "maximal capacity." If a volunteer produces only submaximal muscle contractions, his or her performance may remain steady for a long time. Obtaining maximal contractions from volunteers, however, is not easy even with continuous encouragement and feedback. An individual's level of muscle contraction can be limited by a lack of motivation, among many other factors (Vollestad, 1997). In some instances, electrical stimulation of the motor neurons or the muscle itself can generate maximal force. This electrical stimulation is independent of central nervous system factors, and the difference between the force it generates and the maximum achievable force by voluntary contraction provides an estimate of "central fatigue" (Vollestad, 1997). Central fatigue in this usage is a broad term that includes factors at or above the level of the upper motor neuron.

Measuring changes in eye blink rate has been posited as measure of fatigue (Stern, Boyer, & Schroeder, 1994). Blink rates appear to increase with the amount of time spent on a task that requires vigilance (Stern et al., 1994). Increases in blink rate, reduction in blink amplitude, and long eye closure rates have also been associated with increasing error rates while performing cognitive tasks (Morris & Miller, 1996). In addition, correlations have been found between eye blink measures and self-reported measures of fatigue in highly trained fighter pilots (Morris et al., 1996).

Another method of assessing the impact of fatigue is to measure an individual's level of overall physical activity with a motion-sensing device (Vercoulen et al., 1997). Differences in overall activity have been documented between healthy individuals and those with the fatiguing disorders of MS (in patients with low-level physical disability) and CFS (Vercoulen et al., 1997). This study also found significant correlations between overall activity levels and self-reported fatigue in CFS patients but not in MS patients or healthy controls (Vercoulen et al., 1997).

Cognitive Measures of Performance Decrement

Healthy persons with induced fatigue (e.g., through performance of cognitively demanding task) have been shown to display cognitive declines in planning ability and increases in perseverative errors compared to nonfatigued individuals (van der Linden, Frese, & Meijman, 2003). Healthy persons have also displayed shifts toward lower-effort, higher-risk responses after being fatigued by a simulated workday of mentally demanding tasks (Schellekens, Sijtsma, Vegter, & Meijman, 2000). Others researchers who examined the real-world consequences of long work hours found an increase in operator errors among employees working a 12-hour shift in nuclear power plants (Baker, Olson, & Morisseau, 1994).

Sleep deprivation also induces fatigue-related performance decrements. One study found no correlation between sleep deprivation (≤ 4 hr per night) and objective performance on tests of short-term and long-term verbal recall in medical students and residents (Browne et al., 1994). However, another study found a decline in the cognitive performance of medical residents on a standardized national medical examination with decreased sleep before the examination (Jacques, Lynch, & Samkoff, 1990).

Among clinical populations, much recent work has focused on MS. Patients with this fatiguing disorder have shown declines over time in cognitive performance during mentally challenging tasks (Bryant, Chiaravalloti, & Deluca, 2004; Schwid et al., 2003) or following such tasks (Krupp et al., 2000) compared to healthy controls. However, in direct comparisons between the groups change scores are not always significant (Schwid et al., 2003) or even reported (Bryant et al., 2004).

Studies examining the relationship between declines in cognitive performance and the subjective experience of fatigue have produced inconsistent findings. Some studies of MS patients have found no relation (Bryant et al., 2004; Krupp & Elkins, 2000); in others a relation was found only for some fatigue scales (Schwid et al., 2003). One study correlated increases in subjective mental fatigue with objective cognitive performance in myasthenia gravis patients but not in healthy controls (Paul, Cohen, & Gilchrist, 2002). Still another study examining healthy persons did find correlations between changes in self-reported fatigue and changes in cognitive performance (Schellekens et al., 2000).

Advantages and Disadvantages of Different Approaches to Measuring Fatigue

Fatigue questionnaires have a number of practical advantages over direct measures of performance. They are inexpensive, readily available, and quickly administered. They require little staff training, and place few demands on seriously ill patients, such as those undergoing chemotherapy. In contrast, objective measures of performance decrement, whether based on muscular or cognitive performance, are designed to be demanding and may place an undue burden on some patients. Measures of performance decrement also tend to be more specialized and less widely available, and may require expensive equipment and extensive training to administer.

The important advantage of performance-based measures is that they provide data that is objectively verifiable by outside observers (e.g., a measurable decrease in grip strength over time), whereas subjective reports are directly accessible only to the respondent. Self-report measures are subject to influence by a variety of factors, including mood and recall biases, which can reduce their accuracy. Some methods seek to minimize such bias, for example, reducing recall bias by using handheld organizers (e.g., Palm Pilot) that cue persons to record their momentary fatigue-related symptoms at various points during the day (Whalen, Jamner, Henker, & Delfino, 2001). Recall bias is thus reduced because subjects are required to record their responses soon after the alarm and cannot delay or clump their responses. The possible impact of mood bias can be quantified and at least partially controlled by administering separate mood (Watson, Clark, & Tellegen, 1988) or depression scales (Nyenhuis et al., 1998).

The lack of correlation between direct measurement of performance declines and subject reporting of fatigue is a concern, but it is important to note that it is not proof of the superiority of "objective" performance-based measures. Self-reported measures may reflect, in part, the greater effort required to maintain a given level of performance. For example, patients may require greater effort to maintain a given level of performance than do healthy individuals; the self-reported fatigue scores may be higher even though there is no appreciable difference in the direct measurement of fatigue through performance decrement.

Neurophysiological Correlates

Functional neuroimaging studies have begun to shed light on neural correlates of various fatigue measures. Recent functional magnetic resonance imaging (fMRI) studies demonstrate reliable changes in brain activity in response to maximal and submaximal muscle fatigue in healthy persons (Liu et al., 2003; Liu, Dai, Sahgal, Brown, & Yue, 2002). For example, during sustained voluntary submaximal handgrip contraction, contralateral sensorimotor cortical activity increased sharply and then plateaued (Liu et al., 2003); sustained maximal contractions also led to an initial increase, but this was followed by a decline (Liu et al., 2002). The authors suggest that the initial increased activation may reflect an effort to strengthen the descending command of motor activity to compensate for the force-loss, and the later decreased activity during maximal contraction reflects subsequent inhibition by sensory feedback as fatigue worsens.

Fatigue in MS patients has probably received the most attention in neuroimaging studies among clinical populations. An fMRI study comparing healthy persons to MS patients on a simple motor task found that patients with elevated fatigue scores on the FSS showed lower activation of cortical and subcortical areas involved in motor planning and execution (Filippi et al., 2002). An earlier positron emission tomographic (PET), study of MS patients found hypometabolism in the frontal cortex and basal ganglia were correlated with higher FSS scores (Roelcke et al., 1997).

Though much remains to be learned, functional neuroimaging appears to hold the potential of enriching our understanding and improving our measurement of fatigue. In addition, the positive results from functional imaging contrast with the common failure to identify structural neuroimaging correlates of fatigue, particularly in most MS studies to date (Bakshi et al., 1999; Codella et al., 2002b; Codella et al., 2002c; Codella et al., 2002a; but see Colombo et al., 2000).

Acknowledgments

I would like to thank Lauren Krupp, William MacAllister, and Patricia Melville for their helpful comments, and Dawn Canfora for her invaluable editorial assistance.

References

Ahsberg, E., & Gamberale, F. (1998). Perceived fatigue during physical work: an experimental evaluation of a fatigue inventory. *International Journal of Industrial Ergonomics, 21,* 117–131.

Ahsberg, E., Gamberale, F., & Gustafsson, K. (2000). Perceived fatigue after mental work: an experimental evaluation of a fatigue inventory. *Ergonomics, 43,* 252–268.

Ahsberg, E., Gamberale, F., & Kjellberg, A. (1997). Perceived quality of fatigue during different occupational tasks: development of a questionnaire. *International Journal of Industrial Ergonomics, 20,* 121–135.

Baker, K., Olson, J., & Morisseau, D. (1994). Work practices, fatigue, and nuclear power plant safety performance. *Human Factors, 36,* 244–257.

Bakshi, R., Miletich, R. S., Henschel, K., et al. (1999). Fatigue in multiple sclerosis: cross-sectional correlation with brain MRI findings in 71 patients. *Neurology, 53,* 1151–1153.

Bartley, S. H., & Chute, E. (1947). *Fatigue and Impairment in Man.* New York: McGraw-Hill.

Belza, B. L. (1995). Comparison of self-reported fatigue in rheumatoid arthritis and controls. *Journal of Rheumatology, 22,* 639–643.

Borg, G. (1970). Perceived exertion as an indicator of somatic stress. *Scandinavian Journal of Rehabilitation Medicine, 2,* 92.

Borg, G. (1982a). A Category Scale with Ratio Properties for Intermodal and Interindividual Comparisons. In H. G. Geissler & P. Petzold, eds. *Psychophysical Judgment and the Process of Perception.* Pp. 25–34. New York: North-Holland Publishing Company.

Borg, G. A. (1982b). Psychophysical bases of perceived exertion. *Medical Science of Sports and Exercise, 14,* 377–381.

Browne, B. J., Van Susteren, T., Onsager, D. R., Simpson, D., Salaymeh, B., & Condon, R. E. (1994). Influence of sleep deprivation on learning among surgical house staff and medical students. *Surgery, 115,* 604–610.

Bryant, D., Chiaravalloti, N. D., & Deluca, J. (2004). Objective measurement of cognitive fatigue in multiple sclerosis. *Rehabilitation Psychology, 49,* 213–218.

Chalder, T., Berelowitz, G., Pawlikowska, T., et al. (1993). Development of a fatigue scale. *Journal of Psychosomatic Research, 37,* 147–153.

Codella, M., Rocca, M. A., Colombo, B., Martinelli-Boneschi, F., Comi, G., & Filippi, M. (2002a). Cerebral grey matter pathology and fatigue in patients with multiple sclerosis: a preliminary study. *Journal Neurologic Science, 194,* 71–74.

Codella, M., Rocca, M. A., Colombo, B., Rossi, P., Comi, G., & Filippi, M. (2002b). A preliminary study of magnetization transfer and diffusion tensor MRI of multiple sclerosis patients with fatigue. *Journal of Neurology, 249,* 535–537.

Codella, M., Rocca, M. A., Colombo, B., Rossi, P., Comi, G., & Filippi, M. (2002c). A preliminary study of magnetization transfer and diffusion tensor MRI of multiple sclerosis patients with fatigue. *Journal of Neurology, 249*, 535–537.

Colombo, B., Martinelli, B. F., Rossi, P., et al. (2000). MRI and motor evoked potential findings in nondisabled multiple sclerosis patients with and without symptoms of fatigue. *Journal of Neurology, 247*, 506–509.

Filippi, M., Rocca, M. A., Colombo, B., et al. (2002). Functional magnetic resonance imaging correlates of fatigue in multiple sclerosis. *Neuroimage, 15*, 559–567.

Fisk, J. D., Ritvo, P. G., Ross, L., Haase, D. A., Marrie, T. J., & Schlech, W. F. (1994). Measuring the functional impact of fatigue: initial validation of the fatigue impact scale. *Clinical Infectious Disease, 18 (Suppl 1)*, S79–S83.

Fukuda, K., Straus, S. E., Hickie, I., Sharpe, M. C., Dobbins, J. G., & Komaroff, A. (1994). The chronic fatigue syndrome: a comprehensive approach to its definition and study. International Chronic Fatigue Syndrome Study Group. *Annals of Internal Medicine, 121*, 953–959.

Grant, S., Aitchison, T., Henderson, E., et al. (1999). A comparison of the reproducibility and the sensitivity to change of visual analogue scales, Borg scales, and Likert scales in normal subjects during submaximal exercise. *Chest, 116*, 1208–1217.

Grohar-Murray, M. E., Sears, J. H., Hubsky, E. P., & Becker, A. (1994). Development and testing of a fatigue scale for myasthenia gravis. Unpublished paper, St. Louis University, St. Louis MO.

Hann, D. M., Denniston, M. M., & Baker, F. (2000). Measurement of fatigue in cancer patients: further validation of the Fatigue Symptom Inventory. *Quality of Life Research, 9*, 847–854.

Hartz, A., Bentler, S., & Watson, D. (2003). Measuring fatigue severity in primary care patients. *Journal Psychosomatic Research, 54*, 515–521.

Haylock, P. J., & Hart, L. K. (1979). Fatigue in patients receiving localized radiation. *Cancer Nursing, 2*, 461–467.

Hockenberry, M. J., Hinds, P. S., Barrera, P., et al. (2003). Three instruments to assess fatigue in children with cancer: the child, parent and staff perspectives. *Journal Pain Symptomatology Management, 25*, 319–328.

Iriarte, J., Katsamakis, G., & de Castro, P. (1999). The Fatigue Descriptive Scale (FDS): a useful tool to evaluate fatigue in multiple sclerosis. *Multiple Sclerosis, 5*, 10–16.

Jacques, C. H., Lynch, J. C., & Samkoff, J. S. (1990). The effects of sleep loss on cognitive performance of resident physicians. *Journal Family of Practice, 30*, 223–229.

Kittiwatanapaisan, W., Gauthier, D. K., Williams, A. M., & Oh, S. J. (2003). Fatigue in myasthenia gravis patients. *Journal of Neuroscience Nursing, 35*, 87–93, 106.

Kogi, K., Saito, Y., & Mitsuhashi, T. (1970). Validity of three components of subjective fatigue feelings. *Journal of the Science of Labour, 46,* 251–270.

Krupp, L. B., & Elkins, L. E. (2000). Fatigue and declines in cognitive functioning in multiple sclerosis. *Neurology, 55,* 934–939.

Krupp, L. B., LaRocca, N. G., Muir-Nash, J., & Steinberg, A. D. (1989). The fatigue severity scale. Application to patients with multiple sclerosis and systemic lupus erythematosus. *Archives of Neurology, 46,* 1121–1123.

Lee, K. A., Hicks, G., & Nino-Murcia, G. (1991). Validity and reliability of a scale to assess fatigue. *Psychiatry Research, 36,* 291–298.

Liu, J. Z., Dai, T. H., Sahgal, V., Brown, R. W., & Yue, G. H. (2002). Nonlinear cortical modulation of muscle fatigue: a functional MRI study. *Brain Research, 957,* 320–329.

Liu, J. Z., Shan, Z. Y., Zhang, L. D., Sahgal, V., Brown, R. W., & Yue, G. H. (2003). Human brain activation during sustained and intermittent submaximal fatigue muscle contractions: an FMRI study. *Journal of Neurophysiology, 90,* 300–312.

McNair, D. M., Lorr, M., & Droppleman, L. F. (1992). *Profile of Mood States.* San Diego: Educational and Industrial Testing Service.

Mohr, D. C., Hart, S. L., & Goldberg, A. (2003). Effects of treatment for depression on fatigue in multiple sclerosis. *Psychosomatic Medicine, 65,* 542–547.

Morris, T. L., & Miller, J. C. (1996). Electrooculographic and performance indices of fatigue during simulated flight. *Biological Psychology, 42,* 343–360.

Morrow, G. R., Hickok, J. T., Roscoe, J. A., et al. (2003). Differential effects of paroxetine on fatigue and depression: a randomized, double-blind trial from the university of Rochester cancer center community clinical oncology program. *Journal Clinical of Oncology, 21,* 4635–4641.

Multiple Sclerosis Council for Clinical Practice Guidelines (1998). *Fatigue and Multiple Sclerosis: Evidence-based management strategies for fatigue in multiple sclerosis.* Washington, DC: Paralyzed Veterans of America.

Noble, B. J. (1982). Clinical applications of perceived exertion. *Medical Science of Sports and Exercise, 14,* 406–411.

Nyenhuis, D. L., Luchetta, T., Yamamoto, C., et al. (1998). The development, standardization, and initial validation of the Chicago Multiscale Depression Inventory. *Journal of Personality Assessment, 70,* 386–401.

Paul, R. H., Beatty, W. W., Schneider R., Blanco, C. R., & Hames, K. A. (1998). Cognitive and physical fatigue in multiple sclerosis: relations between self-report and objective performance. *Applied Neuropsychology, 5,* 143–148.

Paul, R. H., Cohen, R. A., & Gilchrist, J. M. (2002). Ratings of subjective mental fatigue relate to cognitive performance in patients with myasthenia gravis. *Journal of Clinical Neuroscience, 9,* 243–246.

Piper, B. F. (1989). Fatigue: current bases for practice. In S. G. Funk, E. M. Tornquist, M. T. Champagne, L. A. Copp, & R. A. Wiese, eds. *Key Aspects of Comfort: Management of Pain, Fatigue, and Nausea*. Pp. 187–240. New York: Springer Publishing Company.

Piper, B. F., Dibble, S. L., Dodd, M. J., Weiss, M. C., Slaughter, R. E., & Paul, S. M. (1998). The revised Piper Fatigue Scale: psychometric evaluation in women with breast cancer. *Oncology Nursing Forum, 25*, 677–684.

Piper, B. F., Lindsey, A. M., Dodd, M. J., Ferketich, S., Paul, S. M., & Weller, S. (1989). The development of an instrument to measure the subjective dimension of fatigue. In S. G. Funk, E. M. Tornquist, M. T. Champagne, L. A. Copp, & R. A. Wiese, eds. *Key Aspects of Comfort: Management of Pain, Fatigue, and Nausea*. Pp. 199–240. New York: Springer Publishing Company.

Roelcke, U., Kappos, L., Lechner-Scott, J., et al. (1997). Reduced glucose metabolism in the frontal cortex and basal ganglia of multiple sclerosis patients with fatigue: a 18F-fluorodeoxyglucose positron emission tomography study. *Neurology, 48*, 1566–1571.

Schellekens, J. M., Sijtsma, G. J., Vegter, E., & Meijman, T. F. (2000). Immediate and delayed aftereffects of long lasting mentally demanding work. *Biological Psychology, 53*, 37–56.

Schwartz, J. E., Jandorf, L., & Krupp, L. B. (1993). The measurement of fatigue: a new instrument. *Journal of Psychosomatic Research, 37*, 753–762.

Schwid, S. R., Covington, M., Segal, B. M., & Goodman, A. D. (2002). Fatigue in multiple sclerosis: current understanding and future directions. *Journal of Rehabilitation Research and Development, 39*, 211–224.

Schwid, S. R., Tyler, C. M., Scheid, E. A., Weinstein, A., Goodman, A. D., & McDermott, M. P. (2003). Cognitive fatigue during a test requiring sustained attention: a pilot study. *Multiple Sclerosis, 9*, 503–508.

Sharma, K. R., Kent-Braun, J., Mynhier, M. A., Weiner, M. W., & Miller, R. G. (1995). Evidence of an abnormal intramuscular component of fatigue in multiple sclerosis. *Muscle Nerve, 18*, 1403–1411.

Sheean, G. L., Murray, N. M., Rothwell, J. C., Miller, D. H., & Thompson, A. J. (1997). An electrophysiological study of the mechanism of fatigue in multiple sclerosis. *Brain, 120 (Pt 2)*, 299–315.

Smets, E. M., Garssen, B., Bonke, B., & De Haes, J. C. (1995). The Multidimensional Fatigue Inventory (MFI) psychometric qualities of an instrument to assess fatigue. *Journal of Psychosomatic Research, 39*, 315–325.

Stein, K. D., Martin, S. C., Hann, D. M., & Jacobsen, P. B. (1998). A multidimensional measure of fatigue for use with cancer patients. *Cancer Practice, 6*, 143–152.

Stern, J. A., Boyer, D., & Schroeder, D. (1994). Blink rate: a possible measure of fatigue. *Human Factors, 36*, 285–297.

van der Linden, D., Frese, M., & Meijman, T. F. (2003). Mental fatigue and the control of cognitive processes: effects on perseveration and planning. *Acta Psychologica, 113,* 45–65.

Vercoulen, J. H., Swanink, C. M., Fennis, J. F., Galama, J. M., van der Meer, J. W., & Bleijenberg, G. (1994). Dimensional assessment of chronic fatigue syndrome. *Journal of Psychosomatic Research, 38,* 383–392.

Vercoulen, J. H. M. M., Bazelmans, E., Swanink, C. M. A., et al. (1997). Physical activity in chronic fatigue syndrome: assessment and its role in fatigue. *Journal of Psychiatric Research, 31,* 661–673.

Vollestad, N. K. (1997). Measurement of human muscle fatigue. *Journal of Neuroscience Methods, 74,* 219–227.

Watson, D., Clark, L. A., & Tellegen, A. (1988). Development and validation of brief measures of positive and negative affect: the PANAS scales. *Journal of Personality and Social Psychology, 54,* 1063–1070.

Wessely, S., Hotopf, M., & Sharpe, D. (1998). *Chronic Fatigue and Its Syndromes.* New York: Oxford University Press.

Whalen, C. K., Jamner, L. D., Henker, B., & Delfino, R. J. (2001). Smoking and moods in adolescents with depressive and aggressive dispositions: evidence from surveys and electronic diaries. *Health Psychology, 20,* 99–111.

3 Fatigue, Cognition, and Mental Effort

John DeLuca

Nothing so fatiguing as the eternal hanging on of an uncompleted task
—William James, 1881

As exemplified throughout this book, fatigue in a clinical setting is typically described as a pervasive complaint of individuals with significant health problems of medical, psychiatric, or neurological origin. A good deal of research has been devoted to elucidating the mechanisms involved in such fatigue, particularly in certain disorders such as multiple sclerosis (MS), traumatic brain injury (TBI), and depression. Despite these efforts, however, fatigue remains a poorly understood symptom whose management strategies, whether behavioral or pharmacological, are only partially effective (Kinkel, 2000). One reason for such a poor level of success is the lack of a widely accepted conceptual framework of fatigue. First, there is no universally accepted definition of fatigue. Second, fatigue continues to be conceptualized as a unitary construct rather than a multifaceted symptom (Brassington & Marsh, 1998; Elkins, Krupp, & Scherl, 2000), with components potentially arising from distinct mechanisms of origin (Iriarte, Subira, & Castro, 2000). For instance, fatigue can be reported in terms of objective physical performance or as a perceived lack of physical or mental stamina (e.g., cognitive fatigue). This multidimensional nature often leads to confusion and miscommunication between professionals as well as with patients.

The primary approach to measuring fatigue today is by subjective patient reporting. To quantify this subjective rating, a variety self-report instruments have been developed (e.g., Krupp, LaRocca, Muir-Nash, & Steinberg, 1989). Some of these instruments provide separate indices of self-reported physical versus mental fatigue (Smets, Garssen, Bonke, & De Haes, 1995); other include subscales designed to measure fatigue severity, distress, timing, and interference (Belza, Henke, Yelin, Epstein, & Gilliss, 1993).

Despite the emphasis on self-report in measuring fatigue, these measures have been known for at least a century to correlate poorly with actual physical performance or measures of disease activity (Mosso, 1904; Wessely, Hotopf & Sharpe, 1998). For

instance, subjective ratings of fatigue in persons with MS show little or no relationship to disease characteristics such as lesion load, disease duration, disease course (e.g.,
relapsing-remitting versus progressive), or functional impairment as measured by the
Expanded Disability Status Scale (EDSS) (Kurtzke, 1983; see also Kinkel, 2000). Even
measures of physiological fatigue (e.g., muscle metabolism) do not correlate with subjective reports of fatigue (Gandevia, Enoka, McComas, Stuart, & Thomas, 1995).

Similarly, no relationship has been found between subjective fatigue and cognitive
dysfunction. For instance, the level of subjective fatigue in MS is not related to a
decline in working memory (Johnson, Lange, DeLuca, Korn, & Natelson, 1997), short-
term memory (Johnson, DeLuca, Diamond, & Natelson, 1998), executive function or
complex attention (Krupp & Elkins, 2000; Rao, Leo, Bernadin, & Unverzagt, 1991),
vigilance (Paul, Beatty, Schneider, Blanco, & Hames, 1998), verbal fluency (Rao et al.,
1991), or verbal memory (Krupp & Elkins, 2000; Paul et al., 1998; Schwartz, Coulthard-
Morris, & Zeng, 1996). In light of these limitations, it is understandable that
researchers have recently focused on developing objective measures of fatigue in MS.

Despite the extensive use of subjective ratings to measure fatigue, a wide array of
techniques have also been developed to objectively measure physical or physiological
manifestations of fatigue (c.f., Gandevia et al., 1995). In contrast, few techniques have
been developed to objectively measure mental or cognitive fatigue. This chapter illus-
trates the attempts at objective measurement of cognitive fatigue, and relates this
objective measurement to cognitive or neuropsychological performance.

Objective Measurement of Cognitive Fatigue

Mental fatigue, or a decrement in performance from excess mental effort, gained widespread attention in the 1880s. However, even today, descriptions of mental or cognitive fatigue are often vague and subjective. One working definition of cognitive or
mental fatigue is a time-related deterioration in the ability to perform certain mental
tasks (Broadbent, 1971). Numerous studies show objective measurement of motor or
muscle fatigue (c.f. Gandevia et al., 1995), but there is a relative dearth of studies quantifying cognitive fatigue in clinical populations. Though a few recent studies have been
reported, for the most part, such studies examined cognitive performance over the
course of an experimental induction of fatigue, using four general approaches. First,
cognitive fatigue can be conceptualized as decreased performance over a *prolonged
period of time*, such as during the course of a work day. Hence, at the end of a long
day one often hears "I am too tired to think anymore." A second approach to cognitive fatigue could be viewed as decreased performance during acute but *sustained
mental effort*. This conception of fatigue is similar to that typically seen in the motor
fatigue literature, in which fatigue is defined as a failure to maintain a required force
or output of power during sustained or repeated muscle contraction (Stokes, Cooper,

& Edwards, 1988). The other two approaches evaluate cognitive fatigue *after* challenging mental exertion and cognitive fatigue after challenging physical exertion. Each approach is explored in the following sections, with special emphasis on clinical populations.

Cognitive Fatigue over an Extended Time (Prolonged Effort)

Not uncommonly, persons report fatigue after a prolonged period of time, such as after a day of work. However, do such self-reported experiences result in cognitive fatigue, which then affects cognitive performance? The following studies examined cognitive functioning after a prolonged period of active mental operations in clinical samples.

Jennekens-Schinkel and colleagues (1988) claimed to be the first to study the effects of fatigue on "mental" functioning in an MS sample. They examined reaction times (RT) before and after a 4-hour neuropsychological evaluation (assumed to measure prolonged effort) in 39 persons with MS and 25 healthy control subjects. Although RT and subjective fatigue changed in both groups after the prolonged effort period, the magnitude of these changes did not differ between the MS and healthy groups.

Johnson and cowokers (1997) used a 3-hour neuropsychological testing session to induce fatigue in persons with MS, chronic fatigue syndrome (CFS), and clinical depression, and in healthy control subjects. Subjects rated their subjective fatigue four times during the 3-hour testing session. Immediately after each rating, subjects completed the Paced Auditory Serial Addition Test (PASAT) (Brittain et al., 1991) to relate subjective ratings of fatigue with objective neuropsychological performance. The PASAT requires subjects to continually monitor a digit string while simultaneously manipulating the digits held in a short-term memory store. The researchers hypothesized that the induced fatigue with prolonged mental activity would result in diminished cognitive performance in the three fatiguing clinical groups relative to controls. However, the three clinical groups and the healthy control subjects exhibited similar degrees of improvement in performance across repeated administrations of PASAT. That is, despite increased levels of subjective fatigue over the 3-hour session, all groups showed the same increase in PASAT performance over time, likely a result of practice effect. There was no relationship between subjective fatigue (or depression, for that matter) and PASAT performance.

Paul and associates (1998) examined MS and healthy subjects in a study similar to the Johnson study (1997). These authors found performance by MS subjects unchanged on grip strength, learning, and vigilance tests from the beginning to the end of a 30-minute testing session, relative to the healthy control group.

Krupp and Elkin (2000) administered a neuropsychological test battery twice over a 4-hour period. In contrast to the previous studies, these authors observed that MS subjects displayed a decline in performance during the second administration whereas the control group improved slightly. However, as I discuss later, it is unclear whether this finding was the result of prolonged effort (the length of the battery) or the acute cognitive fatigue induced by sustained performance of a challenging effortful task by the subjects just before the second test was administered (see next section).

Riese and associates (1999) examined "mental fatigue" in persons with severe TBI on a driving simulator. TBI and healthy control subjects were required to perform several sustained driving-related tasks at either 50 or 80 percent of each individual's maximal performance level, which was established during a separate training session. Pre- and posttest tasks of cognitive performance, subjective distress, and cardiovascular measures (heart rate and blood pressure) were obtained. During the driving simulator task, subjects were required to perform three single tasks simultaneously—lane tracking, dot counting and peripheral detection—over a 50-minute period of sustained performance. Results showed no performance differences on these three behavioral indicators between the TBI and healthy control groups. However, to maintain a level of performance comparable to that of the controls, the TBI subjects displayed elevated levels of subjective distress as well as altered physiological state (i.e., elevated systolic blood pressure). These authors suggested that TBI subjects pay "higher physiological costs" for sustained performance on the dual-task paradigm.

From a survey of 146 polio survivors, Bruno, Galski, and DeLuca (1993) examined six carefully screened individuals with postpolio sequelae (PPS), three reporting severe fatigue and three reporting mild fatigue. The authors hypothesized that fatigue in PPS was associated with neuropsychological impairment in attention, concentration, and processing speed, but not necessarily in higher-level cognitive functions. These subjects were given a 3-hour battery of neuropsychological tests while subjective fatigue was monitored every 45 minutes. Results showed that only PPS subjects reporting severe fatigue demonstrated deficits (relative to normative values) on tests of attention, concentration, and processing speed. Subjective fatigue was not associated with neuropsychological performance. The authors suggest that these cognitive deficits were characteristic of PPS with severe fatigue because the deficits were observed even when subjective levels of fatigue were low (i.e., during the early portion of the testing session). Although intriguing, given the very small sample size and the selective nature of the PPS subjects included, these results must be considered very preliminary and should await replication with a much larger sample.

Taken together, studies of prolonged effort in clinical samples show little to no discernable effect on actual cognitive performance. While prolonged cognitive effort produced an increase in the subjective experience of fatigue in these samples, this increase did not translate into observable cognitive performance deficits.

Cognitive Fatigue During Sustained Mental Effort

Cognitive fatigue can also be conceptualized as similar to how motor or muscle fatigue has been examined, that is, during mental effort that is sustained (i.e., maintaining constant cognitive vigilance) rather than prolonged (performing tasks over a long period of time such as a work day, but not with sustained effort). Objective measures of motor or muscle fatigue examine the deterioration of performance during sustained or repetitive motor activity. The analogy in the cognitive domain would be reduced performance during sustained cognitive work. Few studies have actually used these paradigms in clinical populations, other than studies examining "vigilance," which have conceptualized such deterioration not as fatigue but difficulty in sustained attention (Broadbent, 1971).

Krupp and Elkins (2000) demonstrated diminished performance over the course of a sustained working memory task. They observed that performances of MS and control subjects did not differ during the first half of an alpha-arithmetic test. However, relative to the first half of the alpha-arithmetic task (the A-A Test), MS subjects showed significantly slowed reaction time during the second half of the test than healthy control subjects. Unfortunately, Krupp and Elkins (2000) do not report whether the actual performance levels (i.e., number correct) declined in their MS subjects relative to healthy controls over the course of the A-A Test. Self-reported fatigue was unrelated to cognitive performance.

Kujala, Portin, Revonsuo, and Ruutiainen (1995) reported findings similar to those of Krupp and Elkins (2000). They found that a group of cognitively "preserved" MS subjects exhibited slowness in performance (i.e., reaction time) only toward the end of a longlasting visual vigilance task, whereas a cognitively deteriorated group was slow throughout the test. The authors interpreted these data as the effect of fatigue from sustained cognitive effort.

Bryant, Chiaravalloti, and DeLuca (2004) examined fatigue in 56 persons with MS and 39 healthy controls matched for age and educational level. MS subjects were further subdivided into those with cognitive impairment ($n = 27$) and those not cognitively impaired ($n = 29$). This determination was based on neuropsychological test performance, using a technique from prior studies focusing on cognitive performance in MS patients (e.g., Rao et al., 1991; Schultheis, Garay, & DeLuca, 2001). In this study, cognitive fatigue was conceptualized as "the inability to sustain performance throughout the duration of a continuous complex information processing task," the PASAT. Cognitive fatigue was operationally defined as a decrease in the number of correct responses generated in the second half ("later responses") compared to the first half ("earlier responses") of a PASAT trial. It was hypothesized that although both MS and healthy control subjects experience cognitive fatigue, MS subjects would demonstrate a greater fatigue effect as the sustained cognitive load increased (i.e., with increased difficulty on the PASAT trials, operationalized by faster presentation of stimuli).

When the mean number of correct responses was examined within each trial of the PASAT, all groups showed a significant fatigue effect (i.e., a reliable drop in performance from the earlier to later responses within each PASAT trial). However, MS subjects, both with and without cognitive impairment, showed no greater fatigue affect than did healthy control subjects.

Although these data show that cognitive fatigue can be objectively measured, they do not show the hypothesized differential effect of cognitive fatigue between MS and healthy control subjects. One reason may be that the sustained cognitive effort was not consistently maintained during performance of the PASAT to sufficiently test the central executive of working memory (Fisk and Archibald, 2001; Snyder, Aniskiewicz, & Snyder, 1993). To test this hypothesis, Bryant and colleagues also examined the proportion of correct responses generated during maximal difficulty or "sustained central executive load." This latter dependent measure was defined as the proportion of correct responses generated immediately following another correct response (a "dyad"), which has been considered a measure of the extent to which subjects continue to hold PASAT digits in working memory while performing the required mathematical operation (see Fisk & Archibald, 2001; Snyder et al., 1993). This ensures that a high working memory load is maintained continuously throughout performance of a PASAT trial.

When the percent Dyad score was examined, once again, all groups showed a significant fatigue effect (reliable drop in performance from the first half to the second half of each PASAT trial) collapsed across the four PASAT trials. However, as the central executive load increased (i.e., across the four PASAT trials), both MS groups showed a relative breakdown in performance at a lesser load (trial 3) than the healthy control (HC) group (trial 4) (figure 3.1). This pattern of results suggests that MS subjects, whether or not they demonstrate cognitive impairment, were reaching the limit of their ability to sustain central executive load at an earlier point in PASAT administration than HC subjects. Subjective fatigue (as well as depression scores) did not correlate with either the number correct or percent dyad score for HC, cognitively impaired, or cognitively nonimpaired MS subjects.

Schwid, Tyler, Scheid, Weinstein, Goodman, and McDermott (2003) also used the PASAT to objectively measure cognitive fatigue in 20 MS and 21 healthy control subjects. They also employed a second test to measure sustained attentional performance, the Digit Ordering Test (DOT). The tests were administered four times over three testing session. Data were analyzed for the fourth administration. Although no significant fatigue effect was observed on the DOT, the authors reported a fatigue effect in the MS group on the PASAT (by either decline in performance from the first third to last third of the PASAT or the slope of the regression line). Though this fatigue effect was not observed in the HC group, the MS subjects did not show a significantly different fatigue effect from the control group. Interestingly, subjective fatigue ratings correlated with the PASAT measure of fatigue in MS subjects, but only in one of the three subjective ratings methods employed, and only in the MS group.

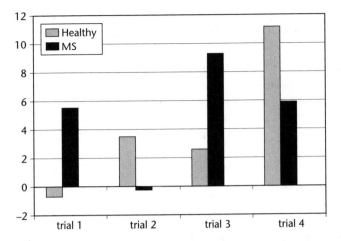

Figure 3.1
Difference score between first half and second half of each PASAT trial on the percent dyad score across PASAT trials for MS and healthy subjects. (Adapted from Bryant, Chiaravalloti, & DeLuca, 2004).

In summary, the method of documenting change in performance during sustained cognitive activity appears to be fruitful in objectively documenting cognitive fatigue and its effect on measures of sustained attention or processing speed. Overall, indices of subjective fatigue are not reliably correlated with objective measures of cognitive fatigue.

Cognitive Fatigue after Challenging Mental Exertion

Another area of study for the influence of fatigue on cognitive performance is performance after carrying out challenging mental operations. The mental effort should result in a "buildup" of fatigue, which then influences cognitive performance. Krupp and Elkins (2000) administered a neuropsychological test battery lasting about 2 hours, followed by a "continuous effortful cognitive task" (the A-A Test), and then repeated the original neuropsychological battery. The notion was that engaging in sustained effortful cognitive activity would have a "carryover" effect on subsequent cognitive performance. The results demonstrated *declining* verbal memory performance and perceptual planning in MS subjects immediately following the A-A test administration, relative to initial performance on the battery. HC subjects showed relative *improved* performance after A-A test administration. Self-reported fatigue was unrelated to the pattern of cognitive decline observed in this study.

It could be argued that, because the entire test session required a 4-hour testing session (i.e., repeat administration of the neuropsychological battery with the A-A test between them), the decline in performance among MS subjects from the initial to the follow-up neuropsychological battery actually supports the first model presented, namely, that prolonged mental effort produces a buildup of fatigue, resulting in a decline in cognitive performance. However, despite this possibility, the authors argued that the decline in cognitive performance in the MS group during the second administration was a result of the "continuous cognitively effortful" nature of the task employed in their study. This suggests that the induced cognitive fatigue due to sustained mental effort had a "spillover" on subsequent cognitive performance. Nevertheless, because the Krupp and Elkins study was conducted over a prolonged period of time, whether the observed decline in cognitive performance was a result of prolonged effort or the effects of a challenging mental exercise (i.e., sustained effort) cannot be determined at this time.

Cognitive Fatigue after Challenging Physical Exertion

Another model that may result in cognitive fatigue and potentially influence neuropsychological performance is the impact of physical exertion. Fatigued patients often report an increase in fatigue following physical exertion, which is also accompanied by a perceived reduction in mental abilities. Because this "postexertional malaise" is part of the working diagnostic criteria for CFS (Fukuda, Straus, Hickie, Sharpe, Dobbins, & Komaroff 1994), several studies specifically examine the effect of physical exertion on cognitive performance in CFS. Up to 70 percent of CFS patients reported symptom exacerbation, including worsening of cognitive functioning, after exertion (Komaroff & Buchwald, 1991).

LaManca and associates (1998) examined the influence of exhaustive exercise on cognitive performance in 19 persons with CFS and 20 healthy controls. A battery of neuropsychological tests of working memory and processing speed was administered before, immediately after, and 24 hours after treadmill exercise to exhaustion. No group difference on the cognitive battery was observed in the preexercise baseline condition. Immediately postexercise, however, the CFS group performed significantly worse than the HC group on the cognitive battery. That is, although the HC subjects showed a significant improvement in cognitive performance after exercise (i.e., practice effect), the CFS subjects did not differ from their own baseline performance post— physical exertion. Interestingly, this lack of improvement in cognitive performance among the CFS group was maintained even 24 hours after the initial baseline testing. The cognitive deficiency in the CFS group after physical exertion was observed in the speed of information processing and not in the overall accuracy of performance. Subjective ratings of fatigue did not correlate with objective cognitive performance. These data support the notion that cognitive processing decreases significantly after physical exertion.

Blackwood, MacHale, Power Goodwin, and Lawrie (1998) conducted a similar study to that of LaManca and colleagues (1998). After exertion, they reporter CFS subjects showed a "greater decrease" than HC subjects on cognitive tests of focused and sustained attention. Interestingly, the CFS group also showed significantly greater cognitive decline post–physical exertion than did a group of patients with major depression.

At least one other study of the effects of physical exertion on cognitive functioning, however, has failed to report an effect on cognitive processing in persons with CFS (Claypoole, Mahurin, Fisher, Goldberg, Schmaling, Schoene, Ashton, & Buchwald, 2001). In this study of 21 monozygotic twins discordant for CFS, the subjects were required to pedal a cycle ergometer to exhaustion. Pre- and postexercise neuropsychological tests of processing speed, attention and concentration, verbal learning, and memory and category fluency (with alternate forms) were administered. Preexercise neuropsychological performance tended to be slightly lower in the CFS twins than the healthy twin group. Compared to the healthy cotwins, however, the CFS twins did not display differential decrements in neuropsychological performance after exercise on three of the four tests. On category fluency, the healthy cotwins showed a significant improvement postexercise relative to the CFS cotwin. As with other studies, perceived rating of exertion during exercise did not correlate with neuropsychological performance. Overall, the authors concluded that exhaustive exercise had no consistent effect on cognitive performance in persons with CFS.

The data suggesting that physical exertion affects later cognitive performance is mixed (at least in CFS), and thus inconclusive. Yet the lack of any relationship between subjective fatigue and objective performance was universal.

Fatigue and Neuropsychological Performance: Clinical and Healthy Samples

The potential detrimental influence of fatigue on neuropsychological performance in clinical populations has long been recognized. One standard neuropsychological text, for instance, suggests fatigue can significantly affect cognitive performance in patients.

The patient who fatigues easily rarely performs well and may experience relatively intact functions as more impaired as they actually are. (Lezak, 1983; p. 127).

In arranging [a] test time, the patient's daily schedule must be considered if the effects of fatigue are to be kept minimal. When necessary, the examiner may insist that the patient take a nap before being tested. (Lezak, 1983, p. 126)

The assumption here is that, at least in "vulnerable patients," neuropsychological performance will be adversely affected by fatigue as the testing session progresses (i.e., prolonged effort model). Lezak (1995) provides a number of recommendations to minimize this purported fatigue effect on neuropsychological performance: shortening test sessions, giving difficult tests early in a session, and allowing many rest periods. Unfortunately, little clinical evidence supports these specific claims regarding fatigue, its effect on neuropsychological performance, or the proposed recommendations to reduce any potential fatigue effect. In fact, several studies in clinical populations with fatigue have yielded results inconsistent with these claims. For instance, Parmenter, Denney, and Lynch (2003) examined 30 persons with MS who experienced "substantial fatigue" and tested them on two occasions: during a period of very high fatigue and again during very low fatigue (counterbalanced across subjects). The MS subjects were tested on a battery of neuropsychological tasks including tests of attention, memory, and executive functions, and completed questionnaires concerning their present state of fatigue. No differences in performance were observed during periods of high versus low fatigue. In fact, these authors state that their data "call into question the necessity of scheduling neuropsychological assessments so as to avoid periods of high fatigue" (p. 11). The studies presented in the section on cognitive fatigue over an extended time (prolonged effort) also generally failed to support the claim that fatigue from prolonged effort results in diminished neuropsychological performance.

In fact, in the vast majority of neuropsychological studies, self-reported fatigue in clinical samples does not correlate with neuropsychological performance. This lack of a relationship between subjective fatigue and neuropsychological performance is observed across a wide variety of clinical samples including MS (Bryant et al., 2004; Johnson et al., 1997; Paul et al., 1998), HIV/AIDS (Millikin, Rourke, Halman, & Power, 2003), CFS (Cluydts, 2001; Johnson et al., 1997), and Parkinson's disease (Abe, Takanashi, & Yanagihara, 2000). The most consistent finding is that subjective fatigue is more closely associated with the degree or severity of psychiatric disturbance (e.g., depression) than with objective cognitive or motor performance (Millikin et al., 2003; see chapter 19). Unfortunately, the lack of relationship between subjective and objective fatigue was observed more than 100 years ago (Mosso, 1904), illustrating how little has been learned since that time.

In contrast with the clinical studies examining the influence of fatigue on neuropsychological performance, a fairly sizeable collection of nonclinical psychological literature shows that fatigue does result in reduced cognitive efficiency in healthy individuals. In industry, accidents are often attributed to mental fatigue resulting from sustained performance (van der Linden, Frese, & Meijman, 2003). The relationship between cognitive fatigue and performance among healthy individuals has been a key area of research. One model suggests that performance on well learned tasks or tasks executed "automatically," can be sustained over long periods of time (i.e., are less susceptible to fatigue) even after sleep deprivation or challenging activities. However, tasks that are more demanding or "require deliberate control of behavior" are more susceptible to factors inducing fatigue. This model suggests that cognitive fatigue is induced by deterioration of "executive control." Executive control can be defined as "the ability to regulate perceptual and motor processes in order to respond in an adaptive way to novel or changing task demands" (van der Linden et al., 2003, p. 47).

Van der Linden and colleagues (2003) conducted a study to test the executive dyscontrol hypothesis of cognitive fatigue. Fatigue was induced by having healthy subjects perform a cognitively demanding task for 2 hours, while controls performed nondemanding activities for the same duration. Following the fatigue-induced challenge, neuropsychological tests of executive functions were administered. The fatigued group displayed significantly more perseverative responses on the Wisconsin Card Sorting Test and significantly prolonged planning time on the Tower of London than the nonfatigued group. Fatigue did not affect performance on relatively simple mental tracking tasks (i.e., digit span forward), and reduced cognitive performance was not related to factors such as mood or motivation. The results were interpreted as supporting the hypothesis that cognitive fatigue influences higher-level executive control of behaviors, resulting in lowered mental flexibility and suboptimal planning, rather than rote, automatic, and well-learned behavior.

Lorist, Kernell, Meijman, and Zijdewind (2003) used a dual-task paradigm to examine the effects of motor fatigue on cognitive performance. Healthy subjects performed an auditory choice reaction time (CRT) task, either alone or simultaneously with a submaximal contraction task. Although performance in single-task conditions were stable over the 15-minute testing interval, in the dual-task condition, reaction time and performance accuracy decreased over time (during the second half of the test only) on the CRT, with increasing motor fatigue. Interestingly, motor task performance also decreased in the dual-task condition, indicating that cognitive fatigue also resulted in diminished motor performance.

Military studies of fatigue and cognitive performance in healthy subjects have examined the influence of fatigue (often defined as prolonged wakefulness) on alertness, for instance, on pilot performance. Morris and Miller (1996) investigated fatigue in partially sleep-deprived pilots performing a 4.5-hour sortie on a flight simulator. Errors on various flight activities such as altitude, air speed, heading, and vertical velocity were recorded. The results showed an overall increase over time in the number of errors committed, with errors positively correlated to subjective fatigue and physiological measures of eye and eyelid movements. Paul, Pigeau, and Weinberg (2001) examined pilot fatigue on actual transatlantic resupply missions in which pilots were airborne for 3 consecutive days. These authors monitored sleep patterns both 5 days before and during the actual flights. Results showed progressively decreasing sleep over the flight period. Decreased sleep was associated with decreased subjective ratings of alertness and increased physical and mental fatigue. Tests of psychomotor functioning and multitask performance showed evidence of "probable" fatigue.

Interestingly, concerning potential methods of diminishing fatigue effects, there is some evidence that interventions such as frequent rest or use of stimulants can diminish the effects of fatigue on cognitive performance. In healthy individuals, for instance, naps have a recooperative effect on alertness and cognitive performance (Tietzel & Lack, 2002). Similarly, brief but regular breaks significantly reduced night-time sleepiness during a 6-hour flight on a Boeing 747 simulator on both physiological and subjective measures (Neri, Oyung, Colletti, Mallis, Tam, & Dinges, 2002). A recent randomized, double-blind, placebo-controlled study examined the effects of slow-release caffeine over a 64-hour period of continuous wakefulness in healthy males. The results showed a significant improvement on tests of vigilance, information processing, working memory, and divided attention (Beaumont, Batejat, Pierard, Coste, Doireau, Van Beers, Chauffard, Chassard, Enslen, Denis, & Lagarde, 2001). Such studies in healthy samples support Lezak's recommendations to reduce the potential effects of fatigue on neuropsychological performance. Unfortunately, results obtained in healthy samples frequently do not generalize to clinical populations (Chiaravalloti, Demaree, Gaudino, & DeLuca, 2003).

There appears to be reasonable evidence that cognitive or mental fatigue is related to reduced cognitive performance in healthy individuals and that short periods of rest can significantly reduce this influence on performance. In contrast, despite increased complaints of cognitive fatigue, little to no evidence supports a relationship between the subjective rating of cognitive fatigue and actual cognitive performance in clinical samples. What explains the discrepancy between healthy individuals and clinical populations? It is possible that the healthy subject and clinical studies are not measuring the same thing. While the clinical studies examine fatigue, many if not most non-clinical studies examine the lack of sleep on performance. Along these lines, Duntley (see chapter 13) argues that "sleepiness" and fatigue are not the same thing, and the terms should not be used synonymously.

Possible Mechanisms of Cognitive Fatigue

Despite the elusive nature of an objective measure of cognitive fatigue in clinical populations, the complaint of cognitive fatigue among these individuals remains pervasive. What are some of the potential mechanisms responsible for the subjective experience of cognitive fatigue in clinical populations? This section focuses primarily on potential mechanisms involving cerebral metabolism and functional organization.

One potential mechanism is metabolic disturbance. For instance, in persons with MS, Krupp and Elkins (2000) suggest a model based on data associated with motor and muscle fatigue, namely, metabolic dysregulation. They speculate that fluctuations in glucose metabolism may be the "final common pathway" leading to cognitive decline. Unfortunately, there is little support for this relationship among persons with MS. Persons with MS have been shown to experience dysregulation of the hypothalamic–pituitary–adrenal (HPA) axis, and HPA axis dysregulation may be related to cognitive performance; however, the relationship with fatigue is fairly low (Heesen, Gold, Raji, Wiedemann, & Schulz, 2002).

A second model of fatigue proposed by Newsholme and Blomstrand (1995) involves a physiological model in which "central fatigue" is caused by an increase in tryptophan levels in the brain (via increased plasma levels due to exercise), leading to an increased level of the neurotransmitter serotonin in the brain. According to this model, because serotonin is known to be involved in sleep, excessive serotonin may also lead to tiredness or fatigue. Specifically, increased serotonin activity in the brain may increase the "mental effort" required to maintain the pace of the fatiguing event (e.g., running). Some evidence supports this theory of central fatigue, but primarily in the motor domain (see Newsholme & Blomstrand, 1995).

A third and more recent potential model for the subjective experience of cognitive fatigue is its association with levels of functional cerebral activity. Recent advances in neuroimaging may shed some light on the potential neural mechanisms responsible for cognitive fatigue.

Functional Imaging Studies in Clinical Samples That Experience Fatigue In a recent series of studies, our laboratory has examined the functional cerebral activity associated with cognitive functioning in persons with TBI, MS, and CFS using functional MRI (fMRI). These studies suggest that the perception of cognitive fatigue may be a result of the increased cerebral effort required to perform the same amount of cognitive work (e.g., maintain the same level of task performance as controls).

Christodoulou and coworkers (2001) examined patterns of brain activation in nine persons with moderate to severe TBI and seven healthy controls performing a complex working memory task during fMRI acquisition. Group activation patterns are presented in figure 3.2. Healthy control subjects showed cerebral activation primarily in the left hemisphere of the brain, involving the frontal and temporal lobes, as well as bilateral parietal lobe activation. In contrast, TBI subjects displayed bilateral activation that was more lateralized, primarily to homologous regions of the right hemisphere relative to controls. In addition, TBI subjects showed a pattern of more dispersed activation within both the ipsilateral (left) and contralateral hemispheres. The authors suggested that the increased right hemisphere recruitment resulted from the TBI subjects' need for more cognitive effort than healthy controls because of damage to the underlying neural substrate that maintains and manipulates information in working memory (presumably normally in the left hemisphere).

One criticism of the Christodoulou and coworkers (2001) study is that the TBI group performed more poorly on the behavioral task than healthy controls. Thus, the group differences in cerebral activation could be a result of actual task difficulty rather than perceived effort. Other recent data suggest this may not be the case. In two studies, McAllister and associates (1999, 2001) examined working memory in

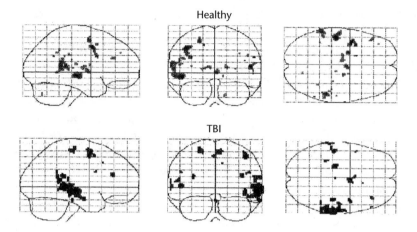

Figure 3.2
Group activation patterns during working memory performance in TBI ($n = 9$) and healthy
control ($n = 7$) groups. Maximum intensity projections in the three orthogonal views of the brain
(sagittal, coronal, axial) depict areas of significant activation. (From Christodoulou et al., 2001,
with permission.)

persons with mild TBI during fMRI. Like the Christodoulou and coworkers (2001)
study, these studies showed increased activation in the right cerebral hemisphere in
regions homologous to left hemisphere activation observed in healthy controls.
However, this activation pattern occurred in the absence of performance differences
between the mild TBI and healthy control groups during the working memory task.
McAllister and colleagues propose that, despite similar objective performance, mild
TBI subjects require additional cerebral resources "to compensate for processing
inefficiencies."

Several recent functional imaging studies in persons with MS (Staffen, Mair, Zauner,
et al., 2002; Hillary et al., 2003; Chiaravalloti et al., 2004) and CFS (Schmaling et al.,
2003; Lange et al., submitted) have reported similar results to those observed in TBI
subjects.

Collectively, these studies suggest that persons with TBI, MS, and CFS require more
cerebral effort than healthy controls to perform a complex cognitive task. What could
account for the increased right hemispheric activity and more dispersed pattern of
cerebral activation among the TBI, MS, and CFS subjects? One reason could be that
the brain reorganizes in response to cerebral damage. Damage to the underlying neural
mechanisms within the left hemisphere that maintain and manipulate information
within working memory may stimulate the brain to seek additional cerebral resources
to solve the cognitive operation. This would engage homologous regions in the

contralateral hemisphere and other remote cerebral regions (Chollet & Weiller, 1994). This extra cerebral activation that may now be required to perform what was previously a routine or more automatic cerebral subroutine, is hypothetically the underlying mechanism for cognitive fatigue. This effect may be due to cerebral overactivation, resulting in less efficient, less accurate, and slower cognitive responses. This decreased efficiency likely results when extensive cortical areas are engaged in information processing for these tasks and cannot simultaneously process other information efficiently (Herndon, 2003).

Functional Imaging Studies during Periods of High and Low Fatigue What do functional neuroimaging studies examining subjects with and without fatigue tell us about brain mechanisms of fatigue? Several functional neuroimaging studies of fatigue have been conducted primarily among persons with MS. However, these studies have been based on subjective fatigue and examined motor performance, not cognitive fatigue. Nonetheless, although structural imaging studies have not shown differences in various conventional MRI metrics between fatigued and nonfatigued MS subjects (Bakshi et al., 1999; Colombo et al., 2000), functional imaging studies have been somewhat more successful.

Using fMRI, Filippi (2002) examined 15 MS subjects with subjective fatigue (based on the fatigue severity scale, or FSS; Krupp et al., 1989), with 14 MS subjects exhibiting no fatigue on a simple motor task. MS subjects with fatigue showed significantly lower activation in cortical and subcortical regions involved in motor planning and execution than MS subjects without fatigue. Roelcke and associates (1997) used PET scanning to compare MS subjects with versus without subjective fatigue. They found that MS subjects with fatigue had reduced glucose metabolism, particularly in the frontal lobes and basal ganglia. Electrophysiological evidence also shows frontal lobe dysfunction in fatigued versus nonfatigued MS subjects using both transcranial magnetic stimulation (Sheean, Murray, Rothwell, Miller, & Thompson, 1997) and electroencephalography (EEG) (Leocani et al., 2001). In fact, this latter study showed a significant correlation between fatigue severity and EEG activity.

It should be reemphasized that all of these studies were conducted while subjects performed motor tasks, which may limit their applicability to fatigue associated with cognitive activity. Sandroni, Walker, and Starr (1992) measured evoked potentials during the performance of an auditory working memory task, and reported that fatigue in MS subjects was associated with shortening of the P_{3a} latency and an increase in P_{3a} and P_{3b} amplitudes compared to when these same subjects were rested. Lorist and colleagues (2000) used behavioral and EEG data to study the effects of cognitive fatigue (i.e., time-on-task) on planning and switching behavior. EEG data showed that increased time-on-task was associated with reduced activity in the frontal lobe, a region known to be associated with executive control. Behavioral data showed an increased number of errors in performance as well as increased reaction time, although cognitive fatigue showed no behavioral effects on executive control per se, a finding similar to that of Parmenter and associates (2003).

Taken together, the functional neuroimaging studies of fatigued participants suggest that self-reported fatigue is associated with frontal lobe and basal ganglia dysfunction and may be related to difficulties with motor programming and response execution. Such evidence suggests that fatigue may be associated with impaired interaction between cortical and subcortical functional systems.

Conclusion

Cognitive fatigue is a multifaceted yet elusive complaint of many individuals with brain damage or dysfunction. Subjective complaints of cognitive fatigue correlate poorly with actual cognitive performance. Recent attempts at objectively measuring cognitive fatigue have been mixed, but they do provide a foundation from which more sophisticated paradigms can be developed. Importantly, even when objective measurement of cognitive fatigue have been observed, no correlations with subjective fatigue ratings were noted.

Fatigue has been associated with higher "physiological costs" both in elevated systolic blood pressure and more widespread cerebral activation. It is suggested that these physiological costs are related to the perception of cognitive fatigue rather than to actual cognitive performance. This suggests that cognitive fatigue and cognitive performance operate on different mechanisms. Evidence for this is provided by Bryant and associates (2004), who observed a cognitive fatigue effect in MS subjects both with and without cognitive impairment.

Functional imaging studies suggest that fatigue may be associated particularly with frontal lobes and the basal ganglia. Specifically, central fatigue (including cognitive fatigue) may be the result of "failure in the integration of limbic input and motor functions within the basal ganglia affecting the striatal-thalamic-frontal cortical system" (Chaudhuri & Behan, 2000). This model is an excellent starting point from which to direct future studies.

In 1971, Broadbent wrote that "there does seem to be some progressive change resulting from continuing exposure to a stimulus situation without opportunity to rest or observe other things. This change takes the form of brief inefficiencies rather than a constant state of inefficiency. We do not know however at this stage whether it takes the form of a failure to select correct input information or not" (p. 58).

Despite the work conducted over the last decade or so, we appear to have progressed little since 1971; yet we presume much in our understanding of the effects of fatigue on cognitive performance.

Acknowledgment

This project was supported in part by NIH grant HD38249, and from the National Multiple Sclerosis Society grant RG 2596B2.

References

Abe, K., Takanashi, M., & Yanagihara, T. (2000). Fatigue in patients with Parkinson's disease. *Behavioural Neurology, 12,* 103–106.

Bakshi, R., Miletich, R. S., Henschel, K., Shaikh, Z. A., Janardhan, V., Wasay, M., Stengel, L. M., Ekes, R., & Kinkel, P. R. (1999). Fatigue in multiple sclerosis: cross sectional correlation with brain MRI findings in 71 patients. *Neurology, 53,* 1151–1153.

Beaumont, M., Batejat, D., Pierard, C., Coste, O., Doireau, P., Van Beers, P., Chauffard, F., Chassard, D., Enslen, M., Denis, J. B., & Lagarde, D. (2001). Slow release caffeine and prolonged (64-h) continuous wakefulness: effects on vigilance and cognitive performance. *Journal of Sleep Research, 10,* 265–276.

Belza, B. L., Henke, C. J., Yelin, E. H., Epstein, W. V., & Gilliss, C. L. (1993). Correlates of fatigue in older adults with rheumatoid arthritis. *Nursing Research, 42,* 93–99.

Blackwood, S. K., MacHale, S. M., Power, M. J., Goodwin, G. M., & Lawrie, S. M. (1998). Effects of exercise on cognitive and motor function in chronic fatigue syndrome and depression. *Journal of Neurology, Neurosurgery and Psychiatrcy, 65,* 541–546.

Brassington, J. C., & Marsh, N. V. (1998). Neuropsychological aspects of multiple sclerosis. *Neuropsychology Review, 8,* 43–77.

Brittain, J. L., LaMarche, J. A., Reeder, K. P., Roth, D. L., & Boll, T. J. (1991). Effects of age and IQ on paced auditory serial addition task (PASAT) performance. *The Clinical Neuropsychologist, 5,* 163–175.

Broadbent, D. E. (1971). *Decision and stress.* New York: Academic Press.

Bruno, R. L., Galski, T., & DeLuca, J. (1993). The neuropsychology of post-polio fatigue. *Archives of Physical Medicine and Rehabilitation, 74,* 1061–1065.

Bryant, D., Chiaravalloti, N. D., & DeLuca, J. (2004). Objective measurement of cognitive fatigue in multiple sclerosis. *Rehabilitation Psychology, 49,* 114–122.

Chaudhuri, A., & Behan, P. O. (2000). Fatigue and basal ganglia. *Journal of Neurological Sciences, 179,* 34–42.

Chiaravalloti, N. D., Demaree, H., Gaudino, E. A., & DeLuca, J. (2003). Can the repetition effect maximize learning in multiple sclerosis? *Clinical Rehabilitation, 17,* 58–68.

Chiaravalloti, N. D., Hillary, F. G., Ricker, J. H., Christodoulou, C., Kalnin, A. J., Liu, W.-C., Steffener, J., & DeLuca, J. (In press). Cerebral activation patterns during working memory performance in multiple sclerosis using fMRI. *Journal of Clinical and Experimental Neuropsychology*.

Chollet, F., & Weiller, C. (1994). Imaging recovery of function following brain injury. *Current Opinion in Neurobiology, 4*, 226–230.

Christodoulou, C., DeLuca, J., Ricker, J. H., Madigan, N., Bly, B. M., Lange, G., Kalnin, A. J., Liu, W. C., Steffener, J., Diamond, B. J., & Ni, A. C. (2001). Functional magnetic resonance imaging of working memory impairment following traumatic brain injury. *Journal of Neurology, Neurosurgery and Psychiatry, 71*, 161–168.

Claypoole, K., Mahurin, R., Fisher, M. E., Goldberg, J., Schmaling, K. B., Schoene, R. B., Ashton, S., & Buchwald, D. (2001). Cognitive compromise following exercise in monozygotic twins discordant for chronic fatigue syndrome: Fact or artifact? *Applied Neuropsychology, 8*, 31–40.

Cluydts, M. V. (2001). Neuropsychological functioning in chronic fatigue syndrome: a review. *Acta Psychiatrica Scandanavica, 103*, 84–93.

Colombo, B., Martineli, F., Rossi, P., Rovaris, M., Maderna, L., Filippi, M., & Comi, G. (2000). MRI and motor evoked potential findings in non-disabled multiple sclerosis patients with and without symptoms of fatigue. *Journal of Neurology, 27*, 506–509.

Elkins, L. E., Krupp, L. B., & Scherl, W. (2000). The measurement of fatigue and contributing neuropsychiatric factors. *Seminars in Clinical Neuropsychiatry, 5*, 58–61.

Filippi, M., Rocca, M. A., Colombo, B., Falini, A., Scotti, G., & Comi, G. (2002). Functional magnetic resonance imaging correlates of fatigue in multiple sclerosis. *NeuroImage, 15*, 559–567.

Fisk, J. D., & Archibald, C. J. (2001). Limitations of the paced auditory serial addition test (PASAT) as a measure of working memory in patients with multiple sclerosis. *Journal of the International Neuropsychological Society, 7*, 363–372.

Fukuda, K., Straus, S. E., Hickie, I., Sharpe, M. C., Dobbins, J. G., & Komaroff, A. (1994). The chronic fatigue syndrome: a comprehensive approach to its definition and study. *Annals of Internal Medicine, 121*, 953–959.

Gandevia, S. C., Enoka, R. M., McComas, A. J., Stuart, D. G., & Thomas, C. K. (1995). *Fatigue: Neural and Muscular Mechanisms*. New York: Plenum Press.

Heesen, C., Gold, S. M., Raji, A., Wiedemann, K., & Schulz, K. H. (2002). Cognitive impairment correlates with hypothalamo-pituitary-adrenal axis dysregulation in multiple sclerosis. *Psychoneuroendocrinology, 27*, 505–517.

Herndon, R. M. (2003). *Multiple sclerosis: Immunology, pathology, and pathophysiology*. New York: Demos.

Hillary, F. G., Chiaravalloti, N. D., Ricker, J. H., Steffener, J., Bly, B. M., Lange, G., Liu, W. C., Kalnin, A. J., & DeLuca, J. (2003). An investigation of working memory rehearsal in multiple sclerosis using fMRI. *Journal of Clinical and Experimental Neuropsychology, 25*, 965–978.

Iriarte, J., Subira, M. L., & Castro, P. (2000). Modalities of fatigue in multiple sclerosis: correlation with clinical and biological factors. *Multiple Sclerosis*, *6*, 124–130.

Jennekens-Schinkel, A., Sanders, E. A. C., Lanser, J. B. K., & Van der Velde, E. A. (1988). Reaction time in ambulant multiple sclerosis patients. Part 1. Influence of prolonged fatigue. *Journal of Neurological Sciences*, 85, 173–186.

Johnson, S. K., DeLuca, J., Diamond, B. J., & Natelson, B. H. (1998). Memory dysfunction in fatiguing illness: examining interference and distraction in short-term memory. *Cognitive Neuropsychiatry*, *3*, 269–285.

Johnson, S. K., Lange, G., DeLuca, J., Korn, L. R., & Natelson, B. H. (1997). The effects of fatigue on neuropsychological performance in patients with chronic fatigue syndrome, multiple sclerosis, and depression. *Applied Neuropsychology*, *4*, 145–153.

Kinkel, R. P. (2000). Fatigue in multiple sclerosis: reducing the impact through comprehensive management. *International Journal of MS Care* (Self-Study Supplement, October).

Komaroff, A. L., & Buchwald, D. (1991). Symptoms and signs of chronic fatigue syndrome. *Review of Infectious Disorders*, *1(Suppl 1)*, S8–S11.

Krupp, L. B., & Elkins, L. E. (2000). Fatigue and declines in cognitive functioning in multiple sclerosis. *Neurology*, *55*, 934–939.

Krupp, L. B., LaRocca, N. G., Muir-Nash, J., & Steinberg, A. D. (1989). The fatigue severity scale: application to patients with multiple sclerosis and systemic lupus erythematosus. *Archives of Neurology*, *46*, 1121–1123.

Kujala, P., Portin, R., Revonsuo A., & Ruutiainen, J. (1995). Attention related performance in two cognitively different subgroups of patients with multiple sclerosis. *Journal of Neurology, Neurosurgery and Psychiatry*, *59*, 77–82.

Kurtzke, J. F. (1983). Rating neurologic impairment in multiple sclerosis: an expanded disability status scale (EDSS). *Neurology*, *33*, 1444–1452.

LaManca, J. J., Sisto, S. A., DeLuca, J., Johnson, S. K., Lange, G., Pareja, J., Cook, S., & Natelson, B. H. (1998). The influence of exhaustive treadmill exercise on cognitive functioning in chronic fatigue syndrome. *American Journal of Medicine*, *105(3A)*, 59S–65S.

Lange, G., Steffener, J., Bly, B. M., Christodoulou, C., Liu, W.-C., DeLuca, J., & Natelson, B. H. (submitted). Chronic fatigue syndrome affects verbal working memory: a BOLD fMRI study.

Leocani, L., Colombo, B., Magnani, G., Martinelli-Boneschi, F., Cursi, M., Rossi, P., Martinelli, V., & Comi, G. (2001). Fatigue in multiple sclerosis is associated with abnormal cortical activation to voluntary movement–EEG evidence. *NeuroImage*, *13*, 1186–1192.

Lezak, M. (1983). *Neuropsychological assessment*, 2nd edition. New York: Oxford University Press.

Lezak, M. (1995). *Neuropsychological assessment*, 3rd edition. New York: Oxford University Press.

Lorist, M. M., Kernell, D., Meijman, T. F., & Zijdewind, I. (2003). Motor fatigue and cognitive performance in humans. *Journal of Physiology, 545(1),* 313–319.

Lorist, M. M., Klein, M., Nieuwenhuis, S., De Jong, R., Mulder, G., & Meijman, T. F. (2000). Mental fatigue and task control: planning and preparation. *Psychophysiology, 37,* 614–625.

McAllister, T. W., Saykin, A. J., Flashman, L. A., Sparling, M. B., Johnson, S. C., Guerin, S. J., Mamourian, A. C., Weaver, J. B., & Yanofsky, N. (1999). Brain activation during working memory 1 month after mild traumatic brain injury. *Neurology, 53,* 1300–1308.

McAllister, T. W., Sparling, M. B., Flashman, L. A., Guerin, S. J., Mamourian, A. C., & Saykin, A. J. (2001). Differential working memory load effects after mild traumatic brain injury. *NeuroImage, 14,* 1004–1012.

Millikin, C. P., Rourke, S. B., Halman, M. H., & Power, C. (2003). Fatigue in HIV/AIDS is associated with depression and subjective neurocognitive complaints but not neuropsychological functioning. *Journal of Clinical and Experimental Neuropsychology, 25,* 201–215.

Morris, T. L., & Miller, J. C. (1996). Electrooculographic and performance indices of fatigue during simulated flight. *Biological Psychology, 42,* 343–360.

Mosso, A. (1904). *Fatigue.* London: Swan Sonnenschein.

Neri, D. F., Oyung, R. L., Colletti, L. M., Mallis, M. M., Tam, P. Y., & Dinges, D. F. (2002). Controlled breaks as a fatigue countermeasure on the flight deck. *Aviation, Space and Environmental Medicine, 73,* 654–664.

Newsholme, E. A., & Blomstrand, E. (1995). Tryptophan, 5-hydroxytryptamine and a possible explanation for central fatigue. In *Fatigue: Neural and muscular mechanisms.* S. C. Gandevia, R. M. Enoka, A. J. McComas, D. G. Stuart, & C. K. Thomas, eds. pp. 315–320. New York: Plenum Press.

Parmenter, B. A., Denney, D. R., & Lynch, S. G. (2003). The cognitive performance of patients with multiple sclerosis during periods of high and low fatigue. *Multiple Sclerosis, 9,* 111–118.

Paul, R. H., Beatty, W. W., Schneider, R., Blanco, C. R., & Hames, K. A. (1998). Cognitive and physical fatigue in multiple sclerosis: relations between self-report and objective performance. *Applied Neuropsychology, 5,* 143–148.

Paul, M. A., Pigeau, R. A., & Weinberg, H. (2001). CC130 pilot fatigue during re-supply missions to former Yugoslavia. *Aviation, Space and Environmental Medicine, 72,* 965–973.

Rao, S. M., Leo, G. J., Bernardin, L., & Unverzagt, F. (1991). Cognitive dysfunction in multiple sclerosis. I. Frequency, patterns, and prediction. *Neurology, 41,* 685–691.

Riese, H., Hoedemaeker, M., Brouwer, W. H., Mulder, L. J. M., Cremer, R., & Veldman, J. B. P. (1999). Mental fatigue after very severe closed head injury: sustained performance, mental effort, and distress at two levels of workload in a driving simulator. *Neuropsychological Rehabilitation, 9,* 189–205.

Roelcke, U., Kappos, L., Lechner-Scott, J., Brunnschweiler, H., Huber, S., Ammann, W., Plohmann, A., Sellas, S., Maguire, R. P., Missimer, J., Radu, E. W., Steck, A., & Leenders, K. L. (1997). Reduced glucose metabolism in the frontal cortex and basal ganglia of multiple sclerosis patients with fatigue: a ^{18}F-fluorodeoxyglucose positron emission tomography study. *Neurology, 48,* 1566–1571.

Sandroni, P., Walker, C., & Starr, A. (1992). "Fatigue" in patients with multiple sclerosis: motor pathway conduction and event-related potentials. *Archives of Neurology, 49,* 517–524.

Schmaling, K. B., Lewis, D. H., Fiedelak, J. I., Mahurin, R., & Buchwald, D. S. (2003). Single-photon emission computerized tomography and neurocognitive function in patients with chronic fatigue syndrome. *Psychosomatic Medicine, 65,* 129–136.

Schultheis, M. T., Garay, E., & DeLuca, J. (2001). The influence of cognitive impairment on driving performance in multiple sclerosis. *Neurology, 56,* 1089–1094.

Schwartz, C. E., Coulthard-Morris, L., & Zeng, Q. (1996). Psychosocial correlates of fatigue in multiple sclerosis. *Archives of Physical Medicine and Rehabilitation, 77,* 165–170.

Schwid, S. R., Tyler, C. M., Scheid, E. A., Weinstein, A., Goodman, A. D., & McDermott, M. P. (2003). Cognitive fatigue during a test requiring sustained attention: a pilot study. *Multiple Sclerosis, 9,* 503–508.

Sheean, G. L., Murray, N. M. F., Rothwell, J. C., Miller, D. H., & Thompson, A. J. (1997). An electrophysiological study of the mechanism of fatigue in multiple sclerosis. *Brain, 120,* 299–315.

Smets, E. M., Garssen, B., Bonke, B., & De Haes, J. C. (1995). The Multidimensional Fatigue Inventory (MFI) psychometric qualities of an instrument to assess fatigue. *Journal of Psychosomatic Research, 39,* 315–325.

Snyder, P. J., Aniskiewicz, A. S., & Snyder, A. M. (1993). Quantitative MRI correlates and diagnostic utility of multi-modal measures of executive control in multiple sclerosis. *Journal of Clinical and Experimental Neuropsychology, 15,* 18.

Staffen, W., Mair, A., Zauner, H., Unterrainer, J., Niederhofer, H., Kutzelnigg, A., Ritter, S., Golaszewski, S., Iglseder, B., & Ladurner, G. (2002). Cognitive function and fMRI in patients with multiple sclerosis: evidence for compensatory cortical activation during an attention task. *Brain, 125,* 1275–1282.

Stokes, M. J., Cooper, R. G., & Edwards, R. H. T. (1988). Normal muscle strength and fatigability in patients with effort syndromes. *British Medical Journal, 297,* 1014–1016.

Tietzel, A. J., & Lack, L. C. (2002). The recuperative value of brief and ultra-brief naps on alertness and cognitive performance. *Journal of Sleep Research, 11,* 213–218.

van der Linden, D., Frese, M., & Meijman, T. F. (2003). Mental fatigue and the control of cognitive processes: effects on perseveration and planning. *Acta Psychologica, 113,* 45–65.

Wessely, S., Hotopf, M., & Sharpe, M. (1998). *Chronic fatigue and its syndromes.* Oxford, England: Oxford University Press.

II Fatigue in Neurological Conditions

4 Multiple Sclerosis and Fatigue

Lauren B. Krupp, Christopher Christodoulou, and Harold Schombert

Fatigue is among the most commonly reported symptoms of multiple sclerosis (MS) (Krupp, Alvarez, LaRocca, & Scheinberg, 1988; Bergamaschi, Romani, Versino, Poli, & Cosi, 1997; Fisk, Pontefract, Ritvo, Archibald, & Murray, 1994). Patients often rate fatigue as the single most troubling aspect of the disorder, and it is frequently the principle presenting symptom at the time of diagnosis (Krupp et al., 1988).

Primary MS fatigue is thought to result from the central nervous system (CNS) and immune dysfunction associated with the disorder, however, additional disease features may contribute to fatigue. A substantial body of data has accumulated regarding both clinical and experimental assessment of fatigue in MS. Understanding how fatigue affects individuals with MS may provide insights that generalize to a broader study of fatigue. This chapter reviews the clinical features of MS fatigue, our current understanding of its pathogenesis, including proposed brain mechanisms, the role of cofactors, and steps used to evaluate and treat the symptom in the clinical setting.

Defining MS-Related Fatigue

MS-related fatigue can be defined in a number of ways, including a feeling of tiredness that is out of proportion to the level of exertion, a feeling of weakness, the lack of capacity to generate sufficient muscle force, or the lack of ability to sustain mental or physical performance (Schwid et al., 1999; Krupp & Elkins, 2000; Multiple Sclerosis Council for Clinical Practice Guidelines, 1998). The Multiple Sclerosis Council for Clinical Practice Guidelines published a consensus definition of fatigue for MS patients (Multiple Sclerosis Council for Clinical Practice Guidelines, 1998). Composed of a wide variety of MS providers including neurologists, psychologists, rehabilitation therapists, and MS nurses, the council defined fatigue as "a subjective lack of physical and/or mental energy that is perceived by the individual or caregiver to interfere with usual and desired activities" (p. 2). This definition has a number of advantages, including its generalizability and understandability for MS patients as well as providers.

Observing that the severity of fatigue waxes and wanes depending on circumstances (e.g., physical exertion, the presence of infection, or hot weather), the council distinguished between chronic and acute fatigue. Chronic persistent fatigue was defined as fatigue present for any amount of time on 50 percent of days for more than 6 weeks, which limits functional activities or quality of life. Acute fatigue was defined as a new or significant increase in feelings of fatigue in the previous 6 weeks, which limits functional activities or quality of life.

Clinical Aspects of MS Fatigue

Fatigue has been studied in individuals with MS for over 20 years. One investigation involving 656 MS patients found that fatigue was the single most commonly reported symptom, cited by 78 percent of patients (Freal, Kraft, & Coryell, 1984). The frequency of fatigue was higher than "typical" MS symptoms such as difficulty in balance, tremor, gait disturbances, weakness, tingling/numbness, and bowel/bladder difficulties (Freal et al., 1984). Twenty-two percent of the patients reported that fatigue caused them to reduce their level of physical activity, 14 percent said it required them to have more rest, and 10 percent said it forced them to quit work (Freal et al., 1984). Others have reported more than two-thirds of MS patients rate fatigue as one of their three worst symptoms (Krupp et al., 1988).

Multiple sclerosis–related fatigue has been contrasted with the fatigue experienced by either healthy adults or individuals with other medical disorders. The fatigue associated with MS differs from that experienced by healthy individuals in its severity and frequency as well as its detrimental impact on activities of daily living, including employment and social relationships (Krupp et al., 1988; Krupp, LaRocca, Muir-Nash, & Steinberg, 1989). Qualitatively, it differs from the fatigue associated with other medical conditions in its particular aggravation by heat (Schwartz, Jandorf, & Krupp, 1993).

MS fatigue tends to be more closely associated with affective state than with clinical measures of neurological impairment and common neuroimaging measures of disease activity (van der Werf et al., 1998; Bakshi et al., 1999; Mainero et al., 1999; Bakshi et al., 2000). The importance of mood in MS fatigue was recently demonstrated in studies showing that behavioral and pharmacological treatments for depression reduced fatigue in MS. This impact resulted primarily from the treatment effects on mood (Mohr, Hart, & Goldberg, 2003).

Pathophysiology

A complete physiologic explanation for MS fatigue is beyond our current level of knowledge of the CNS or of MS. Nonetheless, considerable effort has been made to explain this symptom. A number of pathophysiological mechanisms have been proposed including (1) immune system dysregulation, (2) CNS mechanisms, (3) impaired nerve conduction, (4) neuroendocrine/neurotransmitter dysregulation, (5) autonomic nervous system involvement, and (6) energy depletion. These mechanisms likely interact, with no one pathway serving as the sole cause for MS fatigue.

Immune System Dysregulation   There is strong evidence that alterations in immune system activity substantially contribute to fatigue in MS patients. Fatigue is a significant symptom in a number of autoimmune disorders, such as systemic lupus erythematosus (SLE) (Krupp, LaRocca, Muir, & Steinberg, 1990; Tench, McCurdie, White, & D'Cruz, 2000). In both MS and SLE patients, fatigue can be the first sign of an impending relapse or flare.

Immune activation promoting corticotropin-releasing hormone (CRH), adrenocorticotropic hormone (ACTH), and cortisol secretion may affect MS fatigue through neuroendocrine changes (Wessely, Hotopf, & Sharpe, 1998). An association has also been proposed between fatigue and thyroid function (Jones, Wadler, & Hupart, 1998); a case study of a patient with MS-related fatigue shows the presence of autoimmune thyroid disease following interferon-beta administration (Schwid, Goodman, & Mattson, 1997).

Attempts to correlate MS fatigue with circulating levels of cytokines have had inconsistent results. An association between perceived fatigue and circulating markers of immune activation has been observed in at least one MS study (Iriarte, Subira, & Castro, 2000). However, these findings have not been replicated by others examining inflammatory cytokines and fatigue (Giovannoni, Thompson, Miller, & Thompson, 2001). Given the sensitivity of circulating inflammatory cytokines to many variables and the multiple factors affecting cytokine levels, it is not surprising that associations between circulating levels cytokines and other biologic immune markers and fatigue is difficult to detect.

Another line of evidence that immune system dysregulation is related to fatigue clearly shows fatigue as a side effect of interferon-betas. The interferons have been associated with a flu-like reaction including fatigue, fever, and chills not only in MS but in other disorders such as cancer (Neilley, Goodin, Goodkin, & Hauser, 1996; Quesada, Talpaz, Rios, Kurzrock, & Gutterman, 1986; Gottberg, Gardulf, & Fredrikson, 2000). The precise mechanism by which the interferon-betas induce fatigue is unclear. In one study of healthy individuals, interferon-beta administration was associated with an increase in inflammatory cytokine levels, including tumor necrosis factor alpha (TNF-alpha), interleukin 1 (IL-1), and IL-6 (Goebel et al., 2002). In contrast, another study of healthy volunteers found that interferon-beta administration decreased the levels of cytokines, though fatigue was still a prominent side effect (Rothuizen et al., 1999).

Though there is strong support that immune dysfunction is one underlying mechanism for fatigue, other factors are also important. That fatigue is common even during relapse-free periods or in noninflammatory forms of the disease, suggests that CNS mechanisms also play a key role.

Central Nervous System Mechanisms   Several distinct areas of the CNS are believed to be involved in the pathophysiology of MS-related fatigue. For example, functional imaging studies, including functional magnetic resonance imaging (fMRI) and positron emission tomography (PET), have yielded provocative findings regarding MS fatigue. In one fMRI study of simple motor behavior, MS subjects with higher levels of fatigue displayed reduced activation of several brain areas involved in motor planning and execution, including the thalamus (Filippi et al., 2002). An earlier PET study demonstrated significant hypometabolism in the prefrontal cortex and basal ganglia of fatigued MS patients compared to nonfatigued persons with MS (Roelcke et al., 1997).

The CNS dysfunction identified in these studies may result from immune injury, neuronal dysfunction secondary to demyelination of nerve sheaths and destruction of axons, and other changes resulting from a state of recurrent or chronic CNS inflammation associated with the MS disease process. Hypofunctioning in these CNS regions may lead to decreased motor readiness. Reduced frontal lobe activity has also been associated with fatigue in other progressive CNS disorders such as Parkinson's disease (Abe, Takanashi, & Yanagihara, 2000). Such parallel findings in other neurodegenerative disorders support the importance of CNS perfusion deficits and decreased glucose uptake in fatigue pathophysiology.

Although efforts that tie neuronal function to fatigue have met with some success, investigations directing toward identifying a neuroanatomic locus for fatigue have not been as promising. Several MRI studies have failed to establish an association between MS fatigue and lesion load or brain atrophy, using either T1- or T2-weighted scans (Mainero et al., 1999; Bakshi et al., 1999).

Impaired Nerve Conduction   Demyelination has often been considered a major cause of MS fatigue. The exact mechanism for how demyelination results in fatigue is unclear. One suggestion is that reduced or delayed voluntary muscle innervation requires a compensatory increase in central motor drive excitatory mechanisms, so that affected individuals must expend a greater degree of energy to achieve a given level of motor function (Bakshi, 2003). The increased exertion may also raise body temperature, further exacerbating fatigue symptoms (Bakshi, 2003). Several studies have demonstrated increased central motor drive and delays in voluntary muscle activation associated with impaired conduction along motor pathways (Sheean, Murray, Rothwell, Miller, & Thompson, 1997; Ng & Kent-Braun, 1997).

Neuroendocrine/Neurotransmitter Dysregulation   Endocrinal disturbances, such as abnormal thyroid functioning, may play at least a small role in fatigue development as a consequence of the immune changes with MS or MS therapies (Schwid et al., 1997). In one study linking interferon therapy to cytokines and the endocrine system interferon-beta 1b administered to healthy subjects led to significant increases in the proinflammatory cytokines as well as elevated cortisol, prolactin, and growth hormone plasma levels (Goebel et al., 2002). The strong stimulatory effect cytokines exert on the hypothalamic–pituitary–adrenal (HPA) axis may underlie the link between fatigue and interferon beta in MS patients (Goebel et al., 2002).

The impact of endocrine function on fatigue has received the most attention in the study of chronic fatigue syndrome, focusing primarily on the role of the HPA axis, which is the body's stress regulator. Several studies have been specifically performed on HPA axis dysregulation in MS patients. One such study examining HPA axis activity in 52 patients with clinically definite MS concluded that the HPA axis is activated secondary to inflammation (Wei & Lightman, 1997). Since HPA axis dysregulation has been linked to severe fatigue in other disease states, it may also contribute to the fatigue of MS.

The hypothalamus and pathways involving neurotransmitters such as dopamine, histamine, and serotonin are also likely to contribute to fatigue pathogenesis. For example, it has been argued that disruption in serotonergic pathways interferes with attention, and could lead to cognitive fatigue (Parker, Wessely, & Cleare, 2001; Heilman & Watson, 1997). Effects on the hypothalamus can lead to decreased arousal and hence increased fatigue. Fatigue as a symptom may also depend on defects in both neuroendocrine and neurotransmitter systems as well as the interactions between these systems.

Autonomic Nervous System Involvement   It has been theorized that clinical symptoms of cardiovascular autonomic dysregulation (e.g., dizziness, weakness, neurocognitive complaints, and exhaustion) are similar to symptoms reported by those with fatigue. In a study of 84 MS patients, of whom 64 percent were fatigued, approximately 20 percent had coexistent signs of autonomic failure and fatigue (Merkelbach, Dillmann, Kolmel, Holz, & Muller, 2001). Other studies of MS patients found an association between fatigue and cardiac measures of autonomic functioning, which resembled a hypoadrenergic orthostatic response (Flachenecker et al., 2003). However, a surprising inverse relationship between fatigue and autonomic dysfunction, as measured by pupillary unrest, has also been reported, a result that demonstrates the relation to fatigue and autonomic dysfunction is not straightforward (Egg, Hogl, Glatzl, Beer, & Berger, 2002). Further research is needed to clarify the role of autonomic dysregulation in MS fatigue.

Energy Depletion   Fatigue has been linked to energy depletion in a number of conditions, both chronic (e.g., cancer) and acute (e.g., the postsurgical state) (Holley, 2000; Wessely et al., 1998). Although the impact of energy depletion on fatigue has not been researched directly in MS patients, it is likely that the extreme metabolic demands of battling a chronic illness such as MS contributes to fatigued.

Fatigue Cofactors

A number of factors, while not considered primary causes of MS-related fatigue, may be secondary contributors. These include affective/mood disorders, pain, deconditioning, sleep disorders, and medications for other MS symptoms. As with primary causes of MS-related fatigue, these cofactors can overlap and exacerbate each other, increasing the severity of existing fatigue. For example, the use of sedatives or muscle relaxants can reduce daytime energy and interfere with muscle functioning, leading to decreases in exercise. This, in turn, increases deconditioning and symptoms of fatigue. Because these contributors to fatigue may interfere with efforts to reduce fatigue, the provider should have a high index of suspicion for these problems in the MS patient.

Treatment of MS Fatigue

Nonpharmacologic Treatments

Among the nonpharmacologic treatments, education and support are very important. Patients are directly helped by validating fatigue as a genuine feature of MS. *Exercise* is a powerful method to combat deconditioning and enhance self-esteem. In one study, exercise improved some but not all measures of fatigue (Petajan et al., 1996). Though a graded exercise program is useful, overexertion can be detrimental. Carefully timed rest periods during the work day and avoidance of environmental factors that worsen fatigue (such as heat) can lessen fatigue and enhance productivity.

A multidisciplinary rehabilitation program has also been shown to reduce fatigue and MS symptoms (Di Fabio, Soderberg, Choi, Hansen, & Schapiro, 1998). Behavioral therapy is another means of managing fatigue. Behavioral techniques have been successful for individuals with chronic fatigue syndrome, reducing both depression and fatigue caused by mood disorder (Deale, Husain, Chalder, & Wessely, 2001; Friedberg & Krupp, 1994). Recent evidence suggests that cognitive behavioral therapy for depression in MS may also improve fatigue (Mohr, Boudewyn, Goodkin, Bostrom, & Epstein, 2001; Mohr et al., 2003).

Pharmacologic Treatments

Often nonpharmacologic interventions must be supplemented with medications. Treatments shown to be effective in randomized controlled trials include amantadine, an antiviral agent that also has an antiparkinson effect (Krupp et al., 1995; Murray, 1985; Canadian MS Research Group, 1987), modafinil, a nondopaminergic agent approved for narcolepsy (Rammohan, Rosenberg, Lynn, & Blumenfeld, 2002) and pemoline, a CNS stimulant (Weinshenker, Penman, Bass, Ebers, & Rice, 1992). Other medications for fatigue anecdotally reported to be useful include CNS stimulants such as methylphenidate (Ritalin) and dextroamphetamine. CNS stimulants should be used with caution; in selected cases they have value, but they are contraindicated in patients with abuse potential. A potential future therapy is 4-aminopyridine (4AP). In a study examining its long-term efficacy and safety, fatigue was reported to improve (Polman, Bertelsmann, & van Loenen, 1994). A pilot study in MS with 3,4-diaminopyridine, a related formulation, also reported subjective fatigue improvement in six of eight treated subjects but no change in physiological fatigue measures (Sheean, Murray, Rothwell, Miller, & Thompson, 1998). Unfortunately, 4AP can cause seizures, which has interfered with further development of this therapy for MS.

For patients with current depression and fatigue, the initial treatment of choice is antidepressant medication. Fatigue is likely to be resistant to all therapy if the depression is not treated first. Even patients who deny depressive symptoms may have positive responses to antidepressants, preferably agents with the least sedating properties.

Conclusion

Fatigue is a complex symptom that has long been recognized as a major component of MS. A range of factors contribute to fatigue, including CNS dysfunction, loss of immune regulation, and changes associated with chronic illness. Studies positing a role for the hypothalamus in arousal and fatigue are particularly intriguing, though much of the evidence is still indirect. Functional imaging studies have begun to add to our understanding of fatigue mechanisms. Future functional neuroimaging studies that include physical as well as cognitive fatigue induction may shed further insight on the causes of MS fatigue.

References

Abe, K., Takanashi, M., & Yanagihara, T. (2000). Fatigue in patients with Parkinson's disease. *Behavioral Neurology, 12*, 103–106.

Bakshi, R. (2003). Fatigue associated with multiple sclerosis: diagnosis, impact and management. *Multiple Sclerosis, 9*, 219–227.

Bakshi, R., Miletich, R. S., Henschel, K., et al. (1999). Fatigue in multiple sclerosis: cross-sectional correlation with brain MRI findings in 71 patients. *Neurology, 53*, 1151–1153.

Bakshi, R., Shaikh, Z. A., Miletich, R. S., et al. (2000). Fatigue in multiple sclerosis and its relationship to depression and neurologic disability. *Multiple Sclerosis, 6*, 181–185.

Bergamaschi, R., Romani, A., Versino, M., Poli, R., & Cosi, V. (1997). Clinical aspects of fatigue in multiple sclerosis. *Functional Neurology, 12*, 247–251.

Canadian MS Research Group (1987). A randomized controlled trial of amantadine in fatigue associated with multiple sclerosis. *Canadian Journal of Neural Science, 14*, 273–278.

Deale, A., Husain, K., Chalder, T., & Wessely, S. (2001). Long-term outcome of cognitive behavior therapy versus relaxation therapy for chronic fatigue syndrome: a 5-year follow-up study. *American Journal of Psychiatry, 158*, 2038–2042.

Di Fabio, R. P., Soderberg, J., Choi, T., Hansen, C. R., & Schapiro, R. T. (1998). Extended outpatient rehabilitation: its influence on symptom frequency, fatigue, and functional status for persons with progressive multiple sclerosis. *Archives of Physical Medicine and Rehabilitation, 79*, 141–146.

Egg, R., Hogl, B., Glatzl, S., Beer, R., & Berger, T. (2002). Autonomic instability, as measured by pupillary unrest, is not associated with multiple sclerosis fatigue severity. *Multiple Sclerosis, 8*, 256–260.

Filippi, M., Rocca, M. A., Colombo, B., et al. (2002). Functional magnetic resonance imaging correlates of fatigue in multiple sclerosis. *Neuroimage, 15*, 559–567.

Fisk, J. D., Pontefract, A., Ritvo, P. G., Archibald, C. J., & Murray, T. J. (1994). The impact of fatigue on patients with multiple sclerosis. *Canadian Journal Neurological Science, 21*, 9–14.

Flachenecker, P., Rufer, A., Bihler, I., et al. (2003). Fatigue in MS is related to sympathetic vasomotor dysfunction. *Neurology, 61*, 851–853.

Freal, J. E., Kraft, G. H., & Coryell, J. K. (1984). Symptomatic fatigue in multiple sclerosis. *Archives of Physical Medicine and Rehabilitation, 65*, 135–138.

Friedberg, F., & Krupp, L. B. (1994). A comparison of cognitive behavioral treatment for chronic fatigue syndrome and primary depression. *Clinical Infectious Disease, 18(Suppl. 1)*, S105–S110.

Giovannoni, G., Thompson, A. J., Miller, D. H., & Thompson, E. J. (2001). Fatigue is not associated with raised inflammatory markers in multiple sclerosis. *Neurology, 57*, 676–681.

Goebel, M. U., Baase, J., Pithan, V., et al. (2002). Acute interferon beta-1b administration alters hypothalamic-pituitary-adrenal axis activity, plasma cytokines and leukocyte distribution in healthy subjects. *Psychoneuroendocrinology, 27*, 881–892.

Gottberg, K., Gardulf, A., & Fredrikson, S. (2000). Interferon-beta treatment for patients with multiple sclerosis: the patients' perceptions of the side-effects. *Multiple Sclerosis, 6*, 349–354.

Heilman, K. M., & Watson, R. T. (1997). Fatigue. *Neurology Network Commentary, 1*, 283–287.

Holley, S. (2000). Cancer-related fatigue. Suffering a different fatigue. *Cancer Practice, 8*, 87–95.

Iriarte, J., Subira, M. L., & Castro, P. (2000). Modalities of fatigue in multiple sclerosis: correlation with clinical and biological factors. *Multiple Sclerosis, 6,* 124–130.

Jones, T. H., Wadler, S., & Hupart, K. H. (1998). Endocrine-mediated mechanisms of fatigue during treatment with interferon-alpha. *Seminarsin Oncology, 25,* 54–63.

Krupp, L. B., Alvarez, L. A., LaRocca, N. G., & Scheinberg, L. C. (1988). Fatigue in multiple sclerosis. *Archives of Neurology 45,* 435–437.

Krupp, L. B., Coyle, P. K., Doscher, C., et al. (1995). Fatigue therapy in multiple sclerosis: results of a double-blind, randomized, parallel trial of amantadine, pemoline, and placebo. *Neurology, 45,* 1956–1961.

Krupp, L. B., & Elkins, L. E. (2000). Fatigue and declines in cognitive functioning in multiple sclerosis. *Neurology, 55,* 934–939.

Krupp, L. B., LaRocca, N. G., Muir, J., & Steinberg, A. D. (1990). A study of fatigue in systemic lupus erythematosus. *Journal of Rheumatology, 17,* 1450–1452.

Krupp, L. B., LaRocca, N. G., Muir-Nash, J., & Steinberg, A. D. (1989). The fatigue severity scale. Application to patients with multiple sclerosis and systemic lupus erythematosus. *Archives of Neurology, 46,* 1121–1123.

Mainero, C., Faroni, J., Gasperini, C., et al. (1999). Fatigue and magnetic resonance imaging activity in multiple sclerosis. *Journal of Neurology, 246,* 454–458.

Merkelbach, S., Dillmann, U., Kolmel, C., Holz, I., & Muller, M. (2001). Cardiovascular autonomic dysregulation and fatigue in multiple sclerosis. *Multiple Sclerosis, 7,* 320–326.

Mohr, D. C., Boudewyn, A. C., Goodkin, D. E., Bostrom, A., & Epstein, L. (2001). Comparative outcomes for individual cognitive-behavior therapy, supportive-expressive group psychotherapy, and sertraline for the treatment of depression in multiple sclerosis. *Journal of Consulting and Clinical Psychology, 69,* 942–949.

Mohr, D. C., Hart, S. L., & Goldberg, A. (2003). Effects of treatment for depression on fatigue in multiple sclerosis. *Psychosomatic Medicine, 65,* 542–547.

Multiple Sclerosis Council for Clinical Practice Guidelines (1998). *Fatigue and multiple sclerosis: Evidence-based management strategies for fatigue in multiple sclerosis.* Washington, DC: Paralyzed Veterans of America.

Murray, T. J. (1985). Amantadine therapy for fatigue in multiple sclerosis. *Canadian Journal of Neurology Science, 12,* 251–254.

Neilley, L. K., Goodin, D. S., Goodkin, D. E., & Hauser, S. L. (1996). Side effect profile of interferon beta-1b in MS: results of an open label trial. *Neurology, 46,* 552–554.

Ng, A. V., & Kent-Braun, J. A. (1997). Quantitation of lower physical activity in persons with multiple sclerosis. *Medicine and Science in Sports and Exercise, 29,* 517–523.

Parker, A. J., Wessely, S., & Cleare, A. J. (2001). The neuroendocrinology of chronic fatigue syndrome and fibromyalgia. *Psychological Medicine, 31,* 1331–1345.

Petajan, J. H., Gappmaier, E., White, A. T., Spencer, M. K., Mino, L., & Hicks, R. W. (1996). Impact of aerobic training on fitness and quality of life in multiple sclerosis. *Annals of Neurology, 39,* 432–441.

Polman, C. H., Bertelsmann, F. W., & van Loenen, A. C. (1994). 4-Aminopyridine in the treatment of patients with multipe sclerosis. *Archives of Neurology, 51,* 292–296.

Quesada, J. R., Talpaz, M., Rios, A., Kurzrock, R., & Gutterman, J. U. (1986). Clinical toxicity of interferons in cancer patients: a review. *Journal of Clinical Oncology, 4,* 234–243.

Rammohan, K. W., Rosenberg, J. H., Lynn, D. J., & Blumenfeld, A. M. (2002). Efficacy and safety of modafinil provigil for the treatment of fatigue in multiple sclerosis: a two centre phase 2 study. *Journal of Neurology, Neurosurgery and Psychiatry, 72,* 179–183.

Roelcke, U., Kappos, L., Lechner-Scott, J., et al. (1997). Reduced glucose metabolism in the frontal cortex and basal ganglia of multiple sclerosis patients with fatigue: a 18F-fluorodeoxyglucose positron emission tomography study. *Neurology, 48,* 1566–1571.

Rothuizen, L. E., Buclin, T., Spertini, F., et al. (1999). Influence of interferon beta-1a dose frequency on PBMC cytokine secretion and biological effect markers. *Journal of Neuroimmunology, 99,* 131–141.

Schwartz, J. E., Jandorf, L., & Krupp, L. B. (1993). The measurement of fatigue: a new instrument. *Journal of Psychosomatic Research, 37,* 753–762.

Schwid, S. R., Goodman, A. D., & Mattson, D. H. (1997). Autoimmune hyperthyroidism in patients with multiple sclerosis treated with interferon beta-1b. *Archives of Neurology, 54,* 1169–1190.

Schwid, S. R., Thornton, C. A., Pandya, S., et al. (1999). Quantitative assessment of motor fatigue and strength in MS. *Neurology, 53,* 743–750.

Sheean, G. L., Murray, N. M., Rothwell, J. C., Miller, D. H., & Thompson, A. J. (1997). An electrophysiological study of the mechanism of fatigue in multiple sclerosis. *Brain, 120,* 299–315.

Sheean, G. L., Murray, N. M., Rothwell, J. C., Miller, D. H., & Thompson, A. J. (1998). An open-labelled clinical and electrophysiological study of 3,4 diaminopyridine in the treatment of fatigue in multiple sclerosis. *Brain, 121(Pt 5),* 967–975.

Tench, C. M., McCurdie, I., White, P. D., & D'Cruz, D. P. (2000). The prevalence and associations of fatigue in systemic lupus erythematosus. *Rheumatology. (Oxford), 39,* 1249–1254.

van der Werf, S. P., Jongen, P. J., Nijeholt, G. J., Barkhof, F., Hommes, O. R., & Bleijenberg, G. (1998). Fatigue in multiple sclerosis: interrelations between fatigue complaints, cerebral MRI abnormalities and neurological disability. *Journal of Neurological Science, 160,* 164–170.

Wei, T., & Lightman, S. L. (1997). The neuroendocrine axis in patients with multiple sclerosis. *Brain, 120(Pt 6)*, 1067–1076.

Weinshenker, B. G., Penman, M., Bass, B., Ebers, G. C., & Rice, G. P. (1992). A double-blind, randomized, crossover trial of pemoline in fatigue associated with multiple sclerosis. *Neurology, 42*, 1468–1471.

Wessely, S., Hotopf, M., & Sharpe, D. (1998). *Chronic fatigue and its syndromes*. New York: Oxford University Press.

5 Fatigue after Stroke

Maja Stulemeijer, Luciano Fasotti, and Gijs Bleijenberg

A stroke often results in a sudden and unexpected change in the life of patients as well as their families. Approximately 80 percent (Heugten & Franke, 2001) of stroke survivors experience a broad range of functional disabilities based on underlying changes in cognition, behavior, and emotions. Although much recovery takes place in the first months poststroke, many patients never return completely to their former level of functioning and report a variety of impairments even long after the stroke. A frequently reported symptom in both the acute and postacute phase is fatigue. Studies in other patient populations show that fatigue can have a significant negative effect on functioning and life satisfaction (Staub & Bogousslavsky, 2001; Flechtner & Bottomley 2003).

In the stroke literature only scarce attention has been paid to poststroke fatigue (PSF). Most standard educational handbooks on stroke outcome do not even address fatigue, though this seems to be changing. In the first edition of their handbook, *Stroke: A practical guideline to management* (Warlow, Dennis, van Gijn, Hankey, Sandercock, Bamford, & Wardlaw, 1996), Warlow and associates did not mention PSF, but in the second edition (2001) they dedicate a short paragraph to this topic, recognizing the frequency and impact of the complaint (Warlow et al., 2001). In 2002 Bogousslavsky (Bogousslavsky, 2003) concluded his W. Feinberg Lecture by emphasizing the importance of further study toward, as he put it, "a very intriguing syndrome—which I have classified under pseudo depressive syndromes after stroke, namely, post stroke fatigue." Scientific studies that did focus to this topic confirm what many clinicians already know from their daily practice: fatigue after stroke is common, even in patients who seem to have made a full physical recovery (Warlow et al., 2001), and it can have a debilitating effect on daily living.

The present chapter is devoted to poststroke fatigue. We present overview of how fatigue is assessed, its prevalence, and its impact. Furthermore, we review several theories about its origin and relationship with brain functioning.

Assessment of Fatigue

Concept of Fatigue

No straightforward task, measuring fatigue is complicated by the multidimensional nature of the concept. Most studies dealing directly with PSF have focused on "experienced fatigue," which is based on the person's self-report of general feelings of debilitating tiredness or loss of energy (e.g., in contrast to physiological measures of muscle fatigue). Few to none of these studies, however, actually define fatigue, trusting everyone has an intuitive notion of the concept. Furthermore, most studies do not differentiate between components of the experience of fatigue—physical (e.g., diminished strength, need to rest), cognitive (e.g., diminished concentration or attention), and affective (e.g., decreased motivation or interest). One study examines the presence of "mental fatigue" (Sisson, 1995).

Many studies of poststroke functioning address fatigue within the framework of related subjects such as depression (Stein, Sliwinski, Gordon, & Hibbard, 1996; Fedoroff, Starkstein, Parikh, Price, & Robinson, 1991) or cognition (Van Zandvoort, Kappelle, Algra, & De Haan, 1998), and often among a cluster of other symptoms, sometimes referred to as "diffuse cerebral symptoms" (Hochstenbach, 1999; Leegaard, 1983; Manes, Paradiso, & Robinson, 1999), or within specific lesion types (Sisson, 1995; Manes et al., 1999; Ogden, Mee, & Henning, 1994; Ogden, Utley, & Mee, 1997). In only a handful of original articles is PSF the central focus (Glader, Stegmayr, & Asplund 2002; Ingles, Eskes, & Philips, 1999; Staub, Annoni, & Bogousslavsky, 2002; Van der Werf, Van den Broek, Anten, & Bleijenberg, 2001).

Assessment Approaches

Several approaches have been used to assess PSF using various instruments and instructions.

Instruments   To our knowledge, only one stroke-specific questionnaire is available, the Stroke Specific Quality of Life Scale (SSQOL), which includes questions regarding fatigue (Williams, Weinberger, Harris, Clark, & Biller, 1999). So far, however, no studies on PSF have used this scale. A whole range of validated generic questionnaires measure fatigue, but only three have been used in PSF studies. First, the Fatigue Impact Scale (FIS), a 40-item self-report questionnaire, assesses the frequency, duration, and severity of fatigue during the past month. It also examines the perceived impact of fatigue on cognitive, physical, and psychosocial functioning on a 5-point scale ranging from 0 (no problem) to 4 (extreme problem). The FIS has been shown to have good psychometric qualities (Fisk, Ritvo, Ross, Haase, Marrie, & Schlech, 1994).

The 29-item Fatigue Assessment Instrument was developed to capture both quantitative and qualitative components of a respondent's fatigue in the preceding 2 weeks.

Each of four distinct dimensions underlying these items is scored on a 7-point Likert scale: fatigue severity, situation specificity, consequences of fatigue, and responsiveness to rest/sleep. The sensitivity and specificity of this survey is more than 80 percent in assessing clinically relevant fatigue (Schwartz, 1998).

Finally, the Checklist Individual Strength (CIS) measures different aspects of fatigue. In the "fatigue" subscale, the patient is asked about fatigue severity in the 2 weeks preceding the assessment. The subscale consists of eight items, each scored on a 7-point Likert scale. The three other subscales of the CIS measure concentration problems, reduced motivation, and reduced activity (Vercoulen, Swanink, Galama, Fennis, van der Meer, & Bleijenberg, 1994). The CIS has good reliability and validity and make use of a cutoff for severe fatigue (Beurskens, Bültmann, Kant, Vercoulen, Bleijenberg, & Swaen, 2000; Bültmann, de Vries, Beurskens, Bleijenberg, Vercoulen & Kant, 2000). Both the CIS and the FIS have normative data available from several patient groups and healthy controls.

The largest PSF study so far used one question, "Do you feel tired?," on a 4-point Likert scale (Glader et al., 2002). Several other studies address fatigue in a semistructured interview as part of a symptom checklist, using a dichotomous rating scale (Van Zandvoort et al., 1998; Hochstenbach, 1999; Leegaard, 1983; Manes et al., 1999; Ogden et al., 1997). Some studies on poststroke depression assessed fatigue among other symptoms with a depression-specific questionnaire (Stein et al., 1996; Fedoroff et al., 1991). Furthermore, the "Vitality" subscale from the SF-36, a widely used generic measure of general health, covers four questions regarding energy level and fatigue (Ware, Snow, Kosinski, & Gandek, 1993). Because these latter three studies do not specifically address PSF, their contribution to a broader understanding of PSF is limited. For this reason, we report on only a selection of these studies.

Time Frame Besides using different instruments, studies also differ according to the instructions given. Some studies ask about fatigue only in the past few weeks (Sisson, 1995; Manes et al., 1999; Glader et al., 2002; Ingles et al., 1999; Staub et al., 2002; Van der Werf et al., 2001), whereas others ask subjects to rate present fatigue compared to premorbid fatigue (Van Zandvoort et al., 1998; Hochstenbach, 1999; Leegaard, 1983; Ogden et al., 1994).

Multidimensional Assessment of Fatigue

Because fatigue is a multidimensional experience, assessments should reflect this multidimensionality, for both research and clinical purposes. In patients with chronic fatigue syndrome, Vercoulen (Vercoulen et al., 1994) identified several relatively independent dimensions along which to direct assessment and research. Several of those dimensions can also be thought to relate to poststroke fatigue. Besides "experienced" or subjective fatigue, these are functional impairments in daily life, neuropsychological impairments, sleep disturbances, psychological wellbeing, activity, social functioning, and self-efficacy expectations (e.g., "I think I could positively influence my fatigue").

In summary, PSF is rarely assessed multidimensionally in the literature. However, several reliable and valid instruments are available for assessing fatigue. Future studies can benefit greatly from the use of these instruments.

Prevalence

When examining prevalence rates among studies, two points stand out. First, although rates vary greatly, between 25 and 92 percent, PSF is consistently reported. Second, fatigue is found to be present independent of the time elapsed since stroke within individual studies (Sisson, 1995; Leegaard, 1983; Ingles, Eskes, & Philips, 1999; Van der Werf et al., 2001; Suenkeler, Nowak, Misselwitz, Kugler, Schreiber, Oertel, & Back 2002). However, when the various studies are reviewed together (table 5.1), a trend toward decreasing fatigue seems to occur over time, from about 70 percent in the first year poststroke to 40 percent in the years following. The large variance in prevalence rates is likely due to such factors as the use of different instruments, different time since stroke (TSS), and heterogeneity in patient populations.

These studies show that stroke patients report higher levels of fatigue than healthy adults. Compared to other patient samples, however, the frequency of poststroke fatigue appears similar in magnitude. For example, Leegaard (Leegaard, 1983) assessed the presence of fatigue in patients with a cerebral infarction (CI) versus patients who had suffered a myocardial infarction (MI). The two groups, all of whom were in good health and fully active before the infarction, reported comparable high levels of fatigue.

Gender and Age

Gender   PSF appears to be present equally among men and women. Glader and associates (Glader et al., 2002) reported a small female preponderance; in their sample, 42 percent of all women reported being often or always fatigued compared to 38 percent of men. Other studies did not find significant sex differences (Leegaard, 1983; Ingles et al., 1999; Van der Werf et al., 2001).

Age   Age effects have been found only in Glader's study (Glader et al., 2002). Patients who always felt tired were older at stroke onset than the other patients (74.5 versus 71.5 years). Other studies found no significant age differences (Leegaard, 1983; Ingles et al., 1999; Van der Werf et al., 2001). Overall, despite methodological issues that limit direct comparison of prevalence rates across studies, fatigue is consistently

Table 5.1

Prevalence of poststroke fatigue

Study	N	Age	% Male	Instrument + Scaling	Prevalence Rates % by Time since Stroke			
					<1 Months	<6 Months	6–12 Months	>12 Months
Sisson	13	33–77	46	Neuro Behavioural Rating Scale, Likert	92			
Federoff	205	58,7 ± 13,0	52	Hamilton Depression Rating Scale; Present State Examination, dichotomous	38		85	
Manes	25	≅63	68	Present State Examination, dichotomous		32		
Staub	73	51 ± 14	—	Fatigue Assessment Instrument, Likert			25	
Ingles et al.	88	66,6 ± 13,4	63	Fatigue Impact Scale, adjective		66	75/65	
Stein	189	67,0 ± 11,8	48	Beck Depression Inventory; Hamilton Depression Rating Scale			76/85	
Hochstenbach	172	55,3 ± 10,9	—	Structured interview, dichotomous			74	
Van Zandvoort	16	56,8 ± 12,4	54	Structured interview, dichotomous				38
Leegaard	44	51,0 ± –	66	Structured interview, dichotomous			75	
Glader	3667	71,8	54	Single question, Likert				39
Van der Werf	90	62,1	72	Checklist Individual Strength, Likert				51
Ogden	123	48,8 ± 14,2	34	Structured interview, dichotomous		87		35

observed among stroke survivors. A trend toward decreasing fatigue over time appears compelling as well.

Impact of Fatigue

Fatigue can place a heavy burden on patients' quality of life. A strikingly high percentage of patients, between 29 and 50 percent (Ingles et al., 1999; Staub et al., 2002; Van der Werf et al., 2001), rate PSF as their worst symptom among other poststroke sequalea. Ingles and colleagues (Ingles et al., 1999) found PSF to affect functioning in cognitive, physical, and psychosocial domains. Compared with controls, stroke patients reported a higher total impact of fatigue on their lives, particularly in the latter two domains, and they attributed more functional limitations to their fatigue. Glader and associates (Glader et al., 2002) also found increased fatigue to be highly correlated with other health variables (increased dependency in activities of daily living, worse general health, greater anxiety, depression, and pain). Williams and coworkers (Williams et al., 1999) developed a stroke-specific quality of life (SSQOL) measure based on patient interviews. During these initial interviews, patients reported "energy" to be among the three areas most affected by their stroke. In a larger sample, 65 percent rated the energy domain "a little or a lot worse" than before the stroke.

In addition to its potential negative influence on quality of life, PSF has been associated with worse long-term outcome. Results from the large prospective cohort study of Glader and colleagues (Glader et al., 2002) show that, after adjusting for depression and other important predictors of survival, "always feeling tired" is predictive for activities of daily life (ADL) dependency at 2-year follow-up. Moreover, this study is the first to show that PSF is an independent predictor of death after stroke. Between the follow-up time and 1 year later, significantly more patients who reported feeling "always tired" were deceased. Interestingly, this association between fatigue and mortality has been observed among cardiac patients as well. A state of unusual fatigue, lack of energy, and increased irritability is associated with increased risk of a first MI in apparently healthy males (Appels, Golombeck, Gorgels, de Vreede, & van Breukelen, 2000).

In summary, fatigue can have a tremendous impact on various aspects of quality of life among stroke survivors. The experience of fatigue is often among the most severe symptoms in poststroke seqealae. Moreover, severe PSF is associated with worse long-term outcome and even with greater mortality.

PSF and Stroke Characteristics

To date, findings on associations between lesion characteristics and fatigue are mixed. Several studies report fatigue independent of stroke severity, localization, lateralization, or functional impairment (Leegaard, 1983; Glader et al., 2002; Ingles et al., 1999), whereas others found fatigue to be associated with specific locations in the brain. Staub (Staub, Annoni, & Bogousslavsky, 2002) subdivided 44 nondepressed, nondisabled stroke patients into five anatomical groups. Combined cortical–subcortical and brain-stem lesions tended to be associated with more severe fatigue compared to other anatomical groups. Manes (Manes et al., 1999) found that 8 out of 13 patients (62%) with lesions in the insula reported anergia and tiredness, compared to none in a group of noninsula (cortical) lesion patients. The authors suggested damage to the right insula may lead to disconnections with brain regions such as the anterior cingulate cortex and frontal cortex, possibly disrupting the expression of voluntary motor behavior or affecting the appraisal of affective-motivational content of perceptual experiences. Both processes may give rise to subjective anergia, underactivity, and tiredness.

One study reported an influence of lateralization on the experience of fatigue. Stein (Stein et al., 1996) found fatigue more frequently present among patients with right-sided damage than among patients with left-sided damage. Finally, in a small group of nine female patients 14 weeks after a subarachnoid hemorrhage (SAH), a rare type of cerebrovascular event in which a major cerebral aneurysm ruptures and bleeds into the subarachnoid space, patients reported less fatigue after treatment with tirilazad mesylate than nine placebo-treated controls (Ogden et al., 1998). Because of the presumed neuroprotective effect of this drug, fatigue was hypothesized to be related to and mediated by diffuse neurological damage.

In summary, the findings on the association between lesion characteristics and fatigue are mixed. Several studies found fatigue and lesion characteristics to be unrelated. Future studies need to compare homogeneous groups of patients with clearly defined lesion types (e.g., size, side, site) to determine the roles of specific brain structures in the development of PSF.

Other Factors Related to PSF

Prestroke Characteristics   So far, little is known about premorbid factors that might facilitate the development of PSF. There is some evidence that patients with a less favorable initial condition at stroke onset are at increased risk to develop PSF. Glader and associates (Glader et al., 2002) reported that fatigue 2 years after stroke was more common among patients who were single before stroke, lived in an assisted living facility institution, were dependent on others for primary ADL functions, and experienced a recurrent stroke.

Poststroke Characteristics   Along the way to poststroke recovery, several factors potentially influence fatigue. These factors have been mainly derived from clinical observations.

Functional impairments   Many patients suffer substantial limitations in daily life due to partial paralysis, neglect, muscle weakness, and so on. One study found most of the variance in levels of fatigue to be explained by impaired locomotion (Van der Werf et al., 2001).

Physical deconditioning   Several factors, such as persistent sensorimotor problems or reduced activity, may contribute to physical deconditioning. Deconditioning itself may lead to feelings of fatigue.

Sleep disturbances   More than 50 percent of stroke patients have sleep-disordered breathing and at least 20 percent have sleep–wake disturbances, mainly in the form of hypersomnia or excessive daytime sleepiness (Hermann & Bassetti, 2003). Fatigue induced by sleep disorders is usually characterized by day somnolence rather than loss of drive (Staub & Bogousslavsky, 2001). (See chapter 13.)

Medication use   Medication use is very common even long after stroke. It is important to be aware of fatigue as a possible side effect of regular medications. It is a possible side effect of widely used antihypertensives, for instance (Webster & Koch, 1996). Alterations in drug type or dosage may clarify the role of medication on fatigue.

Reduced capacity for mental effort   Because of subtle limitations in attentional capacity, patients may have to invest more mental effort to reach their premorbid level of cognitive and behavioral functioning (Van Zandvoort et al., 1998). (See chapter 3.)

Psychological factors   Several psychological factors, such as self-efficacy and self-esteem, known to be related to stroke outcome may also be associated with the persistence of fatigue. This effect has been observed in other diseases such as multiple sclerosis, in which a low sense of self-efficacy directly influences severity of fatigue (Van der Werf, Evers, Jongen, & Bleijenberg, 2003). However, psychological factors have yet to be examined systematically in stroke patients.

Social support   As in other populations, satisfactory social support has been found to have a positive effect on outcome in stroke patients (MacKenzie & Chang, 2002). Its direct influence on PSF, however, has not been investigated.

Fatigue versus Depression

Depression   is common after stroke, and fatigue is one of the diagnostic criteria for depression. Fatigue is not only a sign of underlying psychopathology, however, it can constitute a major independent symptom of stroke as well. Studies focusing on PSF share the notion that, although the association between poststroke depression and fatigue is strong, PSF is also often found without depression. Three studies support this dissociation. First, in one-third of the patients in the study of Ingles and coworkers (Ingles et al., 1999), both fatigue and depression were present; however, 39 percent reported fatigue without depression. Second, after excluding depressed patients, Staub and colleagues (Staub et al., 2002) still found that 16 percent of stroke patients had severe fatigue. Finally, using a similar approach, Glader and coworkers (Glader et al., 2002) excluded stroke patients who reported being "always depressed" and still found fatigue present in about 40 percent of the patients.

Other studies show a similar pattern of dissociation between poststroke depression and PSF (Fedoroff et al., 1991; Manes et al., 1999; & Van der Werf et al., 2001). Currently, most studies on depression after stroke do not address fatigue independently, but merely as an accompanying symptom. The previously mentioned distinction shows that fatigue and depression should not be treated as mere equivalents but rather as independent factors.

Interventions

Since the etiology and mechanisms of PSF are not well known, cause-specific treatments have not been developed. Nevertheless, we discuss several possible interventions for PSF, based on current knowledge from literature as well as clinical experience.

Nonpharmacological Interventions

Patient Education   In a review of fatigue after stroke, Michael (Michael, 2002) states that providing patient and family education, such as anticipatory guidance about the likely experience of fatigue, may diminish distress and help the patient maintain feelings of control.

Psychological Interventions   No studies have evaluated PSF–specific treatment programs, yet many hospitals and rehabilitation centers have incorporated fatigue-management modules in their rehabilitation program. One such module aimed at a cognitive-behavioral approach to PSF treatment is the "Dealing with Fatigue" training module, developed by H. Knoop and L. Fasotti of the Sint Maartenskliniek in Nijmegen (the Netherlands). The module is designed to reduce fatigue complaints and anxiety in brain-injured subjects, among which a vast majority are stroke patients. The setting is a day clinic specialized in rehabilitating chronic stroke patients. It offers a comprehensive rehabilitation program, in which graded exercise is devoted to improving the patient's physical condition.

The rationale underlying the fatigue module is that it is impossible to restore energy to the same level as one had before the stroke. With restoration beyond the scope of rehabilitation, all efforts are directed toward teaching patients to make more efficient use of their remaining energy.

The module consists of two distinct parts. First, stroke patients with fatigue complaints are stimulated to register their activities in a log. The purpose is to establish the characteristics of days with extreme fatigue as well as days with less fatigue. The second part involves three compensatory strategies for reducing fatigue complaints: changing activity patterns, planning to compensate for fatigue, and relaxation.

To date, the fatigue module has been evaluated only as part of a cognitive rehabilitation program for brain injury patients. The results of this program are a significant reduction of psychosocial problems and perceived cognitive impairments, measured at the level of subjective judgments.

Graded Exercise   Because of the frequent occurrence of deconditioning after stroke, graded exercise may prove helpful in promoting cardiovascular fitness and thereby diminishing feelings of fatigue. (See chapter 18.) For this reason, the previously mentioned rehabilitation program also offers a module directed at increasing cardiovascular fitness. However, after systematically reviewing the impact of exercise trials poststroke, Meek and associates (Meek, Pollock, Potter, & Langhorn, 2003) found cardiovascular exercise was no better than no exercise with respect to factors such as disability and quality of life.

Pharmacological Interventions

As mentioned earlier, in a small, double-blind trail of a woman with SAH, a neuroprotective drug (tirilazad mesylate) was found to diminish subjective debilitating fatigue (Ogden et al., 1998). In stroke research, no other studies have reported on the effectiveness of pharmacological interventions on PSF. It remains to be seen whether antidepressant medication could benefit some patients by diminishing fatigue.

In summary, both psychobehavioral and pharmacological interventions appear to be potentially effective for PSF treatment. To date, however, systematically evaluated treatment methods for PSF are lacking. Therefore, future research should be directed at determining the applicability and effectiveness of these interventions.

Fatigue and Brain Functioning

Besides its clinical relevance, research on brain mechanisms associated with fatigue after stroke offers scientists an unique opportunity to gain insight into the functional anatomy of the brain and its contribution to the development of PSF. Given the heterogeneity of the population as well as the fact that fatigue is frequently reported after stroke independent of the lesion's site, side, or size, a unimodal model of fatigue is unlikely. Nevertheless, in the absence of a comprehensive theory and in order to generate new hypotheses and guide future studies, several brain mechanisms that may contribute to the experience of PSF have been put forward.

First, fatigue may result from *focal damage* to specific brain structures or circuitry. Several brain regions have been related to fatigue. Based on findings in postpolio survivors, Bruno and colleagues (Bruno, Creange, & Frick, 1998) have hypothesized that alterations within the reticular activating system, located in the brainstem, may lead to fatigue and impaired attention. This view is in accordance with the finding that stroke patients with combined cortical-subcortical and brainstem lesions tend to be associated with higher levels of fatigue. After reviewing neuropathological data of Parkinson's disease, MS, and other disorders, Chaudhuri and Behan (2000) proposed that "central fatigue," as opposed to "peripheral fatigue," may be caused by a failure of the nonmotor component of the basal ganglia (Chaudhuri, & Behan, 2000). Central fatigue, defined as the failure to initiate and sustain attentional tasks and physical activities requiring self-motivation, is experienced without any peripheral motor weakness.

Two mechanisms predispose one to central fatigue: first, damage to striatocortical fibers that channel motivational influences into the motor system; second, a decrease in thalamic activity suppressing frontal activation via the striatocorticofrontal loop. In both cases, the striatal components of the basal ganglia are involved. Since motor weakness and other physical limitations are common after stroke, it seems particularly important to find ways to segregate the physical and cognitive components of PSF. A study examining a large number of older persons found that common symptoms of depression (including fatigue) are associated with small lesions in the basal ganglia. These so-called silent strokes may eventually lead to a full-blown stroke (Steffens Helms, Krishnan, & Burke, 1999). Regarding focal damage, the scarce evidence suggests an association between subcortical areas, particularly the basal ganglia, and centrally induced fatigue. To ascertain the role of other brain areas in this kind of fatigue, future studies should compare fatigue levels among patients with highly specific brain lesion types.

Second, in SAH patients there are indications that *diffuse neuronal damage* may contribute to PSF as well. Potential mechanisms include diffuse cortical disruption caused by neurotoxic effects of the hemorrhage or transient ischemia occurring at the time of SAH (Ogden et al., 1998). After traumatic brain injury (TBI), which often results in extensive diffuse neuronal damage, fatigue is a frequently reported residual complaint (Van Zomeren & van den Burg, 1985). Initial measures of brain-specific proteins (BSP) such as S-100 are known to relate to outcome in both stroke and TBI patients (Elting, de Jager, Teelken, Schaaf, Maurits, van der Naalt, Smit Sibinga, Sulter, & de Keyser, 2000). Since BSP levels are a measure of the severity of diffuse neurological damage, they may be applied to test the hypothesis that fatigue is related to this type of damage.

Third, much scientific attention is directed toward hypothalamic–pituitary–adrenal (HPA) axis *abnormalities* and its possible role in the pathogenesis of fatigue. The HPA endocrine axis is one of the major hormonal systems affected by a multitude of stressors in humans. Disregulation of HPA axis activity may play a role in the motor, cognitive, and behavioral function following ischemic stroke (Franceschini, Tenconi, Zoppoli, & Barreca, 2001).

Early after stroke, inflammatory processes are common and increased cortisol production at various levels of the HPS axis have been documented as well. These processes are normal in reaction to brain tissue damage (Danton & Dalton Dietrich, 2003). Proinflammatory cytokines stimulating HPA activation have been found to be associated with fatigue. A group of fatigued breast cancer survivors had significantly higher serum levels of several markers associated with proinflammatory cytokine activity than nonfatigued survivors (Bower, Ganz, Aziz, Fahey, & Cole, 2003). The inflammatory cascade may be prolonged by chronic stress, which often results from a life-threatening event such as a stroke (Miller, Kim Ritchey, & Cohen, 2002). When inflammation levels are increased for a prolonged period, this may lead to such adverse health outcomes as fatigue. Studies investigating the biological mechanisms relating exhaustion and coronary artery disease observed that exhausted subjects have elevated inflammation markers (Appels, 1999).

Conclusion

Fatigue after stroke is very common, often as one of the most disabling symptoms among other poststroke sequelae. It has been found regardless of age or gender, in the absence of depression, and in patients who apparently made a full functional recovery. Its causal mechanisms are not yet known, although in many cases physical factors alone could not explain the persistence of severe fatigue even many years after stroke. Rather, in accordance with a multidimensional model of illness, physiological, psychological, and social factors are likely to interact. This dimensionality should preferably be reflected in assessing PSF.

To advance our knowledge of PSF, future studies should adopt a longitudinal approach, using validated questionnaires and comparing clearly defined lesion types. The high prevalence of poststroke fatigue and its debilitating effect on daily functioning deserve increased attention in the future.

References

Appels, A. (1999). Inflammation and the mental state before an acute coronary event. *Annals of Medicine, 31(Suppl 1)*, 41–44.

Appels, A., Golombeck, B., Gorgels, A., de Vreede, J., & van Breukelen, G. (2000). Behavioral risk factors of sudden cardiac arrest. *Journal of Psychosomatic Research, 48(4–5)*, 463–469.

Beck, A. T., Steer, R. A., & Garbin, M. G. (1988). Psychometric properties of the Beck Depression Inventory: twenty-five years of evaluation. *Clinical Psychology Review, 8(1)*, 77–100.

Beurskens, A. J. H. M., Bültmann, U., Kant, I. J., Vercoulen, J. H. M. M., Bleijenberg, G., & Swaen, G. M. H. (2000). Fatigue amongst working people: validity of a questionnaire measure. *Occupational & Environmental Medicine, 57*, 353–357.

Bogousslavsky, J. (2003). William Feinberg Lecture 2002: emotions, mood, and behavior after stroke. *Stroke, 34*, 1046–1050.

Bower, J. E., Ganz, P. A., Aziz, N., Fahey, J. L., & Cole, S. W. (2003). T-cell homeostasis in breast cancer survivors with persistent fatigue. *Journal of the National Cancer Institute, 95(15)*, 1165–1168.

Bruno, R. L., Creange, S. J., & Frick, N. M. (1998). Parallels between post-polio fatigue and chronic fatigue syndrome: a common pathophysiology? *The American Journal of Medicine, 105(3 Suppl 1)*, 66S–73S.

Bültmann, U., de Vries, M., Beurskens, A. J. H. M., Bleijenberg, G., Vercoulen, J. H. M. M., & Kant, I. J. (2000). Measurement of prolonged fatigue in the working population: determination of a cut-off point for the Checklist Individual Strength. *Journal of Occupational Health Psychology, 5(4)*, 411–416.

Chaudhuri, A., & Behan, P. (2000). Fatigue and basal ganglia. *Journal of Neurological Sciences, 179*, 34–42.

Danton, G. H., & Dalton Dietrich, W. (2003). Inflammatory mechanisms after ischemia and stroke. *Journal of Neuropathology and Experimental Neurology, 62(2)*, 127–136.

Elting, J., de Jager, A. E. J., Teelken, A. W., Schaaf, M., Maurits, N. M., van der Naalt, J., Smit Sibinga, C.T., Sulter, G. A., & de Keyser, J. (2000). Comparison of serum S-100 protein levels following stroke and traumatic brain injury. *Journal of the Neurological Sciences, 181(1–2)*, 104–110.

Fedoroff, J. P., Starkstein, S. E., Parikh, R. M., Price, T. R., & Robinson, R. G. (1991). Are depressive symptoms nonspecific in patients with acute stroke? *American Journal of Psychiatry, 148(9)*, 1172–1176.

Fisk, J. D., Ritvo, P. G., Ross, L., Haase, D. A., Marrie, T. J., & Schlech, W. F. (1994). Measuring the functional impact of fatigue: initial validation of the fatigue impact scale. *Clinical Infectious Disease, 18(Suppl 1)*, S79–83.

Flechtner, H., & Bottomley, A. (2003). Fatigue and quality of life: lessons from the real world. *Oncologist, 8(Suppl 1)*, 5–9.

Franceschini, R., Tenconi, G. L., Zoppoli, F., & Barreca, T. (2001). Endocrine abnormalities and outcome of ischaemic stroke, *Biomedicine and Pharmacotherapy, 55(8)*, 456–465.

Glader, E., Stegmayr, B., & Asplund, K. (2002). Poststroke fatigue; a 2-year follow-up study of stroke patients in Sweden. *Stroke, 33*, 1327–1333.

Hamilton, M. A. (1967). Development of a rating scale for primary depressive illness. *British Journal of Social and Clinical Psychology, 6*, 278–296.

Hermann, D. M., & Bassetti, C. L. (2003). Sleep apnea and other sleep-wake disorders in stroke. *Current Treatment Options Neurology, 5(3),* 241–249.

Heugten, C. M., & Franke, E. A. M. (2001). *Revalidatie na een beroerte: richtlijnen en aanbevelingen voor zorgverleners.* The Hague: University Press, p. 13.

Hochstenbach, J. B. H. (1999). The cognitive, emotional and behavioural consequences of stroke. *Diss. Nijmegen, ISBN 90 80 49 72 15.*

Ingles, J. L., Eskes, G. A., & Philips, S. J. (1999). Fatigue after stroke. *Archives of Physical and Medical Rehabilitation, 80,* 173–178.

Leegaard, O. F. (1983). Diffuse cerebral symptoms in convalescents from cerebral infarction and myocardial Infarction. *Acta Neurologica Scandinavia, 67,* 348–355.

MacKenzie, A. E., & Chang, A. M. (2002). Predictors of quality of life following stroke. *Disability and Rehabilitation, 24(5),* 259–265.

Manes, F., Paradiso, S., & Robinson, R. G. (1999). Neuropsychiatric effects of insular stroke. *The Journal of Nervous and Mental Disease, 187(12),* 707–712.

Meek, C., Pollock, A., Potter, J., & Langhorne, P. (2003). A systematic review of exercise trials post stroke. *Clinical Rehabilitation, 17(1),* 6–13.

Michael, K. (2002). Fatigue and stroke. *Rehabilitation Nursing, 27(3),* 89–94.

Miller, G. E., Kim Ritchey, A., & Cohen, S. (2002). Chronic psychological stress and the regulation of pro-inflammatory cytokines: a glucocorticoid-resistance model. *Health Psychology, 21(6),* 531–541.

Ogden, J. A., Mee, E. W., & Henning, M. (1994). A prospective study of psychosocial adaptation following subarachnoid haemorrhage. *Neuropsychological Rehabilitation, 4(1),* 7–30.

Ogden, J. A., Mee, E. W., & Utley, T. (1998). Too little, too late: Does tirilazad mesylate reduce fatigue after subarachnoid hemorrhage? *Neurosurgery, 43(4),* 782–787.

Ogden, J. A., Utley, T., & Mee, E. W. (1997). Neurological and psychological outcome 4 to 7 years after subarachnoid hemorrhage. *Neurosurgery, 41(1),* 25–34.

Schwartz, A. (1998). The Schwartz Cancer Fatigue Scale: testing reliability and validity. *Oncology Nursing Forum, 25,* 711–717.

Sisson, R. A. (1995). Cognitive status as a predictor of right hemispere stroke outcomes. *Journal of Neuroscience Nursing, 27(3),* 152–155.

Staub, F., Annoni, J. M., & Bogousslavsky, J. (2002). Post-stroke fatigue: a major problem in "non-disabling" stroke. *Cerebrovascular Disease, 13(Suppl 3),* O416.

Staub, F., & Bogousslavsky, J. (2001). Fatigue after stroke: a major but neglected issue. *Cerebrovascular Diseases, 12,* 75–81.

Staub, F., & Bogousslavsky, J. (2001). Post-stroke depression or fatigue? *European Neurology, 45,* 3–5.

Steffens, D. C., Helms, M. J., Krishnan, K. R., & Burke, G. L. (1999). Cerebrovascular disease and depression symptoms in the cardiovascular health study. *Stroke, 30(10)*, 2159–2166.

Stein, P. N., Sliwinski, M. J., Gordon, W. A., & Hibbard, M. R. (1996). Discriminative properties of somatic and nonsomatic symptoms for post stroke depression. *The Clinical Neuropsychologist, 10(2)*, 141–148.

Suenkeler, I. H., Nowak, M., Misselwitz, B., Kugler, C., Schreiber, W., Oertel, W. H., & Back, T. (2002). Time-course of health-related quality of life as determined 3, 6 and 12 months after stroke; relationship to neurological deficit, disability and depression. *Journal of Neurology, 249*, 1160–1167.

Van der Werf, S. P., Evers, A., Jongen, P. J. H., & Bleijenberg, G. (2003). The role of helplessness as mediator between neurological disability, emotional instability, experienced fatigue and depression in patients with multiple sclerosis. *Multiple Sclerosis, 9*, 89–94.

Van der Werf, S. P., Van den Broek, H. L. P., Anten, H. W. M., & Bleijenberg, G. (2001). The experience of severe fatigue long after stroke and its relation with depressive symptoms and disease characteristics. *European Neurology, 45*, 6–12.

Van Zandvoort, M. J. E., Kappelle, L. J., Algra, A., & De Haan, E. H. F. (1998). Decreased capacity for mental effort after single supratentorial lacunar infarct may affect performance in everyday life. *Journal of Neurology Neurosurgery and Psychiatry, 65*, 697–702.

Van Zomeren, A. H., & van den Burg, W. (1985). Residual complaints of patients two years after severe head injury. *Journal of Neurology, Neurosurgery, and Psychiatry, 48*, 21–28.

Vercoulen, J. H. H. M., Swanink, C. M. A., Galama, J. M. D., Fennis, J. F. M., van der Meer, J. W. M., & Bleijenberg, G. (1994). Dimensional assessment in chronic fatigue syndrome. *Journal of Psychosomatic Research, 38*, 383–392.

Ware, J. E. Jr., Snow, K. K., Kosinski, M., & Gandek, B. (1993). *SF-36 Health Survey Manual and Interpretation Guide*. Boston: Nimrod Press.

Warlow, C. P., Dennis, M. S., van Gijn, J., Hankey, G. J., Sandercock, P. A. G., Bamford, J., & Wardlaw, J. (1996). *Stroke: A Practical Guide to Management*. 1st ed. Malden, MA: Blackwell Science.

Warlow, C. P., Sandercock, P. A. G., Hankey, G. J., van Gijn, J., Dennis, M. S., Bamford, J., & Wardlaw, J. (2001). *Stroke: A Practical Guide to Management, 2nd ed*. Malden, MA: Blackwell Science, p. 420.

Webster, J., & Koch, H. F. (1996). Aspects of tolerability of centrally acting antihypertensive drugs. *Journal of Cardiovascular Pharmacology, (Suppl 3)*, S49–54.

Williams, L. S., Weinberger, M., Harris, L. E., Clark, D. O., & Biller, J. (1999). Development of a stroke-specific quality of life scale. *Stroke, 30(7)*, 1362–1369.

Wing, J. K., Cooper, J. E., & Sartorius, N. (1974). *The Measurement and Classification of Psychiatric Symptoms: An instructional manual for the PSE and CATEGO programs*. New York: Cambridge University Press.

6 Fatigue after Traumatic Brain Injury

Elie P. Elovic, Nino M. Dobrovic, and Jonathan L. Fellus

Fatigue is one of the major problems encountered after traumatic brain injury (TBI), and it can have a tremendous impact on an individual's quality of life. Its incidence in TBI has been reported to range between 21 and 73 percent (Middleboe, Andersen, Birket-Smith, & Friis, 1992; Hillier, Sharpe, & Metzer, 1997; Olver, Ponsford, & Curran, 1996). Fatigue after TBI affects not only an individual's emotional wellbeing but also potential functional recovery from brain injury. Kreutzer, Seel, and Gourley (2001) reported an incidence of 46 percent among persons in an outpatient TBI clinic, suggesting that further information is needed regarding prognosis and the efficacy of treatment alternatives.

Although fatigue is commonly associated with TBI, it is both poorly understood and difficult to treat. This is in part because TBI encompasses a heterogeneous collection of injuries that can result in various physical, cognitive, or emotional dysfunctions. Fatigue itself has also been difficult to define and, as a result, the overall burden it places on the TBI population is still unknown. Nonetheless, the combination of fatigue with cognitive, physical, and emotional difficulties can further reduce quality of life and activities of daily living after TBI. The added limitation in functioning with fatigue may be especially problematic for the patient's ability to sustain purposeful goal-directed mental effort, a key requirement for independent functioning.

Clinicians caring for such individuals are often faced with a vexing, poorly delineated, diagnostic and therapeutic approach to fatigue. Recently, however, a number of new and sophisticated neuroimaging tools and techniques have become available to help unravel the underlying pathophysiology of TBI-induced fatigue. The following discussion reviews the available knowledge concerning fatigue in the TBI population. The authors' intention is to simultaneously educate and increase readers' interest and understanding of fatigue; to promote research in this critical area leading to multidisciplinary efforts to address the problem of fatigue; and to promote the development of treatment protocols through identification of possible fatigue-generating mechanisms.

TBI is a staggering "silent epidemic" in modern society because of the large number of human lives affected and the tremendous economic burden to the healthcare system. For the following discussion the TBI Model Systems Task Force definition of TBI will be used: "damage to brain tissue caused by an external mechanical force, as evidenced by loss of consciousness due to brain trauma, post traumatic amnesia, skull fracture, or objective neurological findings that can be reasonably attributed to TBI on physical examination or mental status examination" (Harrison-Felix et al., 1998). According to the Center for Disease Control's (CDC) Annual Report to Congress on Traumatic Brain Injury from 1999, each year there are an estimated 1.5 million victims of TBI. Of this number, 230,000 are hospitalized, 50,000 die, 80,000 to 90,000 suffer long-term disability, and the vast majority of cases are deemed "mild." TBI is considered a "silent epidemic" because of its low profile and the limited awareness of the problem among of the lay and professional populations. Currently employed surveillance methods for its "disease" burden do not collect information beyond the total number of emergency room visits and hospitalizations. Consequently, the magnitude of the problem of fatigue among all TBI survivors or the subset that is "permanently disabled" is not directly known. Disappointingly, even data bases developed through the comprehensive Traumatic Brain Injury Model Systems overlook fatigue surveillance. TBI is a persistent public health burden that, despite primary prevention, will likely continue to be a major cause of disability in our society.

Definition of Fatigue

Lezak (1995) stated that fatigue required no definition. However, after over 100 years of scientific and clinical inquiry, no consensus on its definition has been found (see chapter 19). As many contributors to this volume have recognized, even a working definition of fatigue can be difficult to develop. This is partly because of the lay terminology often used to describe fatigue (Krupp, 2003). For instance, fatigue is often used synonymously for phrases such as decreased physical or mental endurance, deceased motivation, or a sense of lassitude. Clinicians even define fatigue differently based on the particular population they are treating (Krupp, 2003). For the purposes of the current discussion of TBI, fatigue is divided into "peripheral" fatigue, which is primarily physical or muscular in nature, and "central" fatigue, which is believed to be a direct result of neurological injury to the brain. Chaudhuri and Behan (2000) define central fatigue as "the failure to initiate and/or sustain attentional tasks and physical activities requiring self motivation (as opposed to external stimulation)." Clinical experience echoes this definition in that fatigue affects cognition and the ability to perform instrumental activities of daily living in persons with TBI.

Historically, various surrogates/markers, synonyms, and clinical imitators of fatigue have been delineated in the literature, leading the casual reader astray from the pursuit of a purer characterization of the fatigue that follows TBI. Almost paradoxically, however, the closer we seem to get to the essence of fatigue, the less singular the phenomenon appears to be. Thus, even as one measures and correlates and localizes the fundamental components of fatigue, the syndrome or symptom cannot be appreciated in isolation. Rather, it must be appreciated in its full context, across various domains, and with the understanding that the fatigue experience is not static or constant. As described throughout this volume, there are a multitude of primary and secondary, even tertiary, factors that reliably engender the principle aspects of fatigue for persons with TBI. The current discussion hopes to elucidate the most likely generators of post-TBI fatigue and critique as well as propose an operational definition based on the most appropriate measurement tools for its assessment.

Epidemiology

Self-report has been the primary method for determining the prevalence of fatigue in persons with TBI. The subjectivity of this method makes fatigue susceptible to confusion with other symptoms such as anxiety and depression. A number of investigators over the last several decades have attempted to identify the prevalence of fatigue in the TBI population exclusively through survey-based self-reporting. Lezak (1978) identified fatigue as one of the "subtle" sequelae of brain damage, along with distractibility and perplexity, and compared the incidence of fatigue in those patients seen in consultation (and casual inference) versus those enrolled in careful and in-depth longitudinal research protocols. Among the consulting group of 50 patients post-TBI, 42 percent of those examined once reported fatigue and 60 percent of those examined more frequently. Among TBI patients (46 subjects) in research protocol studies, 98 percent reported symptoms of fatigue. The marked discrepancy in incidence of fatigue in this study suggests that thorough evaluation is vitally important in determining incidence.

Middleboe and associates (1992) noted that, among a cohort of 51 patients with mild TBI, 21 percent reported fatigue 1 year postinjury. Using a longer follow-up period, Olver and coworkers (1996) examined 254 patients with mostly severe TBI at 2 years and 103 at 5 years postinjury, finding fatigue reported by 68 percent and 73 percent, respectively. Masson and associates (1996) studied 231 adults 5 years after TBI, comparing them to a cohort of patients with only lower-limb injury. The sample was stratified by TBI severity, and 30.6 percent of limb injured, 35.1 percent of mild TBI, 32.4 percent of moderate TBI, and 57.7 percent of severe TBI cases reported fatigue, suggesting an association between severity of brain injury and fatigue incidence. Hillier and colleagues (1997) reported fatigue in 37 percent of TBI patients 5 years postinjury, most of whom had severe brain injuries. Kreutzer and coworkers (2001) examined the epidemiology of depression in a cohort of 722 TBI outpatients averaging 2.5 years after injury and with a mean duration of unconsciousness of 10 days. The self-report of fatigue in this severely injured group was 46 percent, and fatigue was the most frequently reported problem.

From these epidemiological reports based on self-report, the incidence of fatigue after TBI ranges from 2 to 98 percent. What these reports do not show is how fatigue affects mentation or function. There has been minimal formal evaluation of the impact of fatigue on cognitive performance in persons with TBI. It is also unclear how fatigue is related to other areas of impairment following TBI. Further, little is known about the natural course of fatigue and its associations with TBI-specific factors such as length of coma, duration of posttraumatic amnesia, and mechanism of injury.

At present, no single measurement instrument has been validated to study fatigue in the TBI population, although instruments discussed elsewhere in this volume may have been used in some TBI studies. LaChapelle and Finlayson (1998) evaluated 30 TBI patients (mean of 44.3 months postinjury) compared to age- and gender-matched healthy controls on measures of both objective and subjective fatigue. Objective fatigue was measured using a continuous thumb pressing task. Over time, both the healthy and TBI groups demonstrated a decline in the number of repetitions per unit of time, and the groups did not differ significantly in performance. Subjective fatigue was quantified on a visual analogue scale along with the fatigue severity score (FSS) and fatigue impact (FIS) scales. Though there were no differences in objective fatigue between healthy control and TBI groups, the TBI group showed significantly increased subjective fatigue scores over the various measures. Similarly, Walker and colleagues (1991) noted that subjective complaint of fatigue did not correlate with physical endurance in TBI cohort. Specifically, they found no difference in quadriceps strength and endurance between the TBI patients complaining of fatigue and either the normal controls or the TBI subjects who did not complain of fatigue.

Peripheral fatigue may have a significant impact on physically challenging factors that are commonly impaired after TBI, such as dressing, grooming, and ambulation. One working definition of peripheral fatigue is "any reduction of maximal force output" (Krupp & Pollina, 1996). A well-known phenomenon post-TBI is the upper motor neuron syndrome (UMNS), with attendant static and dynamic abnormalities in muscle spindle tone. Peripheral fatigue may arise from focal or global impairments in the motor and sensory control systems. In TBI patients with UMNS, ambulation is impaired and the efficiency of gait may be so compromised that fatigue easily occurs after ambulating short household distances. In light of recent advances in measuring energy demands of gait and understanding its determinants, we know that common post-TBI motor system sequelae such as hemiplegia, ataxia, and spasticity lead to increased energy demands for ambulation per unit of distance. While it is possible to separate peripheral from central fatigue in TBI, no such studies have been conducted to date.

Mechanism

Through sleep deprivation, overwork, and overexertion everyone has probably perceived fatigue, but it is easily remediable by sleep, rest, and a period of recovery. The sense of fatigue following TBI appears to be different in that it is usually not fully remedied by sleep or rest. More important, difficulty differentiating fatigue from other factors that are common in TBI such as cognitive impairment, depression, and motor disturbance further complicates determination of the true unique contribution fatigue has on TBI outcome. Thus, the challenge is to distinguish primary from secondary mechanisms producing posttraumatic fatigue (PTF).

Any discussion of fatigue in the TBI population must take into account the underlying neuropathological mechanisms involved in TBI (Rosenthal, Griffith, & Kreutzer, 1999). TBI encompasses a number of injuries to the brain. Including focal and diffuse, hemorrhagic and nonhemorrhagic, coup and contracoup, contusions, and compressive (epi- and subdural) lesions. The unifying mechanism of injury is sufficient transfer of energy to the brain to result in altered consciousness as defined by the widely used Glasgow Coma Scale. Although considerable controversy exists at the milder end of the injury spectrum (e.g., when whiplash is associated with brain trauma), altered consciousness is almost always associated with moderate to severe TBI. Therefore, at the most basic level, TBI begins with a disruption, typically via shearing forces, of the central nervous system (CNS) structures maintaining arousal. TBI-related central fatigue can be conceptualized as a higher-order deficit resulting from altered levels of neurotransmitters release by more caudal structures.

The differential brain destruction wrought by traumatic forces damages individual pathways subserving separate cognitive functions to variable degrees. Because TBI always involves some combination of pathways or systems, producing a potentially infinite number of permutations of causes underperformance by the fatigued brain.

Anatomy

The system in the brain responsible for maintaining arousal is called the ascending reticular activating system (ARAS), originating in the brainstem and represented in each of its three divisions by the following major nuclei, proceeding from caudal to rostral:

Medulla   Raphe and reticularis ventralis (serotonergic)

Pons   Parabrachialis (cholinergic), locus ceruleus (adrenergic), reticularis pontis oralis and caudalis, and the gigantocellularis

Midbrain   PPT/LDT (cholinergic), raphe (serotonergic), and ventral tegmental area (VTA; dopaminergic)

These structures converge or coalesce into two pathways, the ventral and dorsal branches of the ARAS. The ventral branch terminates in the subthalamus and posterior hypothalamus, which in turn send histaminergic fibers to a broad array of cortical targets. In addition, the medial forebrain bundle (MFB) projects into the septal nucleus and basal forebrain, which send a broad array of cholinergic fibers to the cortex. The dorsal pathway projects to the interlaminar nucleus of the thalamus, from which glutaminergic tracts reach a variety of cortical and striatocortical targets (Carpenter, 1985).

The ARAS is a fundamental structure subserving arousal, explaining why bilateral injuries in the brainstem nuclei result in impaired consciousness (Plum & Posner, 1980). This system is also a part of a larger and more complex system that integrates sensory attention and tonic arousal (Heilman & Valenstein, 2003).

The notion that this superstructure is implicated in PTF is partially supported in the recent review article by Chaudhuri and Behan (2000), who postulate that the basal ganglia are the neuroanatomical loci of fatigue following neurological impairment. Specifically, they identify the disruption of two functional loops—the striatocortical fibers and the striatothalamocortical fibers—as being responsible for central fatigue. The interaction of the ARAS and basal ganglia is well-known (Carpenter, 1985) and likely plays a significant role in PTF. This conceptual framework dovetails with the concept of the ARAS as mediating not only arousal but also the ability to "phasically" turn on cortical tissue efficiently. This point is emphasized by Heilman and Valenstein (2003), who state that "brain regions . . . are essentially silent unless and until activated by release of the appropriate transmitter" Thus, the increased "fatigue-ability" after brain injury may be conceptualized as a decreased ability not only to activate but also to efficiently sustain recruited cortical tissue.

Other Factors Contributing to Fatigue

Beyond the ARAS, a number of factors occurring post-TBI are likely to contribute to the clinical entity we know as fatigue. Unfortunately, their specific relationship to fatigue after TBI has largely not been formally studied. In the following sections, we examine psychiatric, biochemical, endocrine, and sleep contributions to the PTF experience.

Psychology/Psychiatry In considering central fatigue, motivational, psychological, and psychiatric contributions are important. Mood disturbance such as depression is commonly associated with fatigue, and current prevailing theories of depression suggest a deficiency of neurotransmitters such as serotonin and norepinephrine. Few studies, if any, clarify the relationship between fatigue and psychological distress in the TBI population. It is an important omission because depression has a high prevalence after TBI, with fatigue often reported as the most common symptom (Kreutzer et al., 2001; Seel & Kreutzer, 2003).

Biochemistry of Fatigue   As mentioned earlier, the ARAS produces numerous neuro-transmitters that directly affect arousal and fatigue. Acetylcholine and catecholamine agents act as stimulants and may influence fatigue. For example, medications such as methylphenidate or donepezil can increase arousal and attention and potentially improve fatigue symptoms.

On the other hand, certain amino acids and neurotransmitters have been associated with increased fatigue. Blomstrand and colleagues (1989) showed that sustained exercise to the point of fatigue resulted in an increase in concentration of tryptophan (a precursor to the neurotransmitter serotonin) by 36 percent across various regions of the brain. Levels of serotonin (5-HT) and its metabolite, 5-HIAA, increased during exercise throughout the brain. Dopamine increased in the brainstem (56%) and hypothalamus (46%), and noradrenaline increased in the striatum (59%). Blomstrand (2001) reported a decrement in human performance when 5-HT was elevated, and rats ran more efficiently when 5-HT levels were lowered.

Tryptophan is regulated by the ratio (through competitive binding for transport proteins) of tryptophan to other large neutral amino acids including branched-chain amino acids (BCAA). During exercise, the ratio of tryptophan to BCAA has been shown to increases. Administration of BCAA reduces perceived exertion and mental fatigue during exercise and improves cognitive performance after exercise (Blomstrand, 2001). Dwyer and Browning (2000) demonstrated that the administration of 5-HT1A (a serotonin agonist) induces fatigue in rats during a running task. As the rats continued to train over 6 weeks, the agents effects diminished. Administration of BCAA was also tested in a placebo-controlled trial during a long-distance race. The authors measured both physical and mental performance. The treatment group was noted to have a superior cognitive performance over the placebo group. Regarding physical performance, the lesser trained runners performed better with BCAA, but the more experienced runners showed no difference between BCAA and placebo. (Blomstrand et al., 1991).

Endocrine Factors   Endocrine or hormonal abnormalities present with a variety of symptoms including fatigue, especially with deficiencies secondary to anterior pituitary dysfunction (Elovic, 2003, 2004; Larsen eL al., 2003). Of course, no singular hormonal deficiency correlates exclusively with fatigue, and numerous other symptoms are manifested as a result. However, the association between endocrine dysfunction and fatigue has been particularly well-documented regarding thyroid hormone, growth hormone (GH), and cortisol deficiencies. GH deficiencies in particular have been associated with decreased bone mineral densities (Colao et al., 1999), aerobic capacity, and muscle strength, lower quality of life, and cognitive impairments in addition to increased fatigue (Deijen et al., 1996; Simpson et al., 2002). Studies of mixed etiologies show that the treatment of endocrine dysfunction is beneficial, reversing the previously described deficits. Treatment of GH insufficiencies has been shown to increase lean body mass and reduce body fat (Newman & Kleinberg, 1998), increase exercise tolerance, improve quadriceps strength (Jørgensen et al., 1994), increase energy and mood (Gibney et al., 1999), increase activity and alertness (Burman et al., 1995), and improve one's sense of wellbeing and quality of life (Carroll et al., 1998).

The importance of this issue, of course, depends on the overall incidence of endocrine dysfunction associated with TBI. It has been known for nearly 100 years that brain injury may produce endocrine dysfunction, but until recently this was considered a relatively rare event (Lieberman et al., 2001). Escamilla and Lisser (1942) reported an incidence of only 0.7 percent (4 of 595 TBI subjects) endocrine dysfunction. Kalisky and coworkers (1985) reported an incidence of only 4 percent and Edwards and Clark (1986) reported only a small percentage of TBI cases were associated with hypopituitarism. However, more recently the magnitude of the problem has become more evident. Benvenga and associates (2000) documented 367 total cases of head trauma associated with hypopituitarism, including their patients and a literature review. Among these patients, 15 percent were not diagnosed with pituitary dysfunction until more than 5 years after injury.

Since the year 2000, researchers have addressed the issue of endocrine dysfunction prospectively, screening TBI patients for endocrine abnormalities, and have demonstrated a much higher incidence of hypopituitarism in the TBI population. Kelly and colleagues (2000) reported that 8 of 22 individuals with TBI undergoing provocative testing had abnormalities. Lieberman and coworkers (2001) studied 70 patients with TBI in a postacute brain injury program and identified endocrine abnormalities in 59 percent of TBI subjects, GH deficiency in 14 percent, hypothyroidism in 21 percent, and low morning basal cortisol in 45 percent.

These TBI studies, however, only identified the presence of endocrine abnormalities. The relationship between endocrine abnormalities and fatigue in TBI individuals is currently under study by the authors. In this pilot work, an inverse relationship has been noted between fatigue and insulin growth factor 1 (IGF-1) in persons with TBI. IGF-1 is commonly used as a screening measure for GH deficiency because of their correlation. Although this work is in its infancy, it suggests that endocrinopathy may be a potential cause of PTF in TBI. If individuals with TBI respond as other populations do, this suggests a potential treatment for some of those suffering from fatigue.

Sleep   In general, sleep disturbances can be characterized as insomnia (deficient sleep initiation or maintenance), hypersomnia (excessive sleep or excessive daytime sleepiness, EDS), and altered sleep–wake cycles (circadian pattern disarray). Sleep disturbances following TBI range in frequency from 36 to 70 percent (McLean et al., 1984; Keshavan et al., 1981). Several key CNS loci regulate sleep patterns, including brainstem, basal forebrain, and hypothalamic nuclei—all areas commonly disrupted in brain trauma. Serotonin and acetylcholine are the two common substances involved. The comprehensive study of posttraumatic sleep disorders is complicated by the frequently encountered comorbidities of depression, anxiety, substance abuse, chronic pain, and medication use, all of which have independent negative influences on normal sleep. Also not to be overlooked is whether a prior (perhaps undiagnosed) sleep disorder may be the proximate cause of the brain injury itself. For instance, falling asleep while driving is not uncommon, especially in persons with sleep apnea.

Controversy exists over whether severity of TBI is directly correlated with increased prevalence of insomnia. Clinchot and coworkers (1998) and Fictenberg and coworkers (2001) showed an *inverse* relationship and Cohen and coworkers (1992) noted increased prevalence with increasing TBI severity. Some researchers have postulated that the severely brain injured likely underreport poor sleep and those with milder brain injury are more aware of their problems and therefore "overreport," or perhaps overly attribute their fatigue to poor sleep. Clinchot and coworkers (1991) examined 100 TBI patients during inpatient rehabilitation and followed them up again 1 year later. These researchers reported that 50 percent of TBI subjects complained of difficulty sleeping. Of this subgroup, 64 percent admitted waking up too early, 25 percent experienced increased sleep time, and 45 percent reported difficulty falling asleep. In this same cohort of 100 patient, 63 percent reported significant problems with fatigue. Interestingly, 80 percent of those admitting to sleeping difficulty also admitted to fatigue as a problem. Cohen and others (1992) have pointed to a temporally differentiated pattern of sleep disruption in which difficulty initiating or maintaining sleep tends to occur soon after TBI and EDS tends to occur more often over the months and years following TBI. Controversy also exists over whether TBI may cause a secondary narcolepsy.

Several varieties of disturbed sleep–wake cycles are seen—the delayed, advanced, and disorganized types—with little literature available specific to the TBI population. Schreiber and coworkers (1998) described sleep–wake disturbance in 15 persons with mild TBI and without a history of apnea syndrome, neurological disorder, or psychiatric illness. Using polysomnography and actigraphy (activity detection device), more than half were found to have delayed-phase and the rest had disorganized type disturbances.

The brain-injured population thus experiences disruption in normal sleep physiology. Busek and Faber (2000) reported a relationship between severity of injury and disturbance of REM sleep, with the more severe injuries causing a greater reduction in REM sleep (Busek and Faber, 2000). Conversely, it has also been found that REM sleep architecture improves as cognition does. There also appears to be an association between cognition and sleep architecture among TBI patients over time, with the former improving along with the latter (Ron et al., 1980).

Overall, though sleep disturbance after TBI is common, little work directly relates this disturbance to fatigue. It is likely, however, that the relationship between sleep and fatigue observed in other populations (see chapter 13) also applies to persons with TBI.

Fatigue and Cognitive Dysfunction

As indicated earlier, the primary focus of this chapter is on TBI-induced central fatigue. Clinical experience suggests that fatigue may contribute to the TBI patients' complaint of diminished mental performance. TBI survivors may present with a broad spectrum of deficits in cognition, such as decreased attention, slower processing speed, memory deficits, and executive dysfunction. Most studies have not correlated fatigue with neuropsychological performance in TBI, however, or when they do, fatigue is based on self-report.

An exception is a study by Riese and colleagues (1999) that examined the impact of central (mental) fatigue on cognition. These investigators studied eight young severely injured TBI patients more than 9 months postinjury. The mean length of coma was 18.4 days and the mean duration of posttraumatic amnesia was 51.1 days. All of the patients studied had suffered not only severe but also diffuse injury; in fact, one inclusion criterion was "no documented focal lesions." The authors did not rate fatigue by self-report, but rather assessed the ability to sustain workload by administering a "continuous dynamic divided attention task." The study findings revealed no difference between control and TBI subject groups in the effect of "task load" on performance, but the TBI cohort required an increased amount of mental effort to maintain the task. The finding of increased mental effort among the TBI cohort was corroborated through both subjective and physiological indicators of distress. Perceived effort was assessed through self-report. (See chapter 3 for more on fatigue, cognition, and mental effort.)

Underlying Riese's research is a "coping" hypothesis that "even when task difficulty is adapted to the cognitive capacities of closed head injury patients, increased effort and distress will be found in this group." The authors hypothesized that the TBI patients' need for increased effort is related to impaired ability to "phasically" recruit and activate sufficient cortical resources to perform a given task. Such an impairment is but one of multiple brain behavior alterations after TBI, and efforts to sustain performance may one day be associated with neuropathologic factors such as shearing of specific axonal pathways as well as to self-reported fatigue.

A recent study by Christodoulou and colleagues (2001) may lend support to Riese's hypothesis. Christodoulou examined cerebral activation in nine persons with TBI and seven controls using functional magnetic resonance imaging (fMRI) while the subjects performed a working memory task. The TBI subjects exhibited an altered pattern of cerebral activation compared to controls, marked by increased right hemisphere activation (healthy subjects showed more left hemisphere activation) as well as a more dispersed pattern of activation throughout the brain. Decreased performance was associated with greater and more dispersed brain activation among the TBI subjects. The authors hypothesized that the TBI subjects' need for additional cerebral resources to conduct the task could be the result of the extra mental effort required due to cerebral inefficiency after TBI. This condition may well result in greater mental fatigue as one works harder to perform cognitive tasks (see chapter 3 for more on this topic). In a related case report by Hillary and others (2003), the TBI participant completed the working memory task in the fMRI, both pre- and posttreatment with stimulant medication (methylphenidate and modafinil). Improved performance was observed with stimulant medication, which also resulted in decreased cerebral activation on fMRI, correlating with the patients self-report of greater ease in performing the task.

Treatment Issues

A separate chapter is devoted to treatment, so this discussion is limited to issues particularly relevant to TBI. The first treatment approach is to address reversible factors that may produce fatigue. This includes removal of potentially deleterious medications. Anticonvulsants, for example, are taken by many individuals with TBI without documented posttraumatic epilepsy. Temkin and associates (1990, 1999) have laid to rest the idea that dilantin or valproate prophylaxis offers any benefit. When anticonvulsants are required after TBI, one can consider using a less sedating and potentially activating agent such as lamotrigine if fatigue becomes a problem. A host of additional medications have fatigue and sedation as a potential side effects including drugs for spasticity and gastrointestinal symptoms, anxiolytics and antipsychotics. When these agents are medically necessary, it is appropriate to choose the one with the least sedating effect. Clinicians must view all of these medications with suspicion for the fatigued and cognitively impaired patient. Medications must earn their place in the treatment of any patient who has these complaints.

Much knowledge regarding the use of medication to directly stimulate the fatigued individual is borrowed from literature outside of TBI. Numerous papers have reported on the use of methylphenidate, dextroamphetamine, and amantadine to treat cognitive deficits secondary to brain injury and fatigue in other populations. Brietbart and associates (2001) demonstrated the benefit of methylphenidate and pemoline in HIV-related fatigue, whereas Wagner and Rabkin (2000) reported a similar benefit of dextroamphetamine. Emonson and Vanderbeek (1995) reported that dextroamphetamine was also useful for flight crews flying during Desert Storm. Krupp and others (1995) showed that amantadine was useful in the treatment of multiple sclerosis (MS)-related fatigue, and Cohen and Fisher (1989) reported an increase in energy with its use.

A relatively new agent, modafinil, has been reported to be useful in various populations with neurological disorder including stroke, MS, depression, and schizophrenia (Rammohan et al., 2003). It has also been shown to reduce the fatigue associated with certain medications that have a sedative side effect. Finally, often overlooked but far more cost-effective, is the agent that many people already self-administer, caffeine. Caffeine, whose mode of action is the inhibition of the sedating agent adenosine has been shown to be useful in treating fatigue in various populations. It has the potential advantage of ease of access and low cost for patients who may be unable to afford modafinil. Wesensten and coworkers (2002) showed that modafinil was not superior to caffeine for fatigue secondary to sleep deprivation. Its place in the TBI population has yet to be studied.

Patient education is another important aspect of treatment that is often overlooked. Despite the desire to be ambulatory, if fatigue is an issue after a lone time on one's feet, partial reliance on a wheelchair may be appropriate for those with mobility problems. The individual's sleep habits and hygiene are additional issues that may contribute to fatigue. Addressing the medical and psychological issues discussed earlier may be of benefit as well. Given the high frequency of depression in persons with TBI, and that fatigue is often among the most common complaints in postinjury depression, selecting drugs with lesser sedating effects, such as wellbutrin, can be important. Exercise is frequently a part of outpatient and mild TBI programs. Promoting exercise as a part of a fatigue program has met with some success in other populations (see chapter 19), but few studies have addressed this benefit among persons with TBI.

Future Directions

Historically, before the advent of advanced neuroimaging modalities, the psychometric tools developed by neuropsychologists were remarkably successful at locating lesions. No unique anatomic location has yet been identified as the "cause" of fatigue. As the work of Christodoulou and Colleagues (2001) suggests, however, neuroimaging offers the promise of correlating deficits in function with morphology, a benefit that is particularly relevant for TBI because neuropharmacological interventions are predicated on the ability to recruit adjoining and related anatomical structures to complete a task. The potential for imaging modalities in selecting pharmacologic interventions and predicting their effectiveness is an exciting prospect.

Future research will have to introduce fatigue into neuropsychological testing to establish the relationship between fatigue and well-known TBI-related deficits, particularly arousal, attention, vigilance, and memory. A combination of neuroimaging, pharmaceutical interventions, and traditional neuropsychological test batteries holds tremendous promise in uncovering the mechanisms of fatigue generation after TBI.

Finally, numerous medical issues differentiate individuals with TBI from other patients with fatigue. Improvements in treating spasticity, endocrine abnormality, sleep disturbance, and mood disorder are just some of the areas in which better medical management may make a substantial difference in the nebulous area of the treatment of TBI-associated fatigue.

References

Benvenga, S., Campenni, A., Ruggeri, R. M., & Trimarchi, F. (2000). Clinical review 113: hypopituitarism secondary to head trauma. *Journal of Clinical Endocrinology and Metabolism, 85,* 1353–1361.

Blomstrand, E. (2001). Amino acids and central fatigue. *Amino Acids, 20,* 25–34.

Blomstrand, E., Hassmen, P., & Newsholme, E. A. (1991). Effect of branched-chain amino acid supplementation on mental performance. *Acta Physiologica Scandinavia, 143,* 225–226.

Blomstrand, E., Perrett, D., Parry-Billings, M., & Newsholme, E. A. (1989). Effect of sustained exercise on plasma amino acid concentrations and on 5-hydroxytryptamine metabolism in six different brain regions in the rat. *Acta Physiologica Scandinavia, 136,* 473–481.

Breitbart, W., Rosenfeld, B., Kaim, M., & Funesti-Esch, J. (2001). A randomized, double-blind, placebo-controlled trial of psychostimulants for the treatment of fatigue in ambulatory patients with human immunodeficiency virus disease. *Archives of Internal Medicine, 12;161(3),* 411–420.

Burman, P., Broman, J. E., Hetta, J., et al. (1995). Quality of life in adults with growth hormone (GH) deficiency: response to treatment with recombinant human GH in a placebo-controlled 21-month trial. *Journal of Clinical Endocrinology and Metabolism, 80,* 3585–3590.

Busek, P., & Faber, J. (2000). The influence of traumatic brain lesion on sleep architecture. *Sbovník Lékarský, 101,* 233–239.

Carpenter, M. B. (1985). *Core Text of Neuroanatomy,* 3rd edn. Baltimore: Williams & Wilkins.

Carroll, P. V., Christ, E. R., Bengtsson, B. A., et al. (1998). Growth hormone deficiency in adulthood and the effects of growth hormone replacement: a review. Growth Hormone Research Society Scientific Committee. *Journal of Clinical Endocrinology and Metabolism, 83,* 382–395.

Chaudhuri, A., & Behan, P.O. (2000). Fatigue and basal ganglia. *Journal of Neurological Sciences, 179,* 34–42.

Christodoulou, C., DeLuca, J., Ricker, J. H., et al. (2001). Functional magnetic resonance imaging of working memory impairment after traumatic brain injury. *Journal of Neurology and Neurosurgical Psychiatry, 71,* 161–168.

Clinchot, D. M., Bogner, J., Mysiw, W. J., Fugate, L., & Corrigan, J. (1998). Defining sleep disturbance after brain injury. *American Journal of Physical Medicine & Rehabilitation, 77(4; July/August 1998)*, 291–295.

Cohen, R. A., & Fisher, M. (1989) Amantadine treatment of fatigue associated with multiple sclerosis. *Archives of Neurology, 46(6)*, 676–680.

Cohen, M., Oksenberg, A., Snir, D., Stern, M. J., & Groswasser, Z. (1992). Temporally related changes of sleep complaints in traumatic brain injured patients. *Journal of Neurology and Neurosurgical Psychiatry, 55*, 313–315.

Colao, A., Di Somma, C., Pivonello, R., Loche, S., Aimaretti, G., Cerbone, G., Faggiano, A., Comeli, G., Ghigo, E., & Lombardi, G. (1999). Bone loss is correlated to the severity of growth hormone deficiency in adult patients with hypopituitarism. *Journal of Clinical Endocrinology and Metabolism, 84*, 1919–1924.

Deijen, J. B., de Boer, H., Blok, G. J., & van der Veen, E. A. (1996). Cognitive impairments and mood disturbances in growth hormone deficient men. *Psychoneuroendocrinology, 21*, 313–322.

Dwyer, D., & Browning, J. (2000). Endurance training in Wistar rats decreases receptor sensitivity to a serotonin agonist. *Acta Physiologica Scandinavia, 170(3)*, 211–216.

Edwards, O. M., & Clark, J. D. (1986). Post-traumatic hypopituitarism. Six cases and a review of the literature. *Medicine (Baltimore), 65*, 281–290.

Elovic, E. P. (2003). Anterior pituitary dysfunction after traumatic brain injury, part I. *Journal of Head Trauma Rehabilitation, 18*, 541–543.

Elovic, E. P. (2004). Anterior pituitary dysfunction after traumatic brain injury, part 2. *Journal of Head Trauma Rehabilitation, 19*, 184–187.

Emonson, D. L., & Vanderbeek, R. D. (1995). The use of amphetamines in U.S. Air Force tactical operations during Desert Shield. *Space Environmental Medicine, 66(3)*, 260–263.

Escamilla, R. F., & Lisser, H. (1942). Simmonds disease. *Journal of Clinical Endocrinology, 2*, 65–96.

Fictenberg, N. L., Putnam, S. H., Mann, N. R., Zafonte, R. D., & Millard, A. E. (2001). Insomnia screening in postacute traumatic brain injury: utility and validity of the Pittsburgh Sleep Quality Index. *American Journal of Physical Medicine and Rehabilitation, 80*, 339–345.

Gibney, J., Wallace, J. D., Spinks, T., et al. (1999). The effects of 10 years of recombinant human growth hormone (GH) in adult GH-deficient patients. *Journal of Clinical Endocrinology and Metabolism, 84*, 2596–2602.

Harrison-Felix, C., Zafonte, R., Mann, N., Dijkers, M., Englander, J., & Kreutzer, J. (1998). Brain injury as a result of violence: preliminary findings from the traumatic brain injury model systems. *Archives of Physical Medicine and Rehabilitation, 79(7)*, 730–737.

Heilman, K. M., & Valenstein, E. (2003). *Clinical Neuropsychology*, 4th ed. Oxford: Oxford University Press.

Hillary, F., Elovic, E., & Ricker, J. (2003). Stimulant induced improvement in brain efficiency as documented by functional magnetic resonance imaging: a case report. *American Journal of Physical Medicine and Rehabilitation, 82(3)*, 240.

Hillier, S. L., Sharpe, M. H., & Metzer, J. (1997) Outcomes 5 years post-traumatic brain injury (with further reference to neurophysical impairment and disability). *Brain Injury, 11(9)*, 661–675.

Jørgensen, J. O. L., Thiesen, L., Müller, J., Ovesem, P., & Skakkebæk, N. E., & Christiansen, J. S. (1994). Three years of growth hormone treatment in growth hormone-deficient adults: near normalization of body composition and physical performance. *European Journal of Endocrinology, 130*, 224–228.

Kalisky, Z., Morrison, D. P., Meyers, C. A., & Von Laufen, A. (1985). Medical problems encountered during rehabilitation of patients with head injury. *Archives of Physical Medicine and Rehabilitation, 66*, 25–29.

Kelly, D. F., Gonzalo, I. T., Cohan, P., Berman, N., Swerdloff, R., & Wang, C. (2000). Hypopituitarism following traumatic brain injury and aneurysmal subarachnoid hemorrhage: a preliminary report. *Journal of Neurosurgery, 93*, 743–752.

Keshavan, M. S., Channabasavanna, S. M., & Reddy, G. N. (1981). Post traumatic psychiatric disturbances: patterns and predictions of outcome. *British Journal of Psychiatry, 138*, 157–160.

Kreutzer, J. S., Seel, R. T., & Gourley, E. (2001). The prevalence and symptom rates of depression after traumatic brain injury: a comprehensive examination. *Brain Injury, 15(7)*, 563–576.

Krupp, L. B. (2003). *Fatigue*. Philadelphia: Butterworth Heinmann.

Krupp, L. B., Coyle, P. K., Doscher, C., et al. (1995). Fatigue therapy in multiple sclerosis: results of a double-blind, randomized, parallel trial of amantadine, pemoline, and placebo. *Neurology, 45*, 1956–1961.

Krupp, L. B., & Pollina, D. A. (1996). Mechanisms and management of fatigue in progressive neurological disorders. *Current Opinions in Neurology, 9*, 456–460.

LaChapelle, D. L., & Finlayson, M. A. (1998). An evaluation of subjective and objective measures of fatigue in patients with brain injury and healthy controls. *Brain Injury, 12(8)*, 649–659.

Larsen, P. R., Kronenberg, H. M., Melmed, S., & Polonsky, K. S. (2003). *Williams Textbook of Endocrinology*, 10th ed. Philadelphia: Saunders.

Lezak, M. D. (1978). *Neuropsychological Assessment*, 1st ed. New York: Oxford University Press.

Lezak, M. D. (1995). *Neuropsychological Assessment*, 3rd ed. New York: Oxford University Press.

Lieberman, S. A., Oberoi, A. L., Gilkison, C. R., Masel, B. E., & Urban, R. J. (2001). Prevalence of neuroendocrine dysfunction in patients recovering from traumatic brain injury. *Journal of Clinical Endocrinology and Metabolism, 86*, 2752–2756.

Masson, F., Maurette, P., Salmi, L. R., et al. (1996). Prevalence of impairments 5 years after a head injury, and their relationship with disabilities and outcome. *Brain Injury, 10*, 487–497.

McLean, A., Dikmen, S., & Temkin, N. R. (1984). Psychosocial functioning at one month after head injury. *Neurosurgery, 14*, 393–399.

Middleboe, T., Andersen, H. S., Birket-Smith, M., & Friis, M. L. (1992). Minor head injury: impact on general health after 1 year. A prospective follow-up study. *Acta Neurologica Scandinavia, 85*, 5–9.

Newman, C. B., & Kleinberg, D. L. (1998). Adult growth hormone deficiency. *Endocrinologist, 8*, 178–186.

Olver, J. H., Ponsford, J. L., & Curran, C. A. (1996). Outcome following traumatic brain injury: a comparison between 2 and 5 years after injury. *Brain Injury, 10*, 841–848.

Plum, F., & Posner, J. B. (1980). *The Diagnosis of Stupor and Coma*, 3rd ed. Philadelphia: F.A. Davis Company.

Rammohan, K. W., Rosenberg, J. H., Lynn, D. J., Blumenfeld, A. M., Pollak, C. P., & Nagaraja, H. N. (2003). Efficacy and safety of modafinil (Provigil) for the treatment of fatigue in multiple sclerosis: a two centre phase 2 study. *Journal of Neurology Neurosurgical Psychiatry, 72(2)*, 179–183.

Riese, H., Hoedemaeker, M., Brouwer, W. H., Mulder, L. J. M., Cremer, R., & Veldman, J. B. P. (1999). Mental fatigue after very severe closed head injury: sustained performance, mental effort, and distress at two levels of workload in a driving simulator. *Neuropsychological Rehabilitation, 9*, 189–205.

Ron, S., Algom, D., Hary, D., & Cohen, M. (1980). Time-related changes in the distribution of sleep stages in brain injured patients. *Electroencephalographic Clinical Neurophysiology, 48*, 432–441.

Rosenthal, M., Griffith, E. R., & Kreutzer, J. S. (1999). *Rehabilitation of the Adult and Child with Traumatic Brain Injury*, 3rd ed. Philadelphia: F.A. Davis.

Schreiber, S., Klag, E., Gross, Y., Segman, R. H., & Pick, C. G. (1998). Beneficial effect of risperidone on sleep disturbance and psychosis following traumatic brain injury. *International Clinical Psychopharmacology, 13*, 273–275.

Seel, R. T., & Kreutzer, J. S. (2003). Depression assessment after traumatic brain injury: an empirically based classification method. *Archives of Physical Medicine and Rehabilitation, 84(11)*,1621–1628.

Simpson, H., Savine, R., Sonksen, P., et al. (2002). Growth hormone replacement therapy for adults: into the new millennium. *Growth Hormones and IGF Research, 12*, 1–33.

Temkin, N. R., Dikmen, S. S., Anderson, G. D., Wilensky, A. J., Holmes, M. D., & Cohen, W. (1999). Valproate therapy for prevention of posttraumatic seizures: a randomized trial. *Journal of Neurosurgery, 91(4)*, 593–560.

Temkin, N. R., Dikmen, S. S., Wilensky, A. J., Keihm, J., Chabal, S., & Winn, H. R. (1990). A randomized, double-blind study of phenytoin for the prevention of post-traumatic seizures. *New England Journal of Medicine, 323(8)*, 497–502.

Wagner, G. J., & Rabkin, R. (2000). Effects of dextroamphetamine on depression and fatigue in men with HIV: a double-blind, placebo-controlled trial. *Journal of Clinical Psychiatry, 61(6)*, 436–440.

Walker, G. C., Cardenas, D. D., Guthrie, M. R., McLean, A., Jr., & Brooke, M. M. (1991). Fatigue and depression in brain-injured patients correlated with quadriceps strength and endurance. *Archives of Physical Medicine Rehabilitation, 72*, 469–472.

Wesensten, N. J., Belenky, G., Kautz, M. A., Thorne, D. R., Reichardt, R. M., & Balkin, T. J. (2002). Maintaining alertness and performance during sleep deprivation: modafinil versus caffeine. *Psychopharmacology (Berlin), 159*, 238–247.

7   Fatigue in Other Neurological Conditions

Jonathan L. Fellus and Wahid Rashidzada

Only recently have interested researchers and clinicians reached a critical mass and recognized the broad importance of fatigue as a contributor to the disability found in many disease states. Seemingly, this has occurred along with the advent of more successful therapies (pharmacologic and otherwise) that, in turn, have brought the issue of fatigue into greater focus for and within reach of a larger clinical audience. Although the scope of this chapter precludes discussion of every type of neurological entity not covered elsewhere in this text, we will attempt to touch on several disorders in which fatigue either plays an important role or its presence reveals important features underlying possible mechanisms.

Fatigue is a common symptom of chronic neurological disorders, and it appears to be one of the most underreported, underrecognized, and undertreated symptoms in many of these diseases (de Groot, Phillips, & Eskes, 2003). While the exact neuroanatomic correlates or mechanism remain unknown, the involvement of the limbic system and basal ganglia subcomponents suggests common underlying themes in many neurological diseases in which central fatigue manifests. This chapter discusses the theoretical underpinnings of cognitive fatigue associated with several neurological diseases not otherwise covered in this book, and proposes a theoretical mechanism to explain such neurobehavioral symptomatology.

Background/Definition

Central fatigue (as distinguished from "peripheral," primarily physical or muscular, fatigue) has been defined as the inability to initiate or sustain attentional tasks and physical activities requiring self-motivation (Chaudhuri & Behan, 2000). Some have emphasized different elements of the fatigue experience, namely, *attention* and *vigilance,* and many wide-ranging definitions are found in other chapters. What is clear from the recent debate over fatigue is that our current characterization may be no more sophisticated or less ambiguous than the old label of "neurasthenia" (Layzer,

1998). Though consensus on what constitutes fatigue in normal individuals may be relatively straightforward, it is infinitely more challenging to disentangle abnormal fatigue from the multiple neurophysiological disturbances at work in central nervous system (CNS) disease states.

Thus, it should not be surprising that, in deconstructing fatigue into its discreet components, the debate is between the lumpers and the splitters. Some of the terms that compete for relevance are *attention, selective attention, alertness, vigilance*, and *speed of processing* (Michiels & Cluydts, 2001; Joyce, Blumenthal, & Wessely, 1996; Michiels, de Gucht, Cluydts, & Fischler, 1999; Parmenter, Denney, & Lynch, 2003; Tiersky, Johnson, Lange, Natelson, & DeLuca, 1997). And whether a given element is positioned in a primary or secondary role of prominence depends on where the theorist believes fatigue *originates*. Furthermore, discussions often tend to be discipline-specific, buttressed by operational definitions frequently derived from assessments borrowed from other disease states. Certain discussions also suffer from a tendency to oversimplify the fatigue experience or to define fatigue in a vacuum, thus minimizing its clinical relevance.

Perhaps a more comprehensive definition rests on the notion that a growing number of recognized factors contribute to measurable fatigue and the fatigue experience. This approach is explored further in the section on theory and mechanism. But the current state of research suggests fatigue defies a simple or grand, unifying theory to account for the prodigious number of contributing factors encountered in the clinical fatigue experience.

Assessment

The simple fact is, we can point to few formal statistics relating fatigue to nearly every aspect of the neurological conditions discussed in this chapter. Literature searches yield few formal studies, and most of those cited make only an initial attempt to characterize the problem of fatigue. Fatigue is even less often the major focus of an observational or interventional study. Assessment may generally focus on attempts to characterize the simple prevalence of fatigue, its severity, and its associated elements or markers; or it may focus on the *impact* of fatigue on performance of certain functional tasks or quality of life. From a practical, clinical standpoint, the opportunity to obtain a comprehensive history, probing for disease-specific contributing elements should not be missed.

When we critique studies purporting to characterize fatigue, it is therefore important to note whether they distinguish between fatigue as a symptom (typically by self-report) and fatigue as a sign (objectively measured by tasks or scales, for instance). At a very basic level, even something as simple as self-report may be confounded by patients' inability to reliably distinguish between mental and physical fatigue. As a further pitfall, we were unable to locate a discussion of the apparent dilemma of passive measurement (e.g., vigilance task) versus assessing an individual's active engagement in tasks of self-determined interest.

Fatigue can be measured by either reported experience of the patient or objective changes in motor or cognitive functioning. Frequently cited assessment tools include the Fatigue Severity Scale (FSS), Fatigue Impact Scale (FIS), Multidimensional Assessment of Fatigue (MAF), Multidimensional Fatigue Inventory (MFI), Fatigue Assessment Instrument (FAI), Fatigue Rating Scale (FRS), and Short Form-36 of the Medical Outcome Survey (SF-36). The advantage to these assessment tools is their ease of administration. Their disadvantages include their inherent lack of objectivity and frequent occurrence of retrospective bias (Krupp, 2003). Recently, functional magnetic resonance imaging (fMRI) and positron emission tomography (PET) scans have been used to assess fatigue objectively, at least in traumatic brain injury (TBI), multiple sclerosis (MS), and chronic fatigue syndrome (CFS) populations (see chapter 3). A screening sleep history may prompt investigation with polysomnography, possibly revealing a sleep disorder partly or wholly responsible for generalized or mental fatigue (see chapter 13).

Epidemiology and Scope of the Problem

As alluded to earlier, insufficient reliable data exist to characterize items such as incidence or prevalence of fatigue for most neurological entities in this "other" category. For the reasons laid out here, fatigue is poorly characterized in the vast majority of neurological entities. Friedman and Friedman (2001) candidly admit to not attempting even to define fatigue, relying only on the subjects' interpretation of fatigue-related questions. Most prior and many current efforts have focused mainly on the more clinically simple assessment or measurement of physical (peripheral) fatigue. Thus, researchers are only beginning to assess how often fatigue coexists or predominates and how fatigue affects the clinical course of diseases less classically associated with fatigue. Likewise, attempts to correlate and quantify comorbid or secondary factors are similarly immature.

Given this paucity of basic information, considerable time will pass before researchers and clinicians can consider the *consequences* of untreated fatigue. Finally, the shear number, mechanism, complexity, and impact of such factors as *nutrition* or *cultural differences*, for example, are of such a daunting magnitude that one may be understandably discouraged from any attempt to correlate these potentially important contributing factors.

Theory and Mechanism

The proposed paradigm views centrally mediated fatigue as the result of mutually interdependent or multiple vicious cycles found in numerous neurological disorders in which cognitive fatigue is a product. As discussed in greater detail later under each disease heading, there is a recurring theme of one symptom or system dysfunction reflexively exacerbating another component of the index disease. For example, mood disturbances affect sleep-wake cycles that, when disturbed, tend to amplify mood disorders. Pain, a frequently encountered symptom in CNS disease, puts the individual at higher risk for mood and sleep disturbance; and conversely, those with dysfunctional mood or sleep are more apt to experience magnified pain (Covington, 1991; Manu, Matthews, Lane, Tennen, Hesselbrock, Mendola, & Affleck, 1989; Wessely & Powell, 1989). It is easy to appreciate how these interactions pose a mounting burden that cumulatively impedes optimal cognitive function. At a more basic, neurophysiological level, it takes little more than upsetting the delicate balance of neurotransmitters to generate several potential mechanisms of fatigue. One well-established example is the balance between serotonin and branched-chain amino acids (BCAA). Higher relative amounts of CNS serotonin are associated with greater fatigue, whereas BCAA levels correlate with less fatigue (Wessely & Powell, 1989; Blomstrand, Celsing, & Newsholme, 1988). Simply put, cognitive fatigue represents the final common pathway of impaired neural processing, whether by primary or secondary mechanisms. As with most CNS systems, final output reflects the absolute difference between inhibitory and excitatory inputs.

Another common scenario is predicated on the emerging relationship between stress (of chronic illness) and cognitive decline. This is highlighted in the section on dementia, but it is important to note here that this interaction requires sufficient insight from the patient (the absence of anosognosia) to appreciate the impact of chronic illness.

A third line of reasoning draws the connection between incipient neurological dysfunction magnified by a cascade of subclinical events within multiple systems and pathways subserving optimal cognitive performance. The organism unwittingly accommodates to a lower level of function, with fatigue behavior gradually becoming entrenched as the norm. Underreported, undertreated, and underrecognized central fatigue in chronic brain disorders reflects, at least in part, an epiphenomenon of fatigue sufferers becoming accustomed to a lower level of cognitive and physical activity and adapting to that lower level of functioning. Thus, fatigue begets more fatigue.

Simultaneously, other more clinically or phenomenologically manifest symptoms may emerge, drawing attention away from fatigue. Fatigue usually goes untreated in favor of more predominating aspects of the index disorder that themselves are often blamed for *causing* fatigue (e.g., a gait disorder, depression) rather than being viewed, assessed, or treated independently. Secondary factors that perpetuate fatigue thus become the focus of treatment.

Given this pattern of insidious symptomatology triggering early behavioral adjustment during the course of illness, a kind of dual-stage hypothesis emerges. In the early stages of neurological illness (primary injury), fatigue may alter one's psychological expectations, resulting in diminished actual performance that, in turn, alters later perception (secondary effect) and ultimately results in chronically disabling fatigue (Metzger & Denney, 2002). This conceptualization draws on two of the four states discussed by Bartley and Chute, namely, the interplay between the "feeling state" (perception) and the "behavior state" (cognitive performance) (Bartley & Chute, 1947). Fatigue behavior, therefore, to some degree evolves into a type of learned helplessness. Such a course of events is an example of the aforementioned "vicious cycles" that perpetuate the experience of fatigue. For the many reasons discussed here, fatigue may be very difficult to reverse totally.

Informed speculation leads us to identify motor coordination centers (basal ganglia), executive and motor planning areas (frontal circuits), and internal motivational apparati (hypothalamus and related limbic structures) as the main arbiters of fatigue-associated behavior (Chaudhuri & Behan, 2000). Against this backdrop, it is unlikely that fatigue will be successfully characterized as a unitary construct. The complex interaction between neuroimmunological factors, neurotransmitters, neuroendocrine systems, and actual substrates of energy (ATP) (Krupp, 2003) make it likely that the essence of the fatigue experience will remain elusive. It is nevertheless easy to appreciate the broad impact of CNS disorders in the development of fatigue.

Fatigue in Early or Mild Dementia

Dementia is characterized by progressive intellectual deterioration that is severe enough to interfere with occupational and social activities (Rowland, 2000). Memory, orientation, abstraction, ability to learn, visuospatial perception, language function, constructional praxis, and higher executive functions (e.g., planning, organizing, and sequencing) may all be impaired in dementia. Most dementias are secondary to neurodegenerative processes. Approximately two-thirds of all dementias relate in some way to Alzheimer disease, based on clinical and autopsy criteria.

In its early stages, detection can be challenging as some mild forgetfulness is often seen among the elderly. However, such mild symptoms are rarely disruptive. Aside from neurodegenerative diseases, many other clinical and disease entities can lead to or manifest as dementia. Depression, for instance, is especially common in the elderly and, when severe, may present as "pseudodementia" (Foerstl, 1990; Lee & Lyketsos, 2003). Medications such as sedatives, hypnotics, blood pressure medicines, and arthritis medications may induce, albeit temporarily, dementialike signs. Conditions that result in sensory deprivation, such as cataracts and hearing loss, may also contribute to a dementialike picture.

Multiple strokes, which cumulatively result in bilateral cerebral involvement, may lead to a multi-infarct dementia, occurring in the setting of vascular disease and chronic uncontrolled hypertension. Hypertensive patients with predominantly sub-cortical disease develop Binswanger dementia, characterized by cerebrovascular lesions in the deep white matter of the brain and resulting in loss of memory and cognition, with mood changes (Rowland, 2000). Metabolic causes such as vitamin B_{12} deficiency and hypothyroidism frequently present as dementia. Such infectious diseases as neu-rosyphilis, Creutzfeldt-Jacob, and HIV yield prominent symptoms of dementia. Struc-tural deformities or progressive, space-occupying lesions such as subdural hematomas and normal-pressure hydrocephalus may display dementia, incontinence, and gait apraxia.

The current discussion focuses only on early dementia or what has recently been called mild cognitive impairment (MCI, often preceding Alzheimer) and, even more recently, age-associated memory impairment (AAMI), a form of mild forgetfulness. (It is simply not meaningful to discuss central fatigue in the setting of more severe stages of various dementias.) However, the underlying processes leading to fatigue (final common pathway) inform our understanding of the fatigue experience in virtually any dementing disorder.

Alzheimer Disease

Taking the example of Alzheimer disease (AD), we explore the potential and probable factors contributing to various aspects of fatigue. The failure to endure sustained mental tasks is often an early sign of progressive disorders such as AD (Chaudhuri & Behan, 2000). Although the exact incidence of fatigue in AD is not known, the consequence of characteristic hippocampal atrophy is undoubtedly the increase of mental effort, leading to fatigue. When patients are told of the diagnosis (or not), they are at risk for depression (Rubin, Veiel, Kinscherf, Morris, & Storandt, 2001) and stress, which may further exacerbate hippocampal atrophy (Lee, Ogle, & Sapolsky, 2002). Disease-related depression, anxiety, and stress have all been shown to independently interfere with cognitive processing (Lee & Lyketsos, 2003; Cummings, 2003; Zubenko, Zubenko, McPherson, Spoor, Marin, Farlow, Smith, Geda, Cummings, Petersen, & Sunderland, 2003), and patients typically report greater fatigue and mental effort (see chapter 10). Intermittent disease-related agitation may further produce stress and take a similar toll. Fortunately, the acetylcholinesterase inhibitors have shown a positive effect on various neurobehavioral and neuropsychiatric phenomena (Cummings, 2003).

Through their negative effect on such cognitive functions as processing speed, medication commonly taken for age-related or comorbid disease often contributes further to central fatigue. Examples include anticholinergics for urinary dysfunction, some antihypertensives, older antidepressants (with mainly anticholinergic action), antipsychotics, anticonvulsants, and certain sedative-hypnotics. And not only are sedative-hypnotics potential culprits, but dementia-related sleep disorders themselves or the sleep deprivation and fragmentation they cause, have a particularly potent negative impact on optimal cognition. The disordered sleep may be primary to the dementia or secondary to medications or associated conditions (e.g., pain from diabetic neuropathy or depression). Exacerbating such cognitive dysfunction as processing speed further taxes the already challenged cognitive ability, resulting in the need to call on additional mental resources. This is not to suggest that all individuals with cognitive impairment display or experience mental fatigue, but merely to underscore the additive burden of coexisting phenomena commonly found in the clinical setting.

The dementing brain is thus less cognitively efficient, requiring greater mental effort to accomplish a given task, and this increased effort may require greater cerebral resources, leading to fatigue. Several studies using functional neuroimaging in different clinical populations such as TBI (Christodoulou, DeLuca, Ricker, Madigan, Bly, Lange, Kalnin, Liu, Steffener, Diamond, & Ni, 2001), MS (Hillary, Chiaravalloti, Ricker, Steffener, Bly, Lange, Liu, Kalnin, & DeLuca, 2003), and CFS (chapter 9) suggest a link between mental effort, cerebral resources, and fatigue. That is, more CNS resources are needed to *coordinate* multiple inputs and, when the execution is imperfect, the mistiming leads naturally to increased processing effort or inefficiencies and greater fatigue perception. It follows that the need to repeatedly reapply such cerebral activation as *attention* to the task induces or exacerbates central fatigue (Chollet & Weiller, 1994). Sperling and associates (2003) demonstrated a similar phenomenon using fMRI in AD. AD subjects required increased recruitment of hippocampal regions to perform as the controls did, and "compensatory" activation of nonhippocampal areas was also noted.

The clinical benefit of the acetylcholinesterase inhibitors derives from their direct effect on recent memory but, almost equally important, from their ability to enhance *cognitive or sensory gating* by dampening competing stimuli or background noise. Arciniegas and coworkers make a strong case for this effect in a TBI population (Arciniegas, Adler, Topkoff, Cawthra, Filley, & Reite, 1999). By reducing the intrusion of extraneous information, they hypothesize that cognitive processing is enhanced and fatigue lessened. Interference may also be at work in demyelinating dementia in which ephaptic transmission (commonly known as crosstalk) impairs the fidelity (and, therefore, efficiency) of cognitive processing/neurophysiological signaling. The resulting alteration in sensitivity or gain on filtering processes consumes mental energy, worsening the fatigue experience (Arciniegas et al., 1999; Alexander & Crutcher, 1990). Recent research (Burton, 2004) has raised an intriguing neuroimmunological connection between a reduced risk of AD and use of nonsteroidal antiinflammatory drugs (NSAIDs). It remains to be seen whether an exciting wave of new cognitive enhancing drugs will reduce central fatigue in the dementia population.

Basal Ganglia

Thus far we have noted how individuals fail to execute incremental or serial tasks that require sustained motivation and attention (Chaudhuri & Behan, 2000). Some researchers found subjects with central fatigue have less difficulty performing a task when stimulated externally or cued in advance, though they require a much higher perceived effort to execute the tasks. The failure of focused, sustained attention represents a disconnection between automatic, self-guided effort, performance of sequential motor or cognitive tasks, and sensory inputs. Chaudhuri and Behan (2000) propose that such failure results from impaired nonmotor function circuits of the basal ganglia (BG). These important projections and pathways have been painstakingly delineated over the past century, revealing influential and tight connections between the BG striatum and the archistriatum or amygdala, itself a critical nexus of limbic signaling and processing. The limbic system clearly provides a route for channeling spontaneous, unconscious, emotionally driven motivational forces into the motor system, influencing the likelihood of initiating and sustaining goal-directed action. For instance, the lack of facial expression in those with Parkinson's disease (PD) is a common example of the deficient limbic (emotional) input in spontaneous motor activity.

A lack of drive, initiation, motivation, and ability to make decisions and set goals is seen in patients with bilateral basal ganglia atrophy or damage. Termed abulia when severe, this condition may be misinterpreted or overlooked altogether in milder forms and is usually construed as mere apathy. Most researchers have converged on the understanding that a separate dopaminergic system projecting from the ventral tegmental area of the midbrain to the frontal lobe, especially the cingulate gyrus, drives internal states toward motivated behavior. This pathway has been termed the mesencephalofrontal activating system (MFAS). In any case, under circumstances of normal dopaminergic functioning, initiation and sequential performance of a task requires an internally driven mechanism integrated at the level of the BG to prepare the emotive, motor, and sensory apparatus responsible for the next and subsequent set of responses. Disruption of normal, BG-derived algorithms of the sequential task-processing mechanism would not only delay the initiation, but also prevent the smooth execution, of the intended task, a feature typical of central fatigue.

Parkinson's Disease (PD)

The motor features of Parkinson's disease (PD) including bradykinesia/akinesia, rigidity, resting tremor, and postural/gait abnormalities dominate the classical clinical picture. The underlying pathology is dopamine depletion of projections to the BG and a relative imbalance between acetylcholine and dopamine. The progressive neurodegeneration also affects reticular and autonomic pathways (Hoehn & Yahr, 1967).

Increasingly, more attention is being paid to the nonmotor features such as depression, dementia, and sleep disturbances, all of which have been positively correlated with PD and known to be associated with fatigue (Chen, 1986; Sandroni, Walker, & Starr, 1992; Buchwald, Pascualy, Bombardier, & Kith, 1994). Yet, as recently as 1999, standard texts on PD do not even list fatigue in their indexes (Koller, 1992; Nutt, Hammerstad, & Gancher, 1992). Because of this obvious overlap of symptomas, considerable effort has focused on determining whether fatigue is an independent, although not necessarily ubiquitous, feature of the disease. Aside from what we understand from BG function in general, central fatigue is a common complaint in people suffering specifically from PD. Fatigue remains clinically underdiagnosed in PD and its negative impact on patients' wellbeing underestimated (Karlsen, Larsen, Tandberg, & Jørgensen, 1999) largely because dopamine loss is overwhelmingly manifested in the motor realm, overshadowing less dramatic features of the disease.

One study of fatigue in PD matched 66 PD patients with two control groups, controlling for cognitive and depressive mood disorder. The study found significantly higher Fatigue Severity Scale (FSS) scores in PD patients, further noting that 50 percent of PD subjects compared with 25 percent of controls had total FSS scores of 4 (the threshold for fatigue) or higher (Herlofson & Larsen, 2002). The researchers concluded that fatigue is a common, independent symptom without relation to other motor or nonmotor symptoms of PD. Taking a broader look at nonmotor comorbidity and its clustering, Shulman, Taback, Bean, and Weiner (2001) used several scales and inventories that revealed a 40 percent incidence of fatigue (FSS > 4) among 99 nondemented PD patients.

Using two scales to study 233 PD patients, Karlsen and colleagues (1999) found a 44 percent incidence of fatigue compared with 18 percent among healthy controls. While they found an overlap with depression, they concluded that fatigue stands as an independent symptom in PD. In their study, they reference the work of Van Hilten and coworkers (1993), who found 43 percent of 90 nondepressed patients with PD reporting excessive fatigue; and others have further supported these findings (Lou, Kearns, Oken, Sexton, & Nutt, 2001). Employing the MFI, the latter researchers found that fatigue is common, an independent feature in PD, and strongly correlated with depression, but they cautioned, "Whether the fatigue measured by the MFI is associated with central dopamine deficiency remains to be determined." Abe, Takanashi, and Yanagihara (2000) found no correlation between the severity of depression and the fatigue scale measures in a study of 26 age-matched to controls, cognitively normal (by MMSE) PD patients. Furthermore, single-positron emission computed tomography (SPECT) scans demonstrated significantly correlated reduction of uptake in the frontal lobes of the fatigued subjects. The researchers concluded that the pattern of hypoperfusion in these self-reported fatigue patients suggested a greater role for frontal circuits than BG function in determining the central fatigue generator responsible for the symptoms.

When fatigue occurs in PD, it occurs early, is pervasive, and tends to persist (Friedman & Friedman, 2001). And although depression and cognitive impairment co-exist with fatigue in some, these factors do not account for all fatigue patients experience. Finally, Chaudhuri and Behan (2000) note that in such related syndromes as multisystem atrophy, progressive supranuclear palsy (PSP)/striatonigral degeneration, and olivopontocerebellar atrophy (OPCA)–autonomic insufficiency, parkinsonian features and central fatigue often coexist. Apathy, in its full spectrum, also dominates the clinical picture in these parkinsonian states (Zgaljardic, Borod, Foldi, & Mattis, 2003).

Beyond probing for the more well-studied and clinically apparent psychological dys-function (Menza, Robertson-Hoffman, & Bonapace, 1993; Schiffer, Kurlan, Rubin, & Boer, 1988; Henderson, Kurlan, Kerson, & Como, 1992) affecting optimal cognitive performance (See chapter 18), research must also consider other contributions. Recently, many reports have warned about unintended effects of medications commonly used to treat PD. Certain dopamine agonists are increasingly being recognized as independent contributors to sudden daytime sleepiness episodes (Hobson, Lang, Martin, Razmy, Rivest, & Fleming, 2002). Such phenomena are naturally easily confused with fatigue. Similarly, primary and secondary sleep disorders confound assessment of pure fatigue in PD. Patients and caregivers often complain of stiffness or pain with nighttime awakenings, psychotic agitation related to medications, and supine dysphagia from sialorrhea.

Post-Lyme Encephalopathy

Post-Lyme syndrome has been characterized by severe fatigue, malaise, and cognitive complaints that persist 6 months or more after antibiotic therapy is completed (Guadino, Colye, & Krupp, 1997). The most common neurological symptom in persons with late-stage Lyme disease is mild chronic encephalopathy, which is manifested behaviorally as memory loss, sleep disturbances, fatigue, and depression. Fatigue is observed in up to 74 percent of Lyme disease patients (Logigian, Kaplan, & Steere, 1990), the severity of which is comparable to that observed in persons with chronic fatigue syndrome (Gaudino et al., 1997). Interestingly, fatigue is reported by patients with both normal and abnormal CSF (antibodies to *Borrelia burgdorferi* and increased CSF protein), suggesting that the actual mechanism of fatigue in post-Lyme disease is likely multifactorial. Whether this sense of fatigue is a perceived cognitive dysfunction due to the chronicity of the disease or an actual sequela of residual neurological deficit has yet to be elucidated. Fatigue has been correlated with increased cognitive impairment, while depression shows an inverse relationship with impaired cognition among persons with Lyme disease (Krupp et al., 1991). Synergy of proinflammatory mediators stimulated by production of *B. burgdorferi* antibodies, and hippocampal atrophy due to stress of chronic disease might play some role in the cognitive fatigue of post-Lyme syndrome. Other secondary factors that could lead to fatigue in post-Lyme disease include sleep disturbances, mood disorders such as depression, and the stress of memory impairment in those with concurrent CSF abnormalities.

Up to 70 percent of cases with Lyme disease show MRI abnormalities, mostly punctate white matter lesions. Evidence from quantitative analysis of SPECT scans and regional cerebral blood flow (Fallon, Keilp, Prohovnik, Van Heertum, & Mann, 2003) shows that Lyme encephalopathy patients with measurable memory deficits have reduced perfusion primarily affecting subcortical frontotemporal white matter, BG, and the posterior temporal and parietal lobes, bilaterally (Kaplan & Jones-Woodward, 1997).

Treatment Issues

As with most medical conditions, particularly neurological conditions, a true cure is rarely achievable. Standard rehabilitation instruction in compensatory strategies and other approaches to energy management can be tailored to the specifics of the neurologic condition in question. It is also useful to distinguish the expected clinical course of a neurodegenerative versus a static process, because the therapeutic goals aimed at energy conservation will vary. (See chapter 18 for a general discussion on treatment of fatigue.)

Education about one's illness can help afflicted individuals and their caregivers prioritize their activity to meet the demands or goals of day-to-day functioning. Reasonable expectations may need to be reconciled with perceived abilities. Dietary counseling for both maximum energy production and weight loss is needed, and the importance of counseling on sleep hygiene should not be underestimated. A screening sleep history may prompt investigation with polysomnography, to reveal any associated sleep disorder responsible for generalized or mental fatigue.

Psychological and psychiatric care, when indicated, may help reduce the impact of psychological distress on cognitive function through treatment of anxiety and depressive states (see Natelson's discussion in chapter 18). Nonpharmacological techniques such as cognitive behavioral therapy (CBT) may similarly improve coping and adjustment to disability. Because of the overlap of other "internally distracting" psychiatric states with fatigue, pharmacological interventions for such psychiatric disorders may ameliorate the fatigue experience, at least in part. Exercise not only promotes physical wellbeing and cardiovascular health, but has a reciprocal effect on mood and immune system optimization, which in turn combat several independent aspects of fatigue.

Pharmacological approaches should first attempt to reduce or eliminate agents that contribute to fatigue either directly or indirectly. This is particularly true for patients who have not had the benefit of a medication regimen review since the advent of newer drugs that usually show fewer side effects (e.g., sedation). Such drug categories include antipsychotics (preferring the newer, atypical agents), anticonvulsants (some are highly cognitively disabling), and antidepressants (the older choices usually having anticholinergic effects).

Next, disease-specific comorbid conditions (e.g., sleep disorders, pain) must be optimally treated. As disease progression occurs, one must remain vigilant for sleep-disordered breathing, which may benefit from a nonpharmacologic solution such as a continuous positive airway pressure mask.

Finally, when modifiable components of fatigue have been addressed, one should proceed to trials of stimulants and, when possible, objectively monitor for meaningful clinical response (Hall, 2003). The therapeutic relationship may also be enhanced by trials of complementary and alternative therapies, as long as they are not patently harmful. It is unknown whether aggravating and ameliorating measures typical for healthy individuals reliably affect perceived or measurable fatigue for every disease entity discussed in this chapter.

It is also unclear at this stage of investigation whether treatment with a psychostimulant, for example, directly addresses the problem at the level of the fatigue generator, the perceptual level, or the behavioral or output level or simply eliminates some of the many contributing factors in the fatigue experience. Further confounding treatment decisions, more general features associated with neurological illness, such as pure arousal and basic self-awareness, override the subjective experience of fatigue at some point in the clinical course of a given disease entity.

Dosing is mostly symptomatic and aimed at improving function in the rehabilitation sense of the word. The authors have used methylphenidate, dextroamphetamine, their various long-acting forms, and modafinil (a novel wake-promoting agent) to treat fatigue across many neurological conditions. Unfortunately, because of the classic stimulants' mixed effect on catecholamines, it remains difficult to parse out their relative effect on dopamine (DA) versus norepinephrine (NE). Atomexitine (Strattera), the newest stimulant agent, is noradrenergic-selective. Modafinil has, putatively, no dopaminergic action but seems to stimulate subcortical structures such as the hypothalamus. The newer agents atomexitine and modafinil possess the clinical advantage of being less tightly controlled substances, allowing refills to be written on the prescription pad. The usual caveats, though not borne out by clinical experience, dictate the monitoring of blood pressure and heart rate at a minimum. Ultimately, it may prove fruitful for treatment to address as many components of fatigue as possible, individually or in combination, based on the expected coexisting deficiencies specific to each disease state.

Conclusion

Fatigue is certainly not a new phenomenon, and yet the recent, surprisingly intense interest in fatigue makes one wonder how this ubiquitous behavior could have been so assiduously ignored for so long. Today, fatigue can no longer be conceived of as a purely motor or psychological phenomenon. Nor is it appropriate to blithely accept a cohort's subjective report of fatigue without accounting for objectively measurable aspects of the fatigue experience. And yet, at least for the disease states discussed here, control of many if not most of the related factors mediating clinical fatigue or the fatigue experience, not to mention its underlying neuropathophysiological complexity, appears to be extremely challenging.

The fact that obvious sources of fatigue occur at many levels reinforces this notion. For instance, we have seen how fatigue-producing circumstances operate at the primary level (e.g., neurotransmitter). Deconditioning or sleep disorders are but two examples of secondary factors exacerbating fatigue. And tertiary factors such as the negative impact of drugs treating the underlying disease are frequently present. Even quaternary factors such as patient and caregiver expectations of performance levels mediate the fatigue experience, particularly the way that experience gets reported. Thus, the concept of fatigue as a separate entity or result of dysfunction in one particular brain pathway seems artificial. We are left with the question, "Does pure fatigue exist or must it always occur in the context of a larger syndrome or disease entity?" If the latter, then must not fatigue be defined as a consequence of such dysfunctions or underlying pathophysiologies? Clearly, any attempt to account for fatigue must include both subjective and objective measures.

More work is needed to characterize the incidence of fatigue in various CNS conditions. Once established, functional imaging will likely be of greatest utility in delineating the pathways responsible for fatigue by comparing the brains of those with and without fatigue within a disease category, assuming one can successfully control for all other major contributing factors. Regarding such pathways or regions already identified, one dominant theory focuses on the role of the nonmotor BG, coupled with frontal and limbic integrative circuitry. Whether fatigue behavior is predominantly psychological or neurological in origin (and even *this* distinction may be artificial, in the final analysis), a tantalizing, albeit alternative, explanation may be that such limitations simply represent an adaptive or conditioned response.

To advance our ability to address fatigue, clinicians must be better trained to screen for the presence and impact of fatigue and gain a broader appreciation of the common contributing factors and, where possible, the treatment of those influences. These efforts should lead to more rigorous studies to evaluate the best treatment approach, whether pharmacological or other. Finally, coordinated effort should be made to assess and publicize the consequences and burden to society of untreated fatigue. In such efforts, let us not swoon from neurasthenia, as was common 100 years ago.

References

Abe, K., Takanashi, M., & Yanagihara, T. (2000). Fatigue in patients with Parkinson's disease. *Behavioral Neurology, 12(3)*, 103–106.

Alexander, G. E., & Crutcher, M. D. (1990). Functional architecture of basal ganglia circuits: neural substrates of parallel processing. *Trends in Neurosciences, 13(7)*, 266–271.

Arciniegas, D., Adler, L., Topkoff, J., Cawthra, E., Filley, C. M., & Reite, M. (1999). Attention and memory dysfunction after traumatic brain injury: cholinergic mechanisms, sensory gating, and a hypothesis for further investigation. *Brain Injury, 13(1)*, 1–13.

Bartley, H., & Chute, E. (1947). *Fatigue and Impairment in Man*. New York: McGraw Hill.

Blomstrand, E. (2001). Amino acids and central fatigue. *Amino Acids, 20*, 25–34.

Blomstrand, E., Celsing, F., & Newsholme, E. A. (1988). Changes in plasma concentrations of aromatic and branch-chain amino acids during sustained exercise in man and their possible role in fatigue. *Acta Physiologica Scandanavia, 133*, 115–121.

Buchwald, D., Pascualy, R., Bombardier, C., & Kith, P. (1994). Sleep disorder in patients with chronic fatigue. *Clinical Infectious Disease, 18*, 68–72.

Burton, A. (2004). NSAIDS and Alzheimer's disease: it's only Rock and Rho. *Lancet Neurology, 3(1)*, 6.

Chaudhuri, A., & Behan, P. O. (2000). Fatigue and basal ganglia. *Journal of Neurological Sciences, 179*, 34–42.

Chen, M. K. (1986). The epidemiology of self-perceived fatigue among adults. *Preventive Medicine, 15*, 74–81.

Chollet, F., & Weiller, C. (1994). Imaging recovery of function following brain injury. *Current Opinion in Neurobiology, 4*, 226–230.

Christodoulou, C., DeLuca, J., Ricker, J. H., Madigan, N. K., Bly, B. M., Lange, G., Kalnin, A. J., Liu, W. C., Steffener, J., Diamond, B. J., & Ni, A. C. (2001). Functional magnetic resonance imaging of working memory impairment after traumatic brain injury. *Journal of Neurology Neurosurgery Psychiatry, 71(2)*, 161–168.

Covington, E. C. (1991). Depression and chronic fatigue in the patient with chronic pain. *Primary Care, 18*, 341–358.

Cummings, J. L. (2003). The impact of depressive symptoms on patients with Alzheimer disease. *Alzheimer Disease and Associated Disorders, 17(2)*, 61–62.

Cummings, J. L. (2003). Use of cholinesterase inhibitors in clinical practice: evidence-based recommendations. *American Journal of Geriatric Psychiatry, 11(2)*, 131–145.

de Groot, M. H., Phillips, S. J., & Eskes, G. A. (2003). Fatigue associated with stroke and other neurologic conditions: implications for stroke rehabilitation. *Archives of Physical Medicine and Rehabilitation, 84(11)*, 1714–1720.

Fallon, B. A., Keilp, J., Prohovnik, I, Van Heertum, R., & Mann, J. J. (2003). Regional cerebral blood flow and cognitive deficits in chronic Lyme disease. *Journal of Neuropsychiatry and Clinical Neuroscience, 15*, 326–332.

Foerstl, H. (1990). "Pseudodementia" and "pseudodepression": a short review on the coexistence of cognitive and affective impairment in the elderly. *Ceskoslovenská Neurologie a Neurochirurgie, 53(5)*, 294–304.

Friedman, J. H., & Friedman, H. (2001). Fatigue in Parkinson's disease: a nine-year follow-up. *Movement Disorders, 16(6)*, 1120–1122.

Guadino, E. A., Colye, P. K., & Krupp, L. B. (1997). Post-Lyme syndrome and chronic fatigue syndrome: neuropsychiatric similarities and differences. *Archives of Neurology, 54*, 1372–1376.

Hall, S. S. (2003). The quest for a smart pill. *Scientific America, 289(3)*, 54–57, 60–65.

Henderson, R., Kurlan, R., Kerson, J. M., & Como, P. (1992). Preliminary examination of the comorbidity of anxiety and depression in Parkinson's disease. *Journal of Neuropsychiatric Clinical Neuroscience, 4*, 257–264.

Herlofson, K., & Larsen, J. P. (2002). Measuring fatigue in patients with Parkinson's disease—the Fatigue Severity Scale. *European Journal of Neurology, 9(6)*, 595–600.

Hillary, F. G., Chiaravalloti, N. D., Ricker, J. H., Steffener, J., Bly, B. M, Lange, G., Liu, W. C., Kalnin, A. J., & DeLuca, J. (2003). An investigation of working memory rehearsal in multiple sclerosis using fMRI. *Journal of Clinical and Experimental Neuropsychology, 25(Oct)*, 965–978.

Hobson, D. E., Lang, A. E., Martin, W. R., Razmy, A., Rivest, J., & Fleming, J. (2002). Excessive daytime sleepiness and sudden-onset sleep in Parkinson disease: a survey by the Canadian Movement Disorders Group. *Journal of American Medical Association, 287(4)*, 455–463.

Hoehn, M., & Yahr, M. (1967). Parkinsonism: onset, progression and mortality. *Neurology, 17*, 427–442.

Joyce, E., Blumenthal, S., & Wessely, S. (1996). Memory, attention, and executive function in chronic fatigue syndrome. *Journal of Neurology, Neurosurgery, and Psychiatry, 60(5)*, 495–503.

Kaplan, R. F., & Jones-Woodward, L. (1997). Lyme encephalopathy: a neuropsychological perspective. *Seminars in Neurology, 17*, 31–37.

Karlsen, K., Larsen, J. P., Tandberg, E., & Jørgensen, K. (1999). Fatigue in patients with Parkinson's disease. *Movement Disorders, 14(2)*, 237–241.

Koller, W. C., ed. (1992). *Handbook of Parkinson's Disease*, 2nd ed. New York: Marcel Dekker.

Krupp, L. B. (2003). Fatigue in multiple sclerosis: definition, pathophysiology and treatment. *CNS Drugs, 17(4)*, 225–234.

Krupp, L. B., Masur, D., Schwartz, J., Coyle, P. K., Langenbach, L. J., Fernquist, S. K., Jandorf, L., & Halperin, J. J. (1991). Cognitive functioning in late Lyme borreliosis. *Archives of Neurology, 48,* 1125–1129.

Layzer, R. B. (1998). Asthenia and the chronic fatigue syndrome. *Muscle & Nerve, 21,* 1609–1611.

Lee, A. L., Ogle, W. O., & Sapolsky, R. M. (2002). Stress and depression: possible links to neuron death in the hippocampus. *Bipolar Disorders, 4(2),* 117–128.

Lee, H. B., & Lyketsos, C. G. (2003). Depression in Alzheimer's disease: heterogeneity and related issues, *Biological Psychiatry, 54(3),* 353–362.

Logigian, E. L., Kaplan, R. F., & Steere, A. C. (1990). Chronic neurologic manifestation of Lyme disease. *New England Journal of Medicine, 323,* 1438–1444.

Lou, J. S., Kearns, G., Oken, B., Sexton, G., & Nutt, J. (2001). Exacerbated physical fatigue and mental fatigue in Parkinson's disease. *Movement Disorders, 18(10),* 1108–1114.

Manu, P., Matthews, D. A., Lane, T. J., Tennen, H., Hesselbrock, V., Mendola, R., & Affleck, G. (1989). Depression among patients with a chief complaint of chronic fatigue. *Journal of Affective Disorders, 17,* 165–172.

Menza, M. A., Robertson-Hoffman, D. E., & Bonapace, A. S. (1993). Parkinson's disease and anxiety: comorbidity with depression. *Biological Psychiatry, 34,* 465–470.

Metzger, F. A., & Denney, D. R. (2002). Perception of cognitive performance in patients with chronic fatigue syndrome. *Annals of Behavior Medicine, 24(2),* 106–112.

Michiels, V., & Cluydts, R. (2001). Neuropsychological functioning in chronic fatigue syndrome: a review. *Acta Psychiatrica Scandinavica, 103(2),* 84–93.

Michiels, V., de Gucht, V., Cluydts, R., & Fischler, B. (1999). Attention and information processing efficiency in patients with chronic fatigue syndrome. *Journal of Clinical and Experimental Neuropsychology, 21(5),* 709–729.

Nutt, J. G., Hammerstad, J. P., & Gancher, S. T. (1992). *Parkinson's Disease. 100 Maxims in Neurology.* London: Edward Arnold.

Parmenter, B. A., Denney, D. R., & Lynch, S. G. (2003). The cognitive performance of patients with multiple sclerosis during periods of high and low fatigue. *Multiple Sclerosis, 9(2),* 111–118.

Rowland, L. P. (2000). *Merritt's Textbook of Neurology,* Philadelpitia: Lippincott Willians & Willians.

Rubin, E. H., Veiel, L. L., Kinscherf, D. A., Morris, J. C., & Storandt, M. (2001). Clinically significant depressive symptoms and very mild to mild dementia of the Alzheimer type. *International Journal of Geriatric Psychiatry, 16(7),* 694–701.

Sandroni, P., Walker, C., & Starr, A. (1992). Fatigue in patients with MS. *Archives of Neurology, 49,* 517–524.

Schiffer, R. S., Kurlan, R., Rubin, A., & Boer, S. (1988). Evidence for atypical depression in Parkinson's disease. *American Journal of Psychiatry, 145,* 1020–1022.

Shulman, L. M., Taback, R. L., Bean, J., & Weiner, W. J. (2001). Comorbidity of the nonmotor symptoms of Parkinson's disease. *Movement Disorders, 16(3),* 507–510.

Sperling, R. A., Bates, J. F., Chua, E. F., Cocchiarella, A. J., Rentz, D. M., Rosen, B. R., Schacter, D. L., & Albert, M. S. (2003). fMRI studies of associative encoding in young and elderly controls and mild Alzheimer's disease. *Journal of Neurology Neurosurgury and Psychiatry, 74(1),* 44–50.

Tiersky, L. A., Johnson, S. K., Lange, G., Natelson, B. H., & DeLuca, J. (1997). Neuropsychology of chronic fatigue syndrome: a critical review. *Journal of Clinical and Experimental Neuropsychology, 19(4),*560–586.

Van Hilten, J. J., Weggeman, M., van der Velde, E. A., Kerkhof, G. A., van Dijk, J. G., & Roos, R. A. C. (1993). Sleep, excessive daytime sleepiness and fatigue in Parkinson's disease. *Journal of Neural Transmission, 5,* 235–244.

Wessely, S., & Powell, R. (1989). Fatigue syndromes: a comparison of chronic post viral fatigue with neuromuscular and affective disorders, *Journal of Neurology, Neurosurgery and Psychiatry, 52,* 940–948.

Zgaljardic, D. J., Borod, J. C., Foldi, N. S., & Mattis, P. (2003). A review of the cognitive and behavioral sequelae of Parkinson's disease: relationship to frontostriatal circuitry. *Cognitive Behavioral Neurology, 16(4),* 193–210.

Zubenko, G. S., Zubenko, W. N., McPherson, S., Spoor, E., Marin, D. B., Farlow, M. R., Smith, G. E., Geda, Y. E., Cummings, J. L., Petersen, R. C., & Sunderland, T. (2003). A collaborative study of the emergence and clinical features of the major depressive syndrome of Alzheimer's disease. *American Journal of Psychiatry, 160(5),* 857–866.

III   Fatigue in Psychiatric Conditions

8 The Diagnosis and Treatment of Fatigue in Psychiatry: A Historical Overview

Edward Shorter

"Neurasthenia has been the Central Africa of medicine," wrote the American electrotherapist George Beard, father of the diagnosis of neurasthenia, in 1880. It was, he said, "an unexplored territory into which few men enter, and those few have been compelled to bring reports that have been neither credited nor comprehended" (Beard, 1880).

More than a hundred years later, it is true that neurasthenia is no longer credited nor comprehended in American psychiatry, though the term lives on elsewhere. Yet much of the history of fatigue as a symptom is bound up in the diagnostic term neurasthenia, conceived as a disease. It is also possible to conceive of it as a symptom and as a syndrome.

Today, fatigue has virtually disappeared from psychiatric diagnosis although it remains common in the population. In Britain in the 1980s, among Home Office employees in their twenties, 37 percent of the women and 29 percent of the men said they experienced "fatigue" (Jenkins, 1985); in 1998, 13.5 percent of a random sample of Americans declared that "everything is an effort" either all or some of the time (Pleis & Coles, 2002). The larger story is that, in psychiatry, the concept of fatigue has passed from a separate, eminently treatable disease to a nondisease that is untreatable except in the context of depression or somatization. How has this state of affairs come about?

Getting Fatigue on the Psychiatric Radar

In the long centuries of medical history before the 1870s, fatigue was really a nonsymptom. People complained to their relatives of being tired, but they did not trouble physicians with such problems. For medicine in those days, fatigue was no more a symptom than was, say, multiple chemical sensitivity (Shorter, 1992). Fatigue is not even mentioned in the standard medical dictionaries of France and Germany in the 1840s and 1850s (Voswinckel, 1986–88). Wilhelm Griesinger, the psychiatry professor in Zurich and later Berlin who was the virtual founder of biological psychiatry, barely touches on the subject of fatigue in his 1861 textbook, not mentioning it at all in his discussion of melancholy and conceding merely that "lack of energy" might exist in "depressed psychic states" (Griesinger, 1964).

Then, for reasons that are still somewhat obscure, the latter third of the nineteenth century saw a big increase in the number of fatigue cases coming to medical attention, as well as the amount of attention being paid to fatigue by physicians and psychiatrists. One historian speaks of the "discovery of fatigue" in the 1870s (Rabinbach, 1990). By 1926, British psychiatrist James Crichton-Browne felt able to write, "Fatigue, over-fatigue, is one of the great dangers of our day, and the ease with which it is induced is perhaps one of the signs of our degeneracy" (Crichton-Browne, 1926).

For the induction of this new wave of sensory complaints—such as fatigue (and downplaying the motor complaints once common in "hysteria")—there are various candidates. Historian of psychiatry Simon Wessely has quite reasonably indicted as a coconspirator the rise of a new psychiatric diagnosis itself: neurasthenia, an older term revived by Beard in 1869 and then vastly popularized in his 1880 book (Wessely, 1991). The new diagnosis expressly drew the attention of both patients and physicians to "nerves," and the consequences of nervous exhaustion, in the sense that a storage battery might be exhausted. There is always an interplay between what physicians consider legitimate disease and what patients deem legitimate symptoms (as opposed to "hysteria," an illegitimate symptom in our time), and patients endeavor to produce evidence of real disease to avoid being told, as they fear, it is all in their heads. Subjective perceptions of fatigue thus disseminated widely in the population once Beard's term had legitimated the symptom among physicians.

Neurasthenia was quickly incorporated into psychiatric nosology, but as a disease of its own, not as a symptom of various syndromes or diseases. Every country had a kind of spiritual ambassador who imported Beard's "neurasthenia" for the edification of the local medical community. In France, for example, it fell to psychiatrist Henri Huchard to incorporate a big section on neurasthenia in the 1883 update of Auguste Axenfeld's 1863 textbook on nervous illness. Huchard replaced Axenfeld's term "nervosity" (nervosisme), "that says nothing," with "neurasthenia," defined as "a certain state of nervous weakness." He called neurasthenia the "depressive" form of "irritable weakness of the nervous system" (Axenfeld & Huchard, 1883). Here we encounter the postulated pathophysiology favored by those who considered neurasthenia a disease in itself, not a symptom found across the spectrum of disorders. In nervous irritability, depleted cerebral centers made sufferers highly reactive to stimuli, as opposed to merely depressing all functions.

In Germany and Austria, the first important ambassador of Beard's concept was psychiatry professor Richard von Krafft-Ebing, then in Graz; in 1888 he devoted a long section of his textbook to "the asthenic neuropsychoses," which he viewed as becoming "ever more frequent," causing the "exhausted" central nervous system to produce "general fatigue, dizziness, mental dysphoria and slowed intellectual achievement." Chief among these neuropsychoses were "the neurasthenic psychoses" and "psychoneurosis on the base of a neurasthenic constitution" (Krafft-Ebing, 1888). Krafft-Ebing emphasized a constantly recurring theme among the neurasthenia scholars of his generation: chronic tiredness was a genetic condition, indeed, evidence of degeneration. In Germany, Emil Kraepelin—the Heidelberg alienist whose nosology was famously revived in DSM-III—accepted Beard's notions almost word for word; "chronic nervous exhaustion," otherwise known as neurasthenia, was caused by "overexertion of the brain" plus lessened resistance of the patient. It had to be differentiated from neurosyphilis and depressive psychosis (Kraepelin, 1896).

In the Anglo-Saxon world, the British lacked a real champion of the diagnosis, but neurasthenia was received with open arms by American colleagues. In 1890, M. Allen Starr, professor of diseases of the mind and nervous system at the College of Physicians and Surgeons in New York, wrote that neurasthenia was caused by "unstable vascular tone" and was treatable with lithium carbonate (Starr, 1890). In Beard's homeland, the outpouring of literature was enormous.

Even Sigmund Freud was inclined to view neurasthenia as a disease of its own, caused by masturbation (Freud, 1952) and distinct from anxiety neurosis, which was caused by premature ejaculation (Freud, 1952). To be sure, these were among Freud's earliest writings. He later lost interest in the subject of fatigue.

These were the big German guns. In 1903 Parisian psychologist and psychiatrist Pierre Janet gave tiredness a particularly French spin under the term "psychasthenia." In psychasthenia—or tired mind—all intellectual functions were down, making the mind vulnerable to such aberrations as obsessive-compulsive disorder (OCD). To be sure, neurasthenia was the core of psychasthenia, yet minor depression, somatized depression, any kind of psychic or motor agitation, tics, phobias, and OCD were all caught up in this grab-bag term that was differentiated only from "hysteria" (Janet, 1903). Psychasthenia never really caught on outside of France, however, and neurasthenia as a disease dominated the international stage for a hundred years.

Fatigue and Psychopathology

The disease-of-its-own period came to an end, or slowed dramatically, with the advent of psychopathological thinking in psychiatry. This term may be unfamiliar to an American audience, far removed as it is from current psychiatric thinking in the United States today, but quite simply, it means focusing on individual symptoms rather than on diseases as evidence of broader psychological and biological processes, such as hereditary disposition or stress. The term was popularized by Karl Jaspers's deservedly famous 1913 book of that title (Jaspers, 1913), but psychopathology was a current through much of German psychiatry in those years, not just a creation of

Jaspers. With psychopathology, psychiatry for the first time confronts fatigue as a pervasive condition across the range of diagnoses (or syndromes), not as a nosologically independent disease. Jaspers himself saw fatigue as one of the "basic concepts of neurophysiology" (though he did accept the existence of "irritable weakness"). Jaspers saw two sides to the fatigue coin: tiredness (*Ermüdung*), "the accumulation of disabling metabolic products," and exhaustion (*erschöpfung*), "the excessive consumption of vital substance." These processes could unleash a flood of mental symptoms, among them subjective fatigue (Jaspers, 1973). This actually is a bit disappointing in its conventionality, the reciting of hoary neuropseudophysiology by a writer whose contributions are so numerous. Yet it puts Jaspers's psychopathology, subsequently very useful in this subject, on the map for us.

Often forgotten in discussions of psychopathology is the "syndrome doctrine" of Freiburg psychiatrist Alfred Hoche, whose failure to write a major psychiatry textbook has left him largely in oblivion. Hoche directly challenged the "disease" concepts of Kraepelin, arguing that the symptoms of Kraepelin's so-called diseases were very mixed and inconstant. These diseases ignored the tendency of symptoms to recur across the spectrum of disorders and, under some circumstances, to cluster within syndromes (Hoche, 1912). (In the hierarchy of ailments, the pecking order is disease–syndrome–symptom.) Hoche wrote nothing on the subject of fatigue of which the current author is aware.

Yet Hoche's student Oswald Bumke, professor of psychiatry in Munich from 1924 to 1946, delivered one of the first highly differentiated assessments of fatigue in psychiatry based on Hoche's doctrine. Bumke argued that symptoms such as fatigue appear in a wide range of acquired reactions or constitutional predispositions (*Anlagen*). He alluded to "acquired fatigability" (*Ermüdbarkeit*), inborn through irritable weakness or acquired through various stressors. The symptoms of reactive and endogenous depression included general fatigue and exhaustibility, and fatigue figured among the prodromal symptoms of schizophrenia as well (Bumke, 1924). With Bumke, we are clearly out of the separate-disease school of thinking about fatigue. (Parenthetically, in 1928 German psychiatrist Georg Stertz, who toward the end of World War I had served on Bumke's staff in Breslau, described a kind of toxic-organic "exogenous neurasthenic reaction," commingling neurology and psychiatry [Stertz, 1928].)

Psychopathological thinking dominated central European psychiatry in the middle third of the twentieth century. Suspicious of large disease aggregations such as Kraepelin's, the big gurus of European psychiatry narrowed the concept of neurasthenia to a synonym for tiredness, explaining it in terms of heredity and current life problems. "Irritable weakness" vanished from the scene. Kurt Schneider, director of the Kaiser Wilhelm Psychiatric Research Institute in Munich, said in 1936 that acute neurasthenia was just general exhaustion and constitutional neurasthenia was the same thing as general "nervosity" (Schneider, 1936). Carrying the Heidelberg tradition of psychopathology with him into exile in England, Willi Mayer-Gross, in his famous 1954 textbook (coauthored by Eliot Slater and Martin Roth), wrote that current stresses precipitated a neurasthenic reaction, and moreover hereditary disposition might result in a kind of debilitated anxious constitution. The symptom of tiredness itself was common in many disorders such as depressive illness, anxiety states, and "organic determinations" (Mayer-Gross, Slater, & Roth, 1954).

Psychoanalysis is not thought to have produced a lively interest in psychopathology. Yet in the 1950s, some psychoanalysts of central European origin did take a psychopathological approach to fatigue. Writing in Silvano Arieti's *American Handbook of Psychiatry* in 1959, Gerard Chrzanowski, an emigré psychiatrist from Germany and then Switzerland, smiled rather indulgently at the concepts of both hypochondria and neurasthenia as "awkward, antiquated pieces of furniture, not much good for anything." The terms remained in use only because they "have gained a powerful foothold in psychiatric terminology." What the terms actually represented were "complicated life careers in people" frequently expressed as fatigue. The "warps in the personality" that Chrzanowski saw as the cause of neurotic tiredness did not result from genetics but from development. But fatigue, as such, was manifest across a wide variety of psychiatric conditions (Chrzanowski, 1959). Except for the lack of speculation about "predisposition," this was roughly what most central European psychiatrists believed about chronic tiredness in the middle third of the twentieth century.

Looking back at the preceding discussion, one realizes the extent to which psychiatric theorizing was dominated by the Germans. This German predominance ended with the events of the Second World War and the Holocaust.

Fatigue Vanishes from Psychiatry with DSM-III

In the hands of the American nosologists, who completely dominated the international scene after the publication of DSM-III in 1980 (American Psychiatric Association, 1980), fatigue vanished as a disease. No official diagnoses mentioning tiredness appeared in the manual. How did this happen?

DSM-I, which was published in 1952, called fatigue a "psychophysiologic nervous system reaction," in which general fatigue was said to be the chief complaint. "The term includes many cases formerly called 'neurasthenia'" (American Psychiatric Association, 1952). This definition was a link to past traditions.

Published in 1968 and even more psychoanalytically oriented, DSM-II frankly used the phrase "neurasthenic neurosis (neurasthenia)" as an official diagnosis: "This condition is characterized by complaints of chronic weakness, easy fatigability, and sometimes exhaustion." Only the "moderateness" of the accompanying depression and the chronicity of the tiredness differentiated neurasthenia from depressive neurosis. (In line with psychoanalysts' fondness for personality disorders, DSM-II also added a seldom-used diagnosis of "asthenic personality," which was characterized by easy fatigability. [American Psychiatric Association, 1968.])

In 1980, American psychiatry turned the page completely on fatigue, returning in the DSM-III to a neo-Kraepelinian style of setting up diseases (now called disorders) rather than focusing on the psychopathology of target symptoms (Shorter, 1997). Symptoms and syndromes were bumped up to diseases, but fatigue remained part of the symptom picture of the larger panoply of affective disorders, as the former asthenic personality was collapsed into "dependent personality disorder." (DSM-III, index 484). Simultaneously, interest in constitutions, body build, and temperament was eclipsed with the triumph of the disease route (Healy, 1998). A classic hypothesis of psychopathology simply ceased to be investigated. This was truly a historical irony: the American nosologists had returned psychiatry to the dominance of the nineteenth-century German heavyweights, yet abandoned the concept of neurasthenia, a comforting weasel word of a century's standing. Fatigue, though still very real in the consultation, vanished from nosology.

But in a second more powerful irony, fatigue, in the moment it disappeared as an official diagnosis in psychiatry, started to become epidemic in the patients' world. In the 1980s, patients began attributing feelings of chronic weariness and chronic pain to Epstein-Barr virus (EBV) infection. This supposed epidemic differed from the many similar "epidemic hysterias" across the ages by the fixity and tenacity of patients' belief in a particular pathogen. Although EBV was soon discredited scientifically as the cause of their symptoms, it was replaced by the diagnosis "chronic fatigue syndrome" (CFS), the purported consequence of a breakdown in the immune system or viral infestation (Shorter, 1992). And though these somatizing patients often shunned psychiatric referrals, they nonetheless often landed in the psychiatrist's office (Wessely, Hotopf, & Sharpe, 1998). American psychiatrists, more besieged by chronic fatigue than ever before, had rendered themselves incapable of diagnosing it independently of such larger, and quite questionable, constructs as somatization and major depression. Neurasthenia, however, remains an active diagnosis internationally, and in the World Health Organization's ICD-10 it is even subdivided into mental and physical types (World Health Organization, 1992).

Addendum: The Treatment of Fatigue Syndromes

The prognosis for fatigue syndromes has changed over the years from fair to poor. The physical therapies of the nineteenth century had quite favorable results in neurasthenia because the patients believed their nervous centers were "exhausted" and physical treatments such as hydrotherapy and the rest cure could revive them. These cures had, of course, a suggestive effect. Patients tend to resist the psychological interventions of today, because they are heavily fixated on the supposed infectious nature of their condition.

Placebo treatments have a long history of success in treating chronic fatigue. The French pharmacopoeia once abounded with patent remedies such as Crino-Sthenyl and Musculosine Byla for neurasthenia (Blondeau, 1994). Family physician and author A. J. Cronin remembered treating tired society ladies in the 1920s in London. He came up with the diagnosis of "asthenia," contradicting their own physicians who kept telling them it was "nerves." "Having created a disease, it was essential to produce the remedy." Cronin would give them an intramuscular injection of various tonifying agents, such as strychnine. "Injections for asthenia were now as much the mode and as eagerly sought after as Manuel's new spring gowns. Again and yet again my sharp and shining needle sank into fashionable buttocks, bared upon the finest linen sheets." Cronin had devised a "cure" for chronic fatigue, one successful only as long as he "charged for it an appropriately exorbitant fee" (Cronin, 1952). Such remedies as electromyographic (EMG) feedback for chronic fatigue syndrome come immediately to mind.

Spa therapy is especially important in treating "general weakness and complicated reconvalescence," said German physiatrist Georg Thilenius in 1884. Rather than bracing climes, milder temperatures reinforce the energies of the nervous system, and spa waters rich in carbon dioxide were to be recommended (Thilenius, 1884). To be sure, 5 years later Hermann Weber and his son, F. Parkes Weber, both internists on London's Harley Street specializing in spa referrals, announced that in the treatment of neurasthenia, "Spa treatment in itself is entirely useless." Yet "Weir-Mitchell has shown us that removal from home surroundings is almost indispensable" (Weber & Weber, 1898). Indeed, it was the famous rest cure of Philadelphia neurologist Silas Weir Mitchell—consisting of bedrest, a milk diet, massage, and electrotherapy (Mitchell, 1881)—that facilitated the recovery of many neurasthenia victims, especially female, and gave the spas a golden reputation in the relief of fatigue. The point is, these placebo treatments of yore seem to have been highly effective; they really did make patients better, through the mechanism of suggestion (Shorter, 1990).

The whole world of spa therapy and placebo treatments was blown away, however, by the loss of faith in mineral springs and tonics, patients' own fixed illness beliefs, and the bioethics movement. Thus, in the 1980s and after, medicine found itself confronting the avalanche of chronic fatigue cases with relatively little to offer. Of course, even today French medicine still features a line of "antiasthenics," such as aceglutamide and pyridoxine camsilate (*Effets recherchés des substances: antiasthénique*, www.biam2.org/www). Outside of France, though, these compounds meet with disbelief.

Today, the most effective remedy psychiatry has to offer for chronic fatigue seems to be cognitive behavior therapy (CBT) (Wessely et al., 1998). Yet this technique requires the patient at some level to accept that his symptoms have a psychogenic component. It is, after all, a psychotherapy, and many patients felt more comfortable with the presumption of organicity offered by the spa environment.

Fatigue has thus passed from being a "real" disease, as treatable as constipation, to a nondisease that is treatable only with elaborate programs of psychotherapy that many fear. One is inclined to ask, Is this progress?

Acknowledgments

The author would like to thank Thomas Ban, MD, for comments on an earlier version of this paper.

References

American Psychiatric Association (1952). *Diagnostic and statistical manual of mental disorders.* Washington, DC: American Psychiatric Association, p. 31.

American Psychiatric Association (1968). *Diagnostic and statistical manual of mental disorders*, 2nd ed. (DSM-II). Washington: American Psychiatric Association, pp. 40–41, 43.

American Psychiatric Association. (1980). *Diagnostic and statistical manual of mental disorders*, 3d ed. (DSM-III). Washington, DC: American Psychiatric Association.

Axenfeld, A., & Huchard, H. (1883). *Traité des névroses*, 2nd ed. Paris: Baillière, p. viii.

Beard, G. (1880). *A practical treatise on nervous exhaustion (neurasthenia).* New York: William Wood, p. vi.

Blondeau, A. (1994). *Histoire des laboratoires pharmaceutiques en France, vol. 2.* Paris: Cherche-midi éditeur, pp. 18–20.

Bumke, O. (1924). *Lehrbuch der Geisteskrankheiten*, 2nd ed. Munich: Bergmann, pp. 241, 548, 912.

Chrzanowski, G. (1959). Neurasthenia and hypochondriasis. In Arieti, S., ed. *American handbook of psychiatry.* New York: Basic Books, vol. 1, pp. 258–71.

Crichton-Browne, J. (1926). *Victorian jottings from an old commonplace book.* London: Etchells, p. 244.

Cronin, A. J. (1952). *Adventures in two worlds.* Toronto: Ryerson, pp. 196–97.

Effets recherchés des substances: antiasthénique. http://www.biam2.org/www (last accessed July 2002).

Freud, S. (1895). Über die Berechtigung von der Neurasthenie einen bestimmten Symptomkomplex als "Angstneurose" abzutrennen. In Freud, S. (1952). *Gesammelte Werke*, vol. 1, pp. 315–42. London: Imago.

Freud, S. (1898). Die Sexualität in der Ätiologie der Neurosen. In Freud, S. (1952). *Gesammelte Werke*, vol. 1, pp. 491–516. London: Imago.

Griesinger, W. (1861; reprint 1964). *Die Pathologie und Therapie der psychischen Krankheiten*, 2nd ed. Reprint Amsterdam: Bonset, pp. 214, 233–37.

Healy, D. (1998). *The psychopharmacologists*, vol. 2. London: Chapman & Hall. p. 421.

Hoche, A. (1912). "Die Bedeutung der Symptomenkomplexe in der Psychiatrie." *Zeitschrift für die gesamte Neurologie und Psychiatrie* 12, 540–51.

Janet, P. (1903). *Les obsessions et la psychasthénie, 2 vols*. Paris: Alcan, vol. 1, p. xxii.

Jaspers, K. (1913). *Allgemeine Psychopathologie*. Berlin: Springer.

Jaspers, K. (1959; 1973). *Allgemeine Psychopathologie*, 9th ed. Berlin: Springer, pp. 132, 369, 387–88.

Jenkins, R. (1985). *Sex Differences in Minor Psychiatric Morbidity*. Cambridge: Cambridge University Press, p. 30, table 3.7.

Kraepelin, E. (1896). *Psychiatrie*, 5th ed. Leipzig: Barth, pp. 321, 341–43, 346, 348.

Krafft-Ebing, R. (1888). *Lehrbuch der Psychiatrie*, 3rd ed. Stuttgart: Enke, pp. 508–18.

Mayer-Gross, W., Slater, E., & Roth, M. (1954). *Clinical psychiatry*. London: Cassell, pp. 114–16.

Mitchell, S.W. (1881). *Lectures on diseases of the nervous system especially in women*. London: Churchill.

Pleis, J.R., & Coles, R. (Dec. 2002). Summary health statistics for U.S. adults: National Health Interview Survey, 1998. National Center for Health Statistics. *Vital Health Statistics 10 (209)*. 39, table 14.

Rabinbach, A. (1990). *The human motor: energy, fatigue, and the origins of modernity*. New York: Basic Books, p. 38.

Schneider, K. (1936). *Psychiatrische Vorlesungen für Ärzte* 2nd ed. Leipzig: Thieme, pp. 43–45.

Shorter, E. (1992). *From paralysis to fatigue: a history of psychosomatic illness in the modern era*. New York: Free Press, pp. 307–14.

Shorter, E. (1997). *A history of psychiatry from the era of the asylum to the age of Prozac*. New York: Wiley, pp. 301–03.

Shorter, E. (1990). Private clinics in Central Europe, 1850–1933. *Social history of medicine 3*, 159–95.

Starr, M. A. (1890). *Familiar forms of nervous disease*. New York: William Wood. The 1891 edition was consulted.

Stertz, G. (1928). Die neurasthenische Reaktion. In Bumke, O., ed. *Handbuch der Geisteskrankheiten*, vol. 5 (I). Pp. 19–27. Berlin: Springer.

Thilenius, G. (1884). *Bäder-Almanach*, 2nd ed. Frankfurt: Mosse, pp. xv.

Voswinckel, P. (1986–88). Das "Tagebuch" eines Distrikt-Krankenhauses (1866/67) als Quelle der Sozialgeschichte mit einem Exkurs über den Ermüdungs-Begriff. *Historia hospitalium 17*: 121–34.

Weber, H., & Weber, F. P. (1898). *The mineral waters and health resorts of Europe*. London: Smith, Elder, p. 439.

Wessely, S. (1991). History of postviral fatigue syndrome. *British Medical Bulletin, 47*, 919–41.

Wessely, S., Hotopf, M., & Sharpe, M. (1998). *Chronic fatigue and its syndromes*. Oxford: Oxford University Press.

World Health Organization. (1992). *The ICD-10 classification of mental and behavioural disorders: clinical descriptions and diagnostic guidelines*. Geneva: WHO, pp. 170–71, F48.

9 Chronic Fatigue Syndrome and the Brain

Susan K. Johnson and John DeLuca

Chronic fatigue syndrome (CFS) has received much attention since the 1980s in the media as well as the medical and psychological communities. Complaints of chronic fatigue are frequently observed in medical practice, accounting for 10 to 15 million office visits every year in the United States (Komaroff, 1994). Yet, only a small fraction of these cases fulfill the diagnostic criteria for CFS. This chapter examines how the fatigue experienced by persons with CFS may be related to brain dysfunction.

Conceptualizing and Defining CFS

Though fatigue syndromes have been recognized for more than 200 years (Straus, 1991), some have related the current interest in CFS to the construct of neurasthenia described over 100 years ago (Wessely et al., 1998). Although neurasthenia was originally viewed as a disease of the nervous system resulting from nervous exhaustion due to overwork, over time neurasthenia came to be seen as a psychiatric illness associated with anxiety and depression. Other manifestations of fatigue over the years (often war-related) included Da Costa syndrome, effort syndrome, neurocirculatory asthenia, and Gulf War syndrome. By the early to mid-1900s, the interest in fatigue syndromes faded, only to be revived again by the mid-1980s (see other chapters for more on the history of fatigue and CFS).

CFS is a heterogeneous illness characterized primarily by severe debilitating fatigue as well as rheumatological, infectious, and neuropsychiatric symptoms (Fukuda et al., 1994). It has been referred to by several names including Epstein-Barr virus infection, chronic mononucleosis, myalgic encephalomyelitis, postviral fatigue syndrome, postinfectious neuromyasthenia, chronic fatigue immune deficiency syndrome (CFIDS), and "yuppie flu" (Greenberg, 1990; Holmes et al., 1988; Sharpe et al., 1991). CFS afflicts males and females of all ages, although the typical patient is a women in middle age (Komaroff, 1994). It is found among individuals from a variety of socioeconomic and ethnic backgrounds (Jason et al., 2000).

Table 9.1
CDC case definitions for chronic fatigue syndrome

	1988 Case Definition (Holmes et al. 1988)	1994 Case Definition (Fukuda et al., 1994)
Major symptom criteria	New onset of fatigue that results in at least a 50% reduction of daily activities for 6 months	Unexplained persistent or relapsing fatigue of new or definite onset that results in a substantial reduction of previous levels of functioning
	Exclusion of other medical conditions that produce similar symptoms	
Minor symptom criteria	Fever	—
	Muscle weakness	—
	Sore throat	Sore throat
	Tender lymph nodes	Tender lymph nodes
	Headaches of new type	Headaches of new type
	Myalgia	Myalgia
	Arthralgia	Arthralgia
	Postexertional fatigue	Postexertional fatigue
	Sleep disturbance	Sleep disturbance
	Neuropsychologic complaints	Neuropsychologic complaints
Physical signs	Low-grade fever	—
	Nonexudative pharyngitis	—
	Palpable lymph nodes	—

Note: The 1988 definition requires satisfying the major criteria plus eight signs and symptoms to diagnose CFS. The 1994 definition requires major criteria plus four symptoms.

To aid in identification, a case definition for CFS developed by a number of experts in the field was published in 1988 (Holmes et al., 1988). This case definition was subsequently revised in 1991 (Schluederberg et al., 1992) and again in 1994 (Fukuda et al., 1994) (table 9.1). The diagnosis of CFS is one of exclusion based on the working case definition. Prevalence estimates for CFS vary depending on the case definition used as well as the characteristics of the study sample. For instance, the point prevalence varies from 0.08 percent to 0.3 percent when the 1988 case definition is used among health maintenance organization (HMO) patients (Buchwald et al., 1995). Using the less restrictive 1994 case definition, a UK study found the prevalence to be as high as 2.6 percent among primary care attendees (Wessely, Chalder, Hirsch, Wallace, & Wright, 1997), while others using the 1994 criteria still only reported prevalence rates of 0.4 percent among community-based samples (Jason et al., 1999).

Currently, there are three operational case definitions for CFS. The first, and most widely used, is the American definition (including the subsequent modifications) presented here. A second definition comes from an Australian group (Lloyd, Wakefield, Boughton, & Dwyer, 1988), and a third from Great Britain (Sharpe et al., 1991). The American criteria attach considerable significance to certain somatic symptoms (although less so, in the modification of Fukuda et al., 1994). Somatic symptoms, however, are not emphasized by the British definition (which uses the term myalgic encephalomyelitis, or ME, interchangeably with CFS) that focus primarily on both physical and mental fatigue. Further, although both the British and Australian criteria require new onset of neuropsychological symptoms (i.e., impaired concentration or memory), the American definitions do not. The Fukuda (1994) definition is the most widely used in clinical practice and research.

Although not well understood, the prognosis for CFS is generally poor. For instance, recovery was observed in only 3 percent of cases while 17 percent reported some level of improvement in one longitudinal study that followed persons with CFS for 18 months (Vercoulen et al., 1996a). In a review of the literature, Joyce, Blumenthal, and Wessely (1996) found that fewer than 10 percent of subjects in the five studies defining CFS operationally returned to premorbid levels of functioning. Schmaling and associates (2003) followed 100 patients with CFS or unexplained chronic fatigue and found 21 percent with improvements in symptoms and functioning over 18 months. Those patients who displayed worsening symptoms over time were older, less educated, unemployed, used more sedating and antidepressant medications, and made more somatic attributions for illness than those who improved. Neuropsychological impairment has been found to be related to functional disability (Christodoulou et al., 1998). Overall, despite some level of improvement, the vast majority of persons with CFS remain disabled over time, and that disability is related to illness beliefs, duration of illness, and initial fatigue level (see Tiersky et al., 2001).

Etiology

Two divergent positions regarding the etiology of CFS have emerged. One posits that CFS is a manifestation of a psychiatric disorder and the other maintains that CFS is "organic" in nature or a form of physical or medical illness (Jones et al., 1988; Manu, Affleck, Tennen, Morse, & Escobar, 1996). This dualistic view has led to confusion as to how best diagnostically classify and thus treat the disorder. For instance, the International Classification of Diseases-10 (ICD-10) diagnostic system places CFS-like syndromes with nearly identical descriptions in both psychiatric and neurologic categories (David & Wessely, 1993). These divergent classifications may lead to different treatment strategies, which can range from the use of various medications to the use of behavioral and exercise therapies; (Wessely, Hotopf, & Sharpe, 1998; also see chapter 18; for more on the dualistic views of CFS, see Wessely et al., 1998; DeLuca & Tiersky, 2003).

Nonetheless, neither the "medical" nor the "psychiatric" hypotheses by themselves are sufficient to explain the etiology of all CFS patients. Some have suggested integrating these two hypotheses, as in the biopsychosocial model of CFS (for reviews, see Sharpe, 1996; Johnson, DeLuca, & Natelson, 1999). CFS is a multidimensional illness experience that cannot be conceptualized as a single diagnostic entity (Wesseley, 1996; Afari & Buchwald, 2003). Although CFS remains a controversial entity with an unknown cause and some have expressed doubts regarding any biologic basis, pathophysiological disturbances appear to occur at least in subsets of persons with CFS. These disturbances exist particularly in neurophysiology, and how these findings relate to fatigue is a major focus of this chapter.

CFS and Neuropsychological Performance

A number of studies document objective, albeit modest, neuropsychological impairments in CFS (Tiersky et al., 1997). The most consistently documented impairments are in the areas of complex information processing speed and efficiency, working memory, and initial learning (Michiels & Cluydts, 2001; DeLuca, Christodoulou, Diamond, Rosenstein, Kramer, & Natelson, 2004). General intellectual abilities and higher-order cognitive skills are generally intact. These neuropsychological impairments are particularly observed in persons suffering from CFS who do not have a comorbid illness or history of psychiatric condition (DeLuca et al., 1997). There is preliminary evidence that objective cognitive impairments are related to functional decline (Christodoulou et al., 1998), employment status (Tiersky, et al., 2001), and severity of brain abnormalities on magnetic resonance imaging (MRI) (Lange et al., 1999, see also in following text). Additionally, cognitive complaints are among the most frequent and debilitating symptoms of CFS (Christodoulou et al., 1998; Abbey & Garfinkle, 1991; Komaroff, 1994), with complaints of impaired cognitive function reported in up to 85 to 95 percent of patients (Grafman, 1993; Komaroff & Buchwald, 1991). Emotional factors influence subjective reports of cognitive difficulty (Wearden & Appleby, 1996), whereas little evidence supports a relationship between complaints and objective neuropsychological findings (Tiersky et al., 1997; Metzger & Denney, 2002; Short, McCabe, & Tooley, 2002). Subjective ratings of fatigue severity have not been associated with neuropsychological impairment. However, subjective fatigue has been shown to be related to increased frequency of subjective cognitive impairment complaints (e.g., Cope, Pernet, Kendall, & Davis, 1995; Michiels, Cluydts, & Fischler, 1998; Vercoulen et al., 1998).

The effects of fatigue on neuropsychological performance were examined using repeated testing with a challenging cognitive task (the Paced Auditory Serial Addition

Test, or PASAT) over the course of a demanding testing session (Johnson, Lange, DeLuca, Korn, & Natelson, 1997). If fatigue affects cognitive performance, one would expect to observe "blunting" of the PASAT practice effect with repeated administration. Subjects consisted of 15 CFS, 15 multiple sclerosis (MS), 14 depressed (DEP) subjects, and 15 healthy, sedentary controls. Overall, PASAT performance was significantly reduced for CFS and DEP subjects compared to controls, though mean performance did not differ across the three fatiguing illness groups. The degree of improvement among these groups across trials (i.e., practice effect) did not differ from the controls. Neither subjective fatigue nor depression was significantly related to PASAT performance. These studies indicate that CFS patients report greater cognitive and metacognitive impairment than is detected on objective assessment. Neither this discrepancy nor objective impairments can be explained simply by depression or fatigue levels.

Neuroimaging Studies

Several recent studies have used brain imaging technology to examine whether persons with CFS have structural and functional abnormalities. The results of structural imaging studies are presented first, followed by studies using functional imaging techniques.

Structural Neuroimaging Techniques

Buchwald and coworkers (1992) examined MRI scans of the brain in 144 persons with chronic fatigue (CF; not all subjects met the CFS criteria); significantly more cerebral abnormalities were found on MRI in CF subjects (78%) than healthy controls (21%). Natelson and colleagues (1993) replicated the finding of significantly more cerebral abnormalities on MRI in 52 CFS participants than in 52 controls. However, the number of participants with abnormalities was much lower than that observed in the Buchwald study (27 percent of the CFS group compared to 2 percent of controls showed abnormalities). In both of these studies, the vast majority of cerebral abnormalities observed were punctate areas of high signal intensity primarily in the cerebral white matter. There was little discussion of the clinical significance of the MRI findings in either study. Schwartz and colleagues (1994a) examined 16 CFS subjects and 15 age-matched controls, reporting that 50 percent of the CFS subjects had cerebral abnormalities on MRI compared to 20 percent in controls (not a statistically significant difference perhaps because the study was underpowered). As in previously reported studies, the abnormalities included small areas of signal hyperintensities in the subcortical and periventricular white matter. The authors argued that the type and location of white matter abnormalities in CFS were unlike those observed in persons with MS. In contrast to these studies, Cope and coworkers (1995) found no elevated number of brain abnormalities using MRI among 45 persons with CF versus controls. They reported abnormalities in 8 percent of the CF group, 22 percent of CF with depression, 33 percent of a clinically depressed sample, and 20 percent among controls.

One factor that may significantly influence the detection of brain lesions with MRI is the heterogeneity of the CFS sample. Lange and colleagues (1999) reported cerebral abnormalities in 46.2 percent of 39 CFS participants and 31.6 percent of 19 controls. However, these authors subdivided the CFS sample into CFS participants without concurrent or past history of psychiatric illness (CFS-No Psych, $n = 21$) and those with a concurrent (but no past history of) psychiatric illness (CFS-Psych, $n = 18$). MRI abnormalities were significantly elevated in the CFS-No Psych group (66.7%) compared to the CFS-Psych (22.2%) and healthy controls (31.6%). The most common abnormalities were hyperintensities in subcortical white matter, present in 48 percent of the CFS-No Psych group compared to 17 percent in the CFS-Psych group and 11 percent in the controls ($p = 0.04$). A similar finding was observed by Greco and coworkers (1997), who examined MRI scans of the brain in 43 persons with CFS and 43 controls. They reported a nonsignificant difference in MRI abnormalities in 32 percent of CFS and 28 percent of controls. However, structural abnormalities were observed in CFS subjects without a psychiatric disorder compared to controls ($p < 0.06$).

Cook, Lange, DeLuca, and Natelson (2001) examined the relationship between MRI-identified cerebral abnormalities and self-reported physical functioning (using the Medical Outcomes Study SF-36) in 48 participants with CFS. These authors found that CFS participants with MRI abnormalities reported significantly more impairments in physical functional activity than CFS participants without MRI abnormalities. In a preliminary study, Lange and colleagues (2001) used MRI to assess cerebral ventricular volumes in 28 CFS and 15 healthy controls. CFS subjects had larger lateral ventricle volumes than controls ($p < 0.06$).

Overall, the MRI studies of the brain in persons with CFS have been inconsistent in demonstrating significant abnormalities. When they do occur, abnormalities are observed in the subcortical white matter. Some evidence suggests a greater number of cerebral abnormalities in persons with CFS who do not have concurrent psychopathology than CFS subjects with concurrent psychopathology. This finding is consistent with the neuropsychological data (presented earlier) showing greater neuropsychological impairment in CFS subjects without concurrent psychopathology. Very preliminary evidence indicates the presence of MRI abnormalities may be associated with increased functional disability, although this work requires replication and extension.

Functional Neuroimaging Techniques

Regarding functional neuroimaging, several studies have used single-photon emission computed tomography (SPECT) technology (e.g., Ichise et al., 1992; Schwartz et al., 1994a,b). Schwartz and coworkers (1994a) reported cerebral abnormalities using

SPECT in 13 of 16 (81%) CFS participants compared to 21 percent of healthy controls. The most common sites of involvement in CFS were the lateral frontal cortex, lateral temporal cortex, and basal ganglia. Schwartz's group (1994b) also used SPECT to compare cerebral perfusion in CFS participants with those in subjects with major depression and HIV infection and in healthy controls. The CFS and major depression groups did not differ in the average number of perfusion defects, but both groups had significantly fewer defects than the HIV group. All three clinical groups had significantly increased perfusion in lateral frontal, lateral temporal, and medial temporal lobes than controls. However, the index of "midcerebral uptake" was reduced in the CFS group and HIV group relative to the depressed and healthy groups.

Costa, Tannock, and Brostoff (1995) stratified CFS participants into those with and those without psychopathology, using SPECT to examine brainstem perfusion. The CFS without psychopathology ($n = 16$) showed significant brainstem hypoperfusion compared to participants with major depression ($n = 20$) and healthy controls ($n = 40$). In addition to the brainstem results, CFS subjects showed generalized hypoperfusion throughout the cerebral hemispheres, most prominently in the frontal lobes, but also in other areas such as the basal ganglia and thalamus, consistent with findings of other work (Ichise et al., 1992). Costa and colleagues (1995) suggest that "CFS and major depression may be two distinct clinical entities with different perfusion of the brainstem."

Machale and associates (2000) examined 30 participants with CFS who were not depressed, 12 subjects with current major depression and melancholia, and 15 healthy control subjects. Results showed increased perfusion in the right thalamus, pallidum, and putamen in both the CFS and the depressed groups compared to controls. Little difference between the CFS and depressed groups was observed other than increased perfusion in the left thalamus and left prefrontal cortex of the CFS group relative to the depressed participants. In a cotwin control study of cerebral perfusion on SPECT scanning of monozygotic twins discordant for CFS, no significant difference in cerebral blood flow (CBF) was observed (Lewis et al., 2001). These data were interpreted as not supporting a "major role of resting rCBF abnormalities in CFS."

Tirelli and associates (1998) used 18-fluorodeoxyglucose positron emission tomography (FDG-PET) to study cerebral metabolism in 18 CFS subjects without psychopathology, 6 persons with depression but no CFS, and 6 healthy controls. Both the CFS and depression groups showed significant hypometabolism in the frontal lobes compared to controls. However, CFS subjects showed significant brainstem hypometabolism relative to the depression group, a finding consistent with what has been reported in SPECT studies (Costa et al., 1995) but not replicated in more recent PET studies (Siessmeier, Nix, Hardt, Schreckenberger, Egle, & Bartenstein, 2003).

Siessmeier and coworkers (2003) examined 26 CFS participants using FDG-PET along with psychometric measures of anxiety, depression, and health-related quality of life

(HRQOL). Abnormalities in glucose metabolism were observed in about half (14 of 26) of the CFS participants. In most cases, abnormalities were in the anterior cingulate gyrus/mesial frontal cortex and orbital frontal cortex. No consistent pattern of metabolic activity was observed, consistent with the heterogeneity of the CFS population. Regions activated in prior studies (e.g., the brainstem in Costa et al., 1995; Tirelli et al., 1998; the thalamus in Machale et al., 2000) were not activated in this study. Decreased metabolism was correlated with anxiety, depression, and the "mental" component of HRQOL. Importantly, there was no relationship between reductions in glucose metabolism and severity of perceived fatigue.

Very few studies have related neuropsychological performance (or complaints) with cerebral perfusion. Fischler and associates (1996) examined whether there was a relationship between cerebral perfusion on SPECT and "physical or mental fatigue" and cognition. They examined 16 participants with CFS, 13 without current major depression, and two control groups: a major depression control group ($n = 19$) and 20 healthy individuals. In CFS patients without depression, subjective and objective neuropsychological performance was negatively correlated with frontal lobe perfusion. No relationship was found between subjective fatigue level and cerebral perfusion. The CFS group showed significantly greater right than left hemisphere perfusion index score than were seen the major depression and healthy control groups. Also, the major depression group displayed significant hypoperfusion in the superofrontal region compared to the CFS and healthy control groups.

Schmaling and colleagues (2003) conducted SPECT scans during rest and while subjects performed a complex and speeded working memory task (PASAT) in 15 CFS and 15 healthy control subjects. CFS subjects showed a pattern of more diffuse regional blood flow than controls, who showed a more focal pattern. While CFS subjects showed less activation in the left anterior cingulate, the change in activation in this region during the PASAT relative to the resting state was significantly greater than that observed in healthy controls. CFS subjects also showed more widespread and diffuse activation in the frontal and temporal lobes as well as the thalamus, indicating increased recruitment of cerebral regions needed to perform the challenging cognitive task. These results were not attributed to group differences in mood, cognitive performance, or effort.

Using blood oxygen level–dependent (BOLD) functional MRI (fMRI), Lange and coworkers (2000) examined persons with CFS who had no concurrent psychopathology as they performed a complex working memory task. CFS subjects displayed more diffuse and bilateral cerebral activation on fMRI while performing the complex working memory task than the healthy group. In the healthy control group, activation was primarily in the prefrontal and superior parietal regions of the left hemisphere. In contrast, cerebral activation in the CFS group extended to the right prefrontal and anterior cingulate and the inferior parietal regions bilaterally. The authors suggest that the pattern of fMRI signal change observed in individuals with CFS may a reflect a compensatory mechanism that operates under conditions of increased mental effort. This notion that additional cerebral resources are required to perform the same amount of mental work in CFS (Schmaling et al., 2003) has been observed in other populations as well, including traumatic brain injury (Christodoulou et al., 2000; McAllister, Sparling, Flashman, Guerin, Mamourian, & Saykin, 2001) and multiple sclerosis (Hillary et al., 2003).

Tanaka, Matsushima, Tamai, and Kajimoto (2002) used near-infrared spectroscopy (NIRS) to study cerebral metabolism in 16 young persons with CFS, 12 subjects with idiopathic CFS (Fukuda et al.,1994), and 20 controls during active standing. Abnormal cerebral hemodynamics (measured on the right forehead) were observed in 15 of 16 subjects with CF and orthostatic intolerance, in 6 of 12 subjects with CF without orthostatic intolerance, and only in 2 of 20 controls. Kuratsune and colleagues (2002) showed decreased uptake of acetylcarnitine (purported to be involved in neurotransmitter biosynthesis) in the prefrontal and temporal lobes as well as the anterior cingulate and cerebellum in 8 CFS subjects without psychiatric comorbidity. They suggested that reduced acetylcarnitine may be associated with neurotransmitter synthesis in the brain, which could be related to fatigue. However, this work needs to be replicated and extended.

Chaudhuri and Behan (2000) used proton magnetic resonance spectroscopy (^{1}H MRS) to examine metabolic function in the basal ganglia of persons with CFS. They examined eight CFS participants without a psychiatric disorder and eight healthy controls. CFS participants had significantly increased choline peaks in the basal ganglia relative to controls. These participants showed no evidence of structural abnormalities of the basal ganglia on MRI. The authors suggest that persons with CFS may experience a "neurobiological process affecting neural cell membrane function." A similar finding was observed in the occipital cortex in persons with CFS (Puri et al., 2002).

Overall, evidence of brain pathology in CFS continues to accumulate, particularly among persons with CFS who have no concomitant psychopathology. Structural neuroimaging studies show white matter hyperinstensities in persons with CFS. Functional neuroimaging shows hypometabolism in the frontal lobes and basal ganglia most consistently in persons with CFS. Collectively, these findings suggest that CFS may be mediated, at least in some individuals, by CNS mechanisms.

HPA Axis in CFS

CFS is associated with reductions in hypothalamic-pituitary-adrenal (HPA) axis functioning and neurotransmission, suggesting an altered physiological response to stress. Cleare (2003), in summarizing studies of basal HPA axis function in CFS, notes that about half the studies found evidence for lowered cortisol levels. In their pioneering study Demitrack and associates (1991) found low levels of basal cortisol in CFS subjects, possibly due to a deficit in corticotropin-releasing hormone (CRH). Deficits in cortisol have been linked to lethargy and fatigue in many conditions (Demitrack, 1994), suggesting that the pervasive fatigue reported in CFS and atypical depression is a result of hypocortisolism. Altemus and colleagues (2001) measured the adrenocorticotropic hormone (ACTH) and cortisol response to infusion of vasopressin in patients with CFS and matched healthy volunteers. Persons with CFS had a reduced ACTH response and a more rapid cortisol response to a vasopressin infusion. They interpret this as evidence of reduced hypothalamic CRH secretion in patients with CFS. Several studies (Bakheit, Behan, Dinan, Gray, & O'Keane, 1992; Sharpe, Hawton, Clements, & Cowen, 1997) have shown that serotonin neurotransmission is increased in CFS subjects compared to both healthy and depressed subjects. Cleare and associates (1995) also reported hypocortisolism and increased serotonin neurotransmitter function in CFS, whereas hypercortisolism and decreased serotonin neurotransmitter function was noted in their depressed subjects.

A study examining endocrine hyporesponsiveness to a maximal treadmill exercise test in CFS subjects found the stress-responsive hormones adrenocorticotropin, catecholamines, prolactin, thyrotropin, and insulin were at less than half the level of controls 4 minutes after exercise (Ottenweller, LaManca, Sisto, Guo, & Natelson, 1997). Glucocorticoids can have an inhibitory effect on serotonin (5-HT) function, and CRH release is modulated by 5-HT. CFS has been associated with increased prolactin responses to the 5-HT–releasing agent fenfluramine. Vassallo and colleagues (2001) found that the increased prolactin response to fenfluramine is due to elevated activity of presynaptic 5-HT neurons. Racciatti and coworkers (2001) found an altered cyclicity of HPA axis hormones (particularly ACTH and prolactin) in a circadian rhythm study. These data suggest that abnormalities in the HPA axis function, hormonal stress responses, and serotonin neurotransmission in CFS subjects are in the opposite direction from the pattern observed in patients with clinical (melancholic) depression (for a discussion on CFS versus depression, see chapter 10). Cleare and colleagues (2001) examined ACTH and cortisol responses to challenge agents in patients with CFS without comorbid psychiatric disorder compared to healthy controls. They found a similar ACTH response to all challenges, suggesting that central control of the HPA axis is intact in CFS. However, they found impaired adrenal responsivity in CFS, consistent with several previous studies.

Given that hypocortisolism has been found in some persons with CFS, treatment with hydrocortisone has been attempted. Cleare and associates (1999) found that 28 days of low-dose hydrocortisone treatment that led to a rise in circulating cortisol resulted in significant reductions in self-rated fatigue and disability compared to a placebo group. A group using a higher dose found adrenal suppression, indicating that risks outweighed benefits (McKenzie et al., 1998). More recently, Cleare and coworkers (2001) found about 28 percent of CFS patients responded to hydrocortisone treatment with reduced fatigue levels (similar to the percentage found in the previous two studies). In those who responded to treatment, there was a corresponding normalization of the blunted cortisol response to human CRH challenge.

Some recent data suggest that CFS patients are capable of mounting a sufficient cortisol response to a psychosocial stressor, a standardized exercise test, and an insulin tolerance test (Gaab et al., 2002a). Yet, these researchers also found moderate HPA axis dysfunction with enhanced sensitivity of the adrenals to ACTH, indicative of secondary or tertiary origin. In a follow-up study (Gaab et al., 2002b), they found no response differences for plasma or salivary cortisol between healthy and CFS subjects after administration of low-dose or high-dose ACTH. Hypocortisolism may be mild and subtle in CFS, but the neuroendocrine patterns resemble those observed in atypical depression (see chapter 10 for a more thorough discussion of this topic). Van Hoof, Cluydts, and De Meirleir (2003) noted that among persons with CFS attending their clinic, the most common affective disorder diagnosed was atypical depression.

Overall, persons with CFS tend to show abnormalities in the HPA axis function, hormonal stress responses, and serotonin neurotransmission in the opposite direction from the pattern observed in patients with clinical (melancholic) depression.

Sleep and CFS

Sleep loss can affect immune parameters and may be a fruitful area for CFS etiology (Mullington, Hinze-Selch, & Pollmacher, 2001). Moldofsky, Saskin, and Lue (1988) found that patients with postfebrile fibrositis had nonrestorative sleep disorders and suggested that these patients share symptoms similar to those of patients with CFS. This was the first study to suggest that persons with CFS may have sleep disorders. Krupp, Jandorf, Coyle, and Mendelson (1993) found persons with CFS had significantly higher scores on fatigue and sleep disturbance scales than MS subjects and healthy controls. On polysomnography, 62 percent revealed some sleep disorder including periodic movement disorder, excessive daytime sleepiness, apnea, and narcolepsy. Morriss, Wearden, and Battersby (1997) examined sleep difficulties through self-report and polysomnography in persons with CFS with and without psychiatric disorder compared to depressed patients and healthy controls. They found that difficulty in maintaining sleep was the principal problem in the CFS group with or without psychiatric disorder, and this problem was associated with greater functional impairment. Compared to depressed subjects, persons with CFS reported more naps, more waking by pain, the same level of difficulty maintaining sleep, and less difficulty falling asleep (Morriss et al., 1997). Le Bon and colleagues (2000) examined primary sleep disorders in CFS and found that 46 percent had sleep apnea/hypoapnea and 5 percent had periodic limb movements' syndrome. When more demanding criteria were used for apnea, only 11 percent met the criteria. These authors concluded that CFS could not be reduced to a somatic expression of a primary sleep disorder. Sleep quality exhibits strong heritability, therefore, a study of insomnia in monozygotic twins discordant for chronic fatigue syndrome by Watson and colleagues (2003) is particularly important. These researchers found the CFS twins more frequently endorsed subjective measures of insomnia and poor sleep than their healthy cotwin, but the twins did not differ on objective polysomnographic measures of insomnia, including sleep latency, total sleep time, sleep efficiency, arousal number, arousal index, REM latency, and percentage of stages 1, 2, 3, and 4. They did note a significant increase in REM sleep in CFS compared to the healthy twin. Watson and colleagues (2003) conclude that persons with CFS have inaccurate perceptions of their own sleep state. It appears that a minority of CFS patients may experience sleep dysfunction on polysomnography, with a larger number reporting sleep difficulties, that is, subjective complaints outweigh objective findings.

Although subjective and objective sleep abnormalities are common in depression, they differ from those found in CFS. Compared to depressed patients, CFS patients show significantly more time spent in delta sleep, and a greater percentage of stage 4 sleep. In contrast, depressed patients show reduced REM latency and increased REM density and activity compared to CFS patients, who generally display normal REM sleep (Zubieta, Demitrack, Shipley, Engleberg, Eiser, & Douglass, 1993; Thase, Frank, & Kupfer, 1985).

Overall, while an objective sleep disorder is apparent in a subgroup of persons with CFS, well-controlled studies do not indicate that sleep dysfunction explains the extreme fatigue found in persons with CFS.

Conclusion

All persons with CFS by definition suffer from significant fatigue, but no single pattern or underlying mechanism has yet been identified to explain the phenomenon of fatigue in these individuals. This is likely a result of our poor understanding of the molecular basis of the perception of fatigue, as well as the heterogeneity of the illness, in large part due to the vague definitions now used for its diagnosis. There is ample evidence, however, to suggest cerebral involvement in CFS more generally. Neuropsychological impairment tends to be associated with CFS subjects who do not have a comorbid psychiatric condition. Notions that CFS is nothing more than depression or some other psychiatric condition is too simplistic. MRI studies consistently show white matter hyperintensities in the brain, particularly in CFS subjects without psychiatric comorbidity. Functional neuroimaging studies have been fairly consistent in showing abnormal cerebral metabolism in the frontal lobes and basal ganglia in person with CFS. Chaudhuri and Behan (2000) have proposed that the basal ganglia play a key role in central fatigue. The work on functional neuroimaging in CFS generally supports their hypothesis.

Interestingly, functional imaging studies have shown both increased activation and a pattern of more diffuse activation throughout much of the brain. This has been interpreted as a compensatory mechanism that operates under conditions of increased mental effort (Lange et al., 2000; Schmaling et al., 2003). Though it tempting to suggest the perception of fatigue may be associated with this increased and more widespread cerebral activation, this hypothesis must be tested empirically. Most imaging studies have not correlated cerebral activation with subjective ratings of fatigue, and the few that did have found no relationship (Siessmeier et al., 2003; Fischler et al., 1996).

A fairly strong finding in CFS is abnormalities of the HPA axis. Importantly, these abnormalities, hormonal stress responses, and serotonin neurotransmission in CFS subjects are in the opposite direction from the pattern observed in patients with clinical (melancholic) depression. In both depression and CFS, reports of unrefreshing and disturbed sleep are legion. No consistent pattern of sleep disorders has yet been found in persons with CFS, although findings on polysomnography differentiate CFS from depression on sleep parameters.

This chapter has provided some preliminary notions on the cerebral mechanism involved in fatigue in CFS, but it is clear that much work remains to understand the brain mechanism underling fatigue in this illness.

References

Abbey, S. E., & Garfinkle, P. E. (1991). Chronic fatigue syndrome and depression: cause, effect, or covariate. *Review Infectious Diseases, 13(Suppl 1)*, S73–83.

Afari, N., & Buchwald, D. (2003). Chronic fatigue syndrome: a review. *American Journal of Psychiatry, 160*, 221–236.

Altemus, M., Dale, D. K., Michelson, D., Demitrack, M. A., Gold, P. W., & Straus, S. E. (2001). Abnormalities in response to vasopressin infusion in chronic fatigue syndrome. *Psychoneuroendocrinology, 26*, 175–188.

American Psychiatric Association. (1994). *Diagnostic and statistical manual of mental disorders*, 4th ed. Washington, DC: American Psychiatric Association.

Bakheit, A. M. O., Behan, P. O., Dinan, T. G., Gray, C. E., & O'Keane, V. (1992). Possible upregulation of hypothalamic 5-hydroxytryptamine receptors in patients with postviral fatigue syndrome. *British Medical Journal, 304*, 1010–1012.

Buchwald, D. P. R., Cheney, P. I., Peterson, B., et al. (1992). A chronic illness characterized by fatigue, neurologic and immunologic disorders and active herpesvirus type 6 infection. *Annals of Internal Medicine, 116*, 103–113.

Buchwald, D., Umali, P., Kith, P., Pearlman, T., & Komaroff, A. (1995). Chronic fatigue and the chronic fatigue syndrome: prevalence in a Pacific Northwest Health Care System. *Annals of Internal Medicine, 123*, 81–88.

Chaudhuri, A., & Behan, P. O. (2000). Fatigue and basal ganglia. *Journal of Neurological Sciences, 179*, 34–42.

Christodoulou, C., DeLuca, J., Lange, G., Johnson, S. K., Sisto, S. A., Korn, L., & Natelson, B. H. (1998). Relation between neuropsychological impairment and functional disability in patients with chronic fatigue syndrome. *Journal of Neurology, Neurosurgery & Psychiatry, 64*, 431–434.

Christodoulou, C., DeLuca, J., Ricker, J. H., Madigan, N. K., Bly, B. M., Lange, G., Kalnin, A. J., Liu, W. C., Steffener, J., Diamond, B. J., & Ni, A. C. (2000). Functional magnetic resonance imaging of working memory impairment after traumatic brain injury. *Journal of Neurology, Neurosurgery & Psychiatry, 71*, 161–168.

Clauw, D. J. (2001). Potential mechanisms in chemical intolerance and related conditions. *Annals of New York Academy of Sciences, 933*, 235–253.

Cleare, A. J. (2003). The neuroendocrinology of chronic fatigue syndrome. *Endocrine Reviews, 24(2)*, 236–252.

Cleare, A. J., Bearn, J., McGregor, A., Allain, T., Wessely, S., Murray, R. M., & O'Kane, V. O. (1995). Contrasting neuroendocrine responses in depression and chronic fatigue syndrome. *Journal of Affective Disorders, 35*, 283–289.

Cleare, A. J., Heap, E., Malhi, G. S., Wessely, S., O'Keane, V., & Miell, J. (1999). Low-dose hydrocortisone in chronic fatigue syndrome: a randomized crossover trial. *The Lancet, 353*, 455–458.

Cleare, A. J., Miell, J., Heap, S., Sookdeo, L., Malhi, G. S., & O'Keane, V. (2001). Hypothalamo-pituitary-adrenal axis dysfunction in chronic fatigue syndrome, and the effects of low-dose hydrocortisone therapy. *The Journal of Clinical Endocrinology & Metabolism, 86*, 3545–3554.

Cook, D. B., Lange, G., DeLuca, J., & Natelson, B. H. (2001). Relationship of brain MRI abnormalities and physical functional status in CFS. *International Journal of Neuroscience, 107*, 1–6.

Cope, H., Pernet, A., Kendall, B., & Davis, A. (1995). Cognitive functioning and magnetic resonance imaging in chronic fatigue syndrome. *British Journal of Psychiatry, 167*, 86–94.

Costa, D. C., Tannock, C., & Brostoff, J. (1995). Brainstem profusion is impaired in chronic fatigue syndrome. *Quarterly Journal of Medicine, 88*, 767–773.

David, A., & Wessely, S. (1993). Chronic fatigue, ME and the ICD-10. *Lancet, 342*, 1247–1248.

DeLuca, J., Christodoulou, C., Diamond, B. J., Rosenstein, E. D., Kramer, N., & Natelson, B. H. (2004). Working memory deficits in chronic fatigue syndrome: differentiating between speed and accuracy of information processing. *Journal of the International Neuropsychological Society, 10(1)*, 101–119.

DeLuca, J., Johnson, S. K., Beldowicz, D., & Natelson, B. H. (1995). Neuropsychological impairments in chronic fatigue syndrome, multiple sclerosis, and depression. *Journal of Neurology, Neurosurgery, and Psychiatry, 58*, 38–43.

DeLuca, J., Johnson, S. K., Ellis, S. P., & Natelson, B. H. (1997). Cognitive functioning is impaired in patients with chronic fatigue syndrome devoid of psychiatric disease. *Journal of Neurology, Neurosurgery, and Psychiatry, 62*, 151–155.

DeLuca, J., Johnson, S. K., & Natelson, B. H. (1993). Information processing in chronic fatigue syndrome and multiple sclerosis. *Archives of Neurology, 50*, 301–304.

DeLuca, J., & Tiersky, L. (2003). Neuropsychological assessment. In L. Jason, P. Fennell, & R. Taylor, eds. *Handbook of chronic fatigue syndrome*, pp. 417–437. New York: John Wiley & Sons.

Demitrack, M. A. (1994). Neuroendocrine aspects of chronic fatigue syndrome. In S. E. Straus, ed. *Chronic Fatigue Syndrome.* Pp. 285–308. New York: Marcel Dekker.

Demitrack, M. A., Dale, J. K., Straus, S. E., Laue, L., Listwak, S. J., Kruesi, M. J. P., Chrousos, G. P., & Gold, P. W. (1991). Evidence for the impaired activation of the hypothalamic-pituitary-adrenal axis in patients with chronic fatigue syndrome. *Journal of Clinical Endocrinology and Metabolism, 73*, 1–11.

Fischler, B., D'Haenen, H., Cluydts, R., Michiels, V., Demets, K., Bossuyt, A., Kaufman, L., & DeMeirleir, K. (1996). Comparison of ^{99m}Tc HMPAO SPECT scan between chronic fatigue syndrome, major depression and healthy controls: an exploratory study of clinical correlates of regional cerebral blood flow. *Neuropsychobiology, 34(4)*, 175–183.

Fukuda, K., Straus, S. E., Hickie, I., Sharpe, M. C., Dobbins, J. G., & Komaroff, A. (1994). The chronic fatigue syndrome: a comprehensive approach to its definition and study. *Annals of Internal Medicine, 121*, 953–959.

Gaab, J., Huster, D., Peisen, R., Engret, V., Heitz, V., Schad, T., Schurmeyer, T., & Ehlert, U. (2002a). Hypothalamic-pituitary-adrenal axis reactivity in chronic fatigue syndrome and health under psychological, physiological, and pharmacological stimulation. *Psychosomatic Medicine, 64*, 951–962.

Gaab, J., Huster, D., Peisen, R., Engret, V., Schad, T., Schurmeyer, T., & Ehlert, U. (2002b). Low dose dexamethasone suppression test in chronic fatigue syndrome and health. *Psychosomatic Medicine, 64*, 311–318.

Goldstein, J. A., Mena, I., Jouanne, E., & Lesser, I. (1995). The assessment of vascular abnormalities in late life chronic fatigue syndrome by brain SPECT: comparison with late life major depressive disorder. *Journal of Chronic Fatigue Syndrome, 1*, 55–79.

Grafman, J., Schwartz, V., Dale, J. K., Scheffers, M., Houser, C., & Straus, S. E. (1993). Analysis of neuropsychological functioning in patients with chronic fatigue syndrome. *Journal of Neurology and Neurosurgical Psychiatry, 56*, 684–689.

Greco, A., Tannock, C., Brostoff, J., & Costa, D. (1997). Brain MR in chronic fatigue syndrome. *American Journal of Neuroradiology, 18*, 1265–1269.

Greenberg, D. B. (1990). Neurasthenia in the 1980's: chronic mononucleosis, chronic fatigue syndrome, and anxiety and depressive disorders. *Psychosomatics, 31*, 129–137.

Hillary, F. G., Chiaravalloti, N. D., Ricker, J. H., Steffener, J., Bly, B. M., Lange, G., Liu, W. C., Kalnin, A. J., & DeLuca, J. (2003). An investigation of working memory rehearsal in multiple sclerosis using fMRI. *Journal of Clinical and Experimental Neuropsychology, 25*, 965–978.

Holmes, G. P., Kaplan, J. R., Gantz, N. M., Komaroff, A. L., Schonberger, L. B., Straus, S. E., et al. (1988). Chronic fatigue syndrome: a working case definition. *Annals of Internal Medicine, 108*, 387–389.

Ichise, M., Salit, I. E., Abbey, S. E., Chung, D. G., Gray, B., Kirsch, J. C., & Freedman, M. (1992). Assessment of regional cerebral perfusion by 99Tcm-HMPAO SPECT in chronic fatigue syndrome. *Nuclear Medicine Communications, 13*, 767–772.

Jason, L. A., Richman, J. A., Rademaker, A. W., Jordan, K. M., Plioplys, A. V., Taylor, R. R., McCready, W., Huang, C. F., & Plioplys, S. (1999). A community based study of chronic fatigue syndrome. *Archives of Internal Medicine, 159(18)*, 2129–2137.

Jason, L. A., Taylor, R. R., Kennedy, C. L., Jordan, K., Song, S., Johnson, D. E., & Torres, S. R. (2000). Chronic fatigue syndrome: sociodemographic subtypes in a community-based sample. *Evaluation and the Health Professions, 23(3)*, 243–263.

Johnson, S. K., DeLuca, J., & Natelson, B. H. (1999). Chronic fatigue syndrome: A critical review. *Annals of Behavioral Medicine, 21*, 258–271.

Johnson, S. K., DeLuca, J., Natelson, B. H., Jones, J., Ray, G., Minnich, L., Hicks, M., Kibler, R., & Lucas, D. (1985). Evidence for active Epstein-Barr virus infection in patients with persistent, unexplained illnesses; elevated anti-early antigenantibodies. *Annals of Internal Medicine, 102*, 1–7.

Johnson, S. K., Lange, G., DeLuca, J., Korn, L. R., & Natelson, H. (1997). Effects of fatigue on neuropsychological performance on patients with chronic fatigue syndrome, multiple sclerosis and depression. *Applied Neuropsychology, 4*, 145–153.

Jones, J. F. (1998). Epstein-Barr virus and the chronic fatigue syndrome: a short review. *Microbiological Science, 5(12)*, 366–369.

Joyce, E., Blumenthal, S., & Wessely, S. (1996). Memory, attention, and executive function in chronic fatigue syndrome. *Journal of Neurology, Neurosurgery, and Psychiatry, 60*, 495–503.

Komaroff, A. L. (1994). Clinical presentation and evaluation of fatigue and chronic fatigue syndrome. In S. E. Straus, ed. *Chronic Fatigue Syndrome.* Pp. 61–84. New York: Marcel Deckker, Inc.

Komaroff, A. L., & Buchwald, D. (1991). Symptoms and signs of chronic fatigue syndrome. *Review of Infectious Diseases, 13*, S8–S11.

Komaroff, A. L., Fagioli, L. R., Geiger, A. M., Doolittle, T. H., Lee, J., Kornish, J., Gleit, M. A., & Guerriero, R. T. (1996). An examination of the working case definition of chronic fatigue syndrome. *The American Journal of Medicine, 100,* 56–64.

Krupp, L. B., Jandorf, L., Coyle, P. K., & Mendelson, W. B. (1993). Sleep disturbance in chronic fatigue syndrome. *Journal of Psychosomatic Research, 37,* 325–331.

Kuratsune, H., Yamaguti, K., Lindh, G., et al. (2002). Brain regions involved in fatigue sensation: reduced acetylcarnitine uptake into the brain. *NeuroImage, 17,* 1256–1265.

Lange, G., DeLuca, J., Maldjian, J. A., Lee, H.-J., Tiersky, L. A., & Natelson, B. H. (1999). Brain MRI abnormalities exist in a subset of patients with chronic fatigue syndrome. *Journal of the Neurological Sciences, 171,* 3–7.

Lange, G., Holodny, A., DeLuca, J., Lee, H. J., Yan, X. H. M., Steffener, J., & Natelson, B. H. (2001). Quantitative assessment of cerebral ventricular volumes in CFS. *Applied Neuropsychology, 8(1),* 23–30.

Lange, G., Steffener, J., Christodoulou, C., Liu, W.-C., Bly, B. M., DeLuca, J., & Natelson, B. H. (2000). FMRI of auditory verbal working memory in severe fatiguing illness. *Neuroimage, 11(5),* S95.

Le Bon, O., Fischler, B., Hoffman, G., Murphy, J. R., De Meirleir, K., Cluydts, R., & Pelc, I. (2000). How significant are primary sleep disorders and sleepiness in the chronic fatigue syndrome? *Sleep Research Online, 3,* 43–48.

Lewis, D. H., Mayberg, H. S., Fischer, M. E., Goldberg, J., Ashton, S., Graham, M. M., & Buchwald, D. (2001). Monozygotic twins discordant for chronic fatigue syndrome: regional cerebral blood flow SPECT. *Radiology, 219(3),* 766–773.

Lezak, M. D. (1995). *Neuropsychological Assessment,* 3rd ed. New York: Oxford University Press.

Lloyd, A. R., Wakefield, D., Boughton, C., & Dwyer, J. (1988). What is myalgic encephalomyelitis? *Lancet, 1(8597),* 1286–1287.

Machale, S. M., Lawrie, S. M., Cavanagh, J. T. O., Glabus, M. F., Murray, C. L., Goodwin, G. M., & Ebmeier, K. P. (2000). Cerebral perfusion in chronic fatigue syndrome and depression. *British Journal of Psychiatry, 176,* 550–556.

Manu, P., Affleck, G., Tennen, H., Morse, P. A., & Escobar, J. I. (1996). Hypochondriasis influences quality-of-life outcomes in patients with chronic fatigue. *Psychotherapy & Psychosomatics, 65(2),* 76–81.

Marshall, P. S., Forstot, M., Callies, A., Peterson, P. K., & Schenck, C. H. (1997). Cognitive slowing and working memory difficulties in chronic fatigue syndrome. *Psychosomatic Medicine, 59(1),* 58–66.

McAllister, T. W., Sparling, M. B., Flashman, L. A., Guerin, S. J., Mamourian, A. C., & Saykin, A. J. (2001). Differential working memory load effects after mild traumatic brain injury. *NeuroImage, 14,* 1004–1012.

McKenzie, R., O'Fallon, A., Dale, J., Demitrack, M., Sharma, G., Deloria, M., Garcia-Borreguero, D., Blackwelder, W., & Straus, S. E. (1998). Low-dose hydrocortisone for treatment of chronic fatigue syndrome: comparison with chronic fatigue syndrome. *American Behavior Medicine, 24,* 106–112.

Metzger, F. A., & Denney, D. R. (2002). Perception of cognitive performance in patients with chronic fatigue syndrome. *Annals of Behavioral Medicine, 24(2),* 106–112.

Michiels, V., & Cluydts, R. (2001). Neuropsychological functioning in the chronic fatigue syndrome: a review. *Acta Psychiatric Scandnavia, 103,* 84–93.

Michiels, V., Cluydts, R., & Fischler, B. (1998). Attention and verbal learning in patients with chronic fatigue syndrome. *Journal of the International Neuropsychological Society, 4,* 456–466.

Moldofsky, H., Saskin, P., & Lue, F. A. (1988). Sleep and symptoms in fibrositis syndrome after a febrile illness. *Journal of Rheumatology, 15,* 1701–1704.

Morriss, R. K., Wearden, A. J., & Battersby, L. (1997). The relation of sleep difficulties to fatigue, mood and disability in chronic fatigue syndrome. *Journal of Psychosomatic Research, 42(6),* 597–605.

Mullington, J. M., Hinze-Selch, D., & Pollmacher, T. (2001). Mediators of inflammation and their interaction with sleep. *Annals of the New York Academy of Sciences, 933,* 201–210.

Natelson, B. H., Cohen, J. M., Brassloff, I., & Lee, H. J. (1993). A controlled study of brain magnetic resonance imaging in patients with fatiguing illnesses. *Journal of the Neurological Sciences, 120,* 213–217.

Ottenweller, J., LaManca, J. J., Sisto, S. A., Guo, W., & Natelson, B. (1997). Endocrine hyporesponsiveness to exercise in patients with chronic fatigue syndrome. *Integrative Physiological Behavioral Science, 32,* 189.

Puri, B. K., Counsell, S. J., Zaman, R., Main, J., Collins, A. G., Hajnal, J. V., & Davey, N. J. (2002). Relative increase in choline in the occipital cortex in chronic fatigue syndrome. *Acta Psychiatry Scandinavia, 106,* 224–226.

Racciatti, D., Guagnano, M. T., Vecchiet, J., De Remigis, P. L., Pizzigallo, E., Della Vecchia, R., Di Sciascio, T., Merlitti, D., & Sensi, S. (2001). Chronic fatigue syndrome: circadian rhythm and hypothalamic-pituitary-adrenal (HPA) axis impairment. *International Journal of Immunopathology and Pharmacology, 14(1),* 11–15.

Schluederberg, A., Straus, S. E., Peterson, P., et al. (1992). Chronic fatigue syndrome: definition and medical outcome assessment. *Annals of Internal Medicine, 117,* 325–331.

Schmaling, K. B., Fiedelak, J. I., Katon, W. J., Bader, J. O., & Buchwald, D. S. (2003). Propsective study of the prognosis of unexplained chronic fatigue in a clinic-based cohort. *Psychosomatic Medicine, 65,* 1047–1054.

Schmaling, K. B., Lewis, D. H., Fiedelak, J. I., Mahurin, R., & Buchwald, D. S. (2003). Single-photon emission computerized tomography and neurocognitive function in patients with chronic fatigue syndrome. *Psychosomatic Medicine, 65,* 129–136.

Schwartz, R. B., Garada, B. M., Komaroff, A. L., et al. (1994a). Detection of intracranial abnormalities in patients with chronic fatigue syndrome: comparison of MRI imaging and SPECT. *American Journal of Radiology*, *162*, 935–941.

Schwartz, R. B., Komaroff, A. L., Garada, B. M., Gleit, M., Doolittle, T. H., Bates, D. W., Vasile, R. G., & Holman, B. L. (1994b). SPECT imaging of the brain: comparisons of findings in patients with chronic fatigue syndrome, AIDS dementia complex, and major unipolar depression. *American Journal of Radiology*, *162*, 943–951.

Scott, L. V., & Dinan, T. G. (1998). Urinary free cortisol excretion in chronic fatigue syndrome, major depression and in healthy volunteers. *Journal of Affective Disorders*, *47*, 49–54.

Scott, L. V., Medbak, S., & Dinan, T. G. (1998). The low dose ACTH test in chronic fatigue syndrome and in health. *Clinical Endocrinology*, *48*, 733–737.

Sharpe, M. (1996). Chronic fatigue syndrome. *Psychiatric Clinics of North America*, *19(3)*, 549–573.

Sharpe, M., Archard, L., Banatvala, J., et al. (1991). Chronic fatigue syndrome: guidelines for research. *Journal Royal Society Medicine*, *84*, 118–121.

Sharpe, M., Hawton, K., Clements, A., & Cowen, P. J. (1997). Increased brain serotonin function in men with chronic fatigue syndrome. *British Medical Journal*, *315*, 164–165.

Short, K., McCabe, M., & Tooley, G. (2002). Cognitive functioning in chronic fatigue syndrome and the role of depression, anxiety, and fatigue. *Journal of Psychosomatic Research*, *52*, 475–483.

Siessmeier, T., Nix, W. A., Hardt, J., Schreckenberger, M., Egle, U. T., & Bartenstein, P. (2003). Observer independent analysis of cerebral glucose metabolism in patients with chronic fatigue syndrome. *Journal of Neurology, Neurosurgery & Psychiatry*, *74*, 922–928.

Straus, S. E. (1991). History of chronic fatigue syndrome. *Review Infectious Diseases*, *13(Suppl 1)*, S2–7.

Tanaka, H., Matsushima, R., Tamai, H., & Kajimoto, Y. (2002). Impaired postural cerebral hemodynamics in young patients with chronic fatigue with and without orthostatic intolerance. *Journal of Pediatrics*, *140*, 412–417.

Thase, M. E., Frank, E., & Kupfer, D. J. (1985). Biological processes in major depression. In E. E. Beckham & W. R. Leber, eds. *Handbook of Depression: Treatment, assessment and research*. Pp. 816–819. Homewood, IL: Dorsey Press.

Tiersky, L. A., DeLuca, J., Hill, N., Dhar, S. K., Johnson, S. K., Lange, G., Rappolt, G., & Natelson, B. H. (2001). Longitudinal assessment of neuropsychological functioning, psychiatric status, functional disability and employment status in chronic fatigue syndrome. *Applied Neuropsychology*, *8(1)*, 41–50.

Tiersky, L. A., Johnson, S. K., Lange, G., Natelson, B. H., & DeLuca, J. (1997). Neuropsychology of chronic fatigue syndrome: a critical review. *Journal of Clinical Clinical and Experimental Neuropsychology*, *19*(4), 560–586.

Tirelli, U., Chierichetti, F., Tavio, M., Simonelli, C., Bianchin, G., Zanco, P., & Ferlin, G. (1998). Brian positron emisión tomography (PET) in chronic fatigue syndrome: preliminary data. *American Journal of Medicine, 105*, 54s–58s.

Van Hoof, E., Cluydts, R., & De Meirleir, K. (2003). Atypical depression as a secondary symptom in chronic fatigue syndrome. *Medical Hypotheses, 61(1)*, 52–55.

Vassallo, C. M., Feldman, E., Peto, T., et al. (2001). Decreased tryptophan availability but normal post-synaptic 5-HT receptor sensitivity in chronic fatigue syndrome. *Psychological Medicine, 31*, 585–591.

Vercoulen, J. H. M. M., Bazelmans, C. M. A., Swanick, J. M. D., et al. (1998). Evaluating neuropsychological impairment in chronic fatigue syndrome. *Journal of Clinical and Experimental Neuropsychology, 20*, 144–156.

Vercoulen, J. H. M. M., Swanink, C. M. A., Zitman, F. G., Vreden, S. G. S., Hoofs, M. P. H., Fennis, J. F. M., Galama, J. M. D., van der Meer, J. W. M., & Bleijenberg, G. (1996). Randomized, double-blind, placebo-controlled study of fluoxetine in chronic fatigue syndrome. *Lancet, 347*, 858–861.

Watson, N. F., Kapur, V., Arguelles, L. M., et al. (2003). Comparison of subjective and objective measures of insomnia in monozygotic twins discordant for chronic fatigue syndrome. *Sleep, 26(3)*, 324–328.

Wearden, A. J., & Appleby, L. (1996). Research on cognitive complaints and cognitive functioning inpatients with chronic fatigue syndrome: What conclusions can we draw? *Journal of Psychosomatic Research, 41(3)*, 197–211.

Wessely, S. (1996). Chronic fatigue syndrome. Summary of a report of a joint committee of the Royal Colleges of Physicians, Psychiatrists and General Practioners. *Journal of the Royal College of Physicians (London)*, 497–504.

Wessely, S., Chadler, T., Hirsch, S., Wallace, P., & Wright, D. (1997). The prevalence and morbidity of chronic fatigue and chronic fatigue syndrome: a prospective primary care study. *American Journal of Public Health, 87*, 1449–1455.

Wessely, S., Hotopf, M., & Sharpe, M. (1998). *Chronic Fatigue and Its Syndromes*. New York: Oxford University Press.

Zubieta, J. K., Demitrack, M. A., Shipley, J. E., Engleberg, N. C., Eiser, A., & Douglass, A. (1993). Sleep EEG in chronic fatigue syndrome: comparison with major depression. *Biological Psychiatry, 33*, 74A.

10 Depression and Fatigue

Susan K. Johnson

This chapter examines the relationship between depression and fatigue. We examine the epidemiology of depression and fatigue symptoms, gender differences in depression, melancholic versus atypical depression, as well as the neurobiology, endocrinology, and functional neuroanatomy of depression and fatigue symptoms. The chapter concludes with a discussion of similarities and differences between depression and chronic fatigue.

Depression has traditionally been viewed as a syndrome with an affective core accompanied by disturbances in sleep and appetite, decreased concentration, loss of interest, fatigue, and suicidal behaviors. According to the *Diagnostic and Statistical Manual of Mental Disorders* (DSM-IV), to meet the criteria for depression an individual needs to have at least at least five of the following symptoms (including either symptom 1 or 2):

1. Depressed mood most of the day, nearly every day
2. Markedly diminished interest or pleasure in all, or almost all, activities
3. Significant weight loss when not dieting or weight gain, or decrease or increase in appetite nearly every day
4. Insomnia or sleeping too much (hypersomnia) nearly every day
5. Psychomotor agitation or retardation nearly every day
6. Fatigue or loss of energy nearly every day
7. Feelings of worthlessness or excessive or inappropriate guilt
8. Diminished ability to think or concentrate, or indecisiveness
9. Recurrent thoughts of death, recurrent suicidal ideation, or a suicide attempt or specific plan for committing suicide

Fatigue, sleep, and appetite disturbances are also part of *International Classification of Diseases* criteria. Besides being diagnostic, multiple somatic complaints are common in depression. In a study by Kirmayer and colleagues (1993), 70 to 80 percent of patients with significant depressive symptoms manifested somatic symptoms. Conversely, patients whose presenting problems include fatigue, headache, back pain,

chest pain, dizziness, musculoskeletal complaints, and weakness may have an underlying depression that goes undiagnosed. Posse and Hallstrom (1998) found the recognized frequency of depression in a primary care setting was only 1.8 percent in a
sample of 442 patients, but when 62 individuals with high somatic scores were
assessed for the presence of an affective disorder, 66 percent were found to have a
mood disorder. In an international study of medical clinics conducted in 14 countries
on 5 continents, somatic symptoms were common in each of the centers. An average
of 69 percent of patients with major depression presented only with somatic symptoms. Unexplained physical symptoms were reported by half of the depressed
patients, and 11 percent of the participants denied any symptoms of depression
(Simon, VonKorff, Piccinelli, Fullerton, & Ormel,1999). The number of physical symptoms reported by primary care patients is related to the presence of psychiatric disorders. Primary care studies have shown that the likelihood of anxiety or mood disorder
increases with the number of somatic symptoms (Kroenke et al., 1994; World Health
Organization, 2002).

Of the somatic complaints indicating an underlying depression, one of the most
common is self-reported fatigue. Most epidemiological studies find that two-thirds of
patients with depression present with symptoms of fatigue, low energy, and listlessness. A large-scale pan-European study, the Depression Research in European Society
(DEPRES), found that 17 percent of the general population suffered from major depression, minor depression, or depressive symptoms (Tylee, 2000). In the second phase of
the DEPRES, semistructured interviews were conducted with 1884 of the depressed
adults. The most commonly experienced symptoms were low mood (76%), tiredness
(73%), and sleep problems (63%) (Tylee, Gastpar, Lepine, & Mendlewicz, 1999).

In a survey of 79 general practitioners in France, the most common symptoms
in major depression patients were depressed mood (96%), fatigue or loss of energy
(94%), and loss of pleasure (86%) (Maurice-Tison, Verdoux, Gay, Perez, Salamon, &
Bourgeois, 1998). A study of fatigue in the Danish general population using multiple regression analysis found that respondents with low social status and those
with depression had the highest fatigue scores (Watt et al., 2000). A prospective
population-based sample of the Epidemiologic Catchment Area Program found that
the number of somatization symptoms and a dysphoric history at baseline were the
two strongest predictors of both new onset of fatigue and recurrent/chronic fatigue
over the 13-year follow-up interval. In addition, individuals who reported a history of
unexplained fatigue at baseline as well as during the follow-up were at markedly
increased risk for new-onset major depression (Addington, Gallo, Ford, & Eaton, 2001).
These studies indicate that not only is fatigue a prominent symptom in undiagnosed
and diagnosed depression, but depression predicts fatigue and fatigue predicts depression in the general population.

In a primary care sample, van der Linden et al. (1999) found that although fatigue and psychiatric disorders were closely correlated for most of the sample, a small subset of patients were identified with a "pure" fatigue state persisting over 6 months that was not associated with psychiatric disorder at any time point. Kirk, Hickie, and Martin (1999) measured fatigue, anxiety, and depression in a community-based sample of twins over age 50 years. A two-factor solution of their questionnaire data showed a separate factor of fatigue clearly distinct from a depression/anxiety factor. These findings indicate that although distress and fatigue are frequently comorbid and predictive of each other, they can also occur as independent entities.

Gender, Depression, and Fatigue

Women with unipolar depression outnumber men two to one, and by a similar number they outnumber men with chronic fatigue syndrome (CFS). The gender difference in depression is not fully understood, but it is robust with a female preponderance in prevalence, incidence, and morbidity risk for major depression, dysthymia, atypical depression, and seasonal affective disorder (Piccinelli & Wilkinson, 2000). A consistent factor differentiating female and male depression is the frequency of somatic symptoms in female depression. Women are much more likely than men to report depression with appetite and sleep disturbances and fatigue, but they are not more likely than men to report depression without these symptoms, that is, "pure depression" (Silverstein, 2002). In a study of 201 opposite-sex twin pairs in which both twins fulfilled DSM-III-R criteria for major depression, the female twins reported significantly more fatigue, hypersomnia, and psychomotor retardation than their male twins (Khan, Gardner, Prescott, & Kendler, 2002). In an international study of 14 countries (traditional and industrialized), the gender ratio of 2 : 1 held constant, and females in all of the centers tended to report more somatic symptoms than men (Maier, Gansicke, Gater, Rezaki, Tiemens, & Urzua, 1999).

In a review of gender differences in depression, several social factors were found to contribute to the female preponderance. These factors included adverse events in childhood, depression and anxiety disorders in childhood and adolescence, crises involving children and housing, reproductive problems, and poor coping skills (Piccellini & Wilkinson, 2000). In a series of studies, Silverstein and colleagues have found anxious somatic depression, but not pure depression, was associated with distress over maternal limitations. Adolescent girls and women who reported distress over the achievement and occupational limits their mothers had experienced were much more likely to report anxious somatic depression including headaches, fatigue, sleep problems, and disordered eating (Silverstein, Caceres, Perdue, & Cimarolli, 1995; Silverstein & Blumenthal, 1997; Silverstein & Lynch, 1998).

Girls are more likely than boys to be victims of sexual abuse in childhood, and subsequently are at greater risk for depression and anxiety disorders (Weiss, Longhurst, & Mazure, 1999). Adverse events in childhood, particularly sexual abuse, may activate the hypothalamic-pituitary-adrenal axis (HPA), resulting in a perpetuating negative feedback loop; this hypercortisolism can contribute to symptoms such as fatigue and depression (Kiecolt-Glaser, McGuire, Robles, & Glaser, 2002). Wolkowitz and Reus (1999) found that once cortisol levels rise, they can perpetuate depressive behaviors and symptoms such as anxiety, insomnia, and poor memory.

Recent neurobiological studies on the effects of chronic stress report converging evidence for decreased rather than increased cortisol secretion in a variety of disorders such as posttraumatic stress syndrome (PTSD), CFS, fibromyalgia, chronic pelvic pain, and burnout with physical complaints (Heim, Ehlert, & Hellhammer, 2000). Thus, the risk factors for depression appear to result in divergent HPA axis abnormalities. Early childhood sexual abuse and trauma can result in hypercortisolism in some cases, whereas in others it appears to result in hypocortisolism (Heim et al., 1999). Thus, early abuse can initiate a trajectory whose outcome is depression, anxiety, and a hyperactive HPA axis or PTSD, CFS, other fatigue and pain disorders characterized by a hypoactive HPA axis. Similarly, evidence indicates that one subtype of depression (melancholic) is associated with increased levels of cortisol and another subtype (atypical) is associated with decreased levels of cortisol. We examine these depression subtypes in the next section.

Atypical versus Melancholic Depression

The two major subtypes of unipolar depression are melancholic and atypical depression (Gold, Goodwin, & Chrousos, 1988; Gold & Chrousos, 1998). In particular, atypical depression affords insight into the relationship between depression and fatigue. Melancholic and atypical depression are in some ways antithetical. Melancholic depression symptoms include hyperarousal, anxiety, decreased sleep and appetite, variable energy levels, centrally activated HPA axis, increased autonomic sympathetic activity, and relative immunosuppression (Gold, Goodwin, & Chrousos, 1988). Hyperactivity of the HPA axis and higher production of cortisol is a well-documented event in depression (Carroll, Curtis, & Mendels, 1976; Kalin et al., 1987; Kathol, 1985). A smaller subgroup of depressed patients present with symptoms including hypoarousal, increased sleep and food intake, pronounced inertia and fatigue, hypoactivity of the HPA axis, low locus coeruleus norepinephrine activity, decreased sympathetic activity, and relative immunoactivation (Gold, Goodwin, & Chrousos, 1988; Gold et al., 2002; Tsigos & Chrousos, 2002). This subtype has been labeled atypical depression. The neuroendocrinology of atypical depression differs from melancholic depression. Evidence suggests that the prominent atypical depression features of lethargy, fatigue, hypersomnia, and hyperphagia are associated with hyposecretion of hypothalamic corticotropin-releasing factor (CRF) (Gold, Gabry, Yasuda, & Chrousos, 2002).

Both syndromes include loss of everyday pleasure and diminished libido. Fatigue is more prominent in atypical depression, whereas anxiety, agitation, and hyperarousal are prevalent in melancholic depression. Clinically, many patients do not present with a clearly distinctive subtype but rather a mixture of these characteristics. A community study of 8116 Ontario residents found 653 (8%) people met criteria for current or lifetime major depression. Of these, 53 percent had neither melancholic nor atypical, while 30 percent had only melancholic and 12 percent had episodes with only atypical features; 6 percent had both types of episodes (Levitan, Lesage, Parikh, Goering, & Kennedy, 1997). Physiologically and in symptom presentation, atypical depression looks more like CFS than does melancholic depression, but no research to date has addressed these similarities directly by comparing the two patient groups.

Neurobiology of Depression

Disturbances in the serotonin (5-HT) and norepinephrine (NE) systems and the limbic hypothalamic–pituitary–adrenal (LHPA) axis are the neurobiological alterations most consistently associated with depression (Gold, Goodwin, & Chrousos, 1988; Nemeroff, 1998). The LHPA regulates arousal, sleep, appetite, and the capacity to experience and enjoy pleasure, as well as controlling mood.

The preponderance of somatic symptoms may be partly associated with the underlying neurobiology of depression. Both fatigue and bodily pains, including pain in the abdomen, chest, head, back, and joints, are modulated in part by 5-HT and NE neurotransmission. Many of the cognitive and attention deficits seen in depression are thought to be partly modulated by activity in the prefrontal cortex (Drevets, 2000a, 2000b), which receives strong NE and 5-HT projections. Both 5-HT and NE also send projections to the caudate and cerebellum, which may play roles in the psychomotor retardation common in some forms of depression. 5 NE and 5-HT also appear to have modulatory roles in the spinal cord, where they suppress routine physiological input from the periphery from reaching consciousness. Thus, 5-HT and NE system dysfunction, which often occurs in depression, may allow these peripheral signals that would normally be ignored to reach consciousness, where they are interpreted as pain or fatigue. This results in increased somatic disturbances and subsequent symptom reports of fatigue or pain (Stahl, 2002).

Functional Neurobiology of Depression and Anxiety Symptoms

Only recently have studies attempted to look at the functional neuroanatomy associated with specific symptom factors in depression and anxiety. These studies have examined regional brain functioning through positron emission tomographic (PET) imaging. Neuroimaging studies have found similarities between anxiety and psychomotor retardation/sadness, both of which are associated with increased activity in the ventral prefrontal cortex (VPFC), anterior cingulate gyrus (AC), insula, and anterior temporal lobe. Only psychomotor retardation/sadness has been associated with decreased activity in the dorsolateral prefrontal cortex (DLPFC) (Mayberg et al., 1999; Liotti et al., 2000).

Brody and colleagues (2001) examined the relationship between improvement in specific depression symptom clusters and change in regional brain metabolism in outpatients with major depressive disorder after treatment with either paroxetine or interpersonal psychotherapy. They found that improvement in anxiety, psychomotor retardation, tension, and, fatigue was associated with decreased metabolism in the ventral frontal lobe, improvement in anxiety and tension was also associated with decreasing ventral AC and anterior insula activity. Psychomotor retardation improvement was associated with increasing dorsal AC activity, whereas improvement in cognitive disturbance (guilt, suicidality, agitation, paranoia) was associated with increased DLPFC metabolism. These studies indicate that the AC and the DLPFC are particularly important in the psychomotor slowing and sadness symptoms of depression. Since the AC communicates between the prefrontal cortex and subcortical areas of the limbic system, these findings suggest that a limbic–cortical circuit is critical in modulating depression symptoms.

Depression and Chronic Fatigue Syndrome

This section examines the similarities and differences between CFS and depression (see chapter 9 for a discussion in detail of CFS). The primary symptom in CFS is severe and pervasive fatigue. High levels of somatization in individuals with depression and anxiety (Katon & Russo, 1989; Kirmayer et al., 1993) indicate that CFS may be a somatic depression. Alternatively, high rates of depression and anxiety in CFS may result from overlapping symptomatology, reaction to disability imposed by fatigue, or viral-indicator immune changes in the brain. Although CFS subjects may meet diagnostic criteria for depressive disorder or score in the depressed range on a self-report inventory, they report significantly lower levels of dysphoria and self-reproach symptoms than clinically depressed patients (Johnson et al., 1996; Powell, Dolan, & Wessely, 1990). Patients with CFS are significantly less likely than depressed, MS, or healthy controls to interpret symptoms in terms of negative emotional states (Dendy, Cooper, & Sharpe, 2001). Unlike depressed patients whose cognitions are dominated by a negative view of the self, CFS patients make physical attributions for their symptoms, which helps maintain their self-esteem (Moss-Morris & Petrie, 2001).

HPA axis abnormalities have been widely studied in CFS and generally involve a mild hypocortisolism of central origin, in contrast to the hypercortisolism seen in major depression. CFS symptoms have been noted to be similar to those found in adrenal insufficiency (flulike symptoms, fatigue, malaise, arthralgias, myalgias, sleep problems, and dizziness) (Parker, Wessely, & Cleare, 2001).

CFS subjects generally demonstrate greater impairment than depressed subjects on a variety of measures of functional disability (Natelson et al., 1995; Buchwald, Pearlman, Umali, Schmaling, & Katon, 1996). Despite frequent use of antidepressants for fatigue, Dzurec (2000; Dzurec et al., 2002) concludes that antidepressants provide little long-term amelioration of fatigue in patients with normal laboratory values. In a double-blind, placebo-controlled study, fluoxetine had no beneficial effect in patients with CFS, with or without depression (Vercoulen et al., 1996). Sleep patterns of CFS and depressed patients differ. These studies suggest that CFS can be separated from most subtypes of depression, though it still resembles atypical depression in neuroendocrine responses.

Brain Abnormalities

Several studies have reported significantly more abnormalities on MRI among CFS subjects than in controls (Natelson, Cohen, Brassloff, & Lee, 1993; Buchwald et al., 1992; Lange et al., 1999; Cook, Lange, DeLuca, & Natelson, 2001), while others (Schwartz et al., 1994; Cope & David, 1996) have found no significant differences. Lange and associates (1999) found brain abnormalities clustered in the nonpsychiatric rather than the psychiatric CFS cases. Specifically, there were higher levels of T2 hyperintensities in the subcortical white matter of the frontal lobes among CFS subjects without psychiatric disorders. When MRI abnormalities are found, they consistently occur in the cerebral white matter of CFS patients. Cook and coworkers (2001) found that the most functionally disabled CFS patients had the greatest number of MRI abnormalities.

Similarly, white matter hyperintensity on MRI has been the most consistently replicated finding in structural neuroimaging studies of depression (Schweitzer, Tuckwell, Ames, & O'Brien, 2001). Thus, it is somewhat surprising that nondepressed CFS patients would be more likely to show white matter abnormalities, if such hyperintensities were due solely to depression. Studies have also demonstrated abnormalities on SPECT in CFS. Decreases in global regional cerebral blood flow (rCBF) throughout the brain have been reported in CFS groups compared to healthy controls (Ichise et al., 1992; Schwartz et al., 1994). Moreover, significantly greater brainstem hypoperfusion on SPECT has been found in patients with CFS than in controls and depressed patients (Costa, Tannock, & Brostoff, 1995); hypoperfusion was also greater in CFS patients without psychiatric disturbance. Machale and colleagues (2000) compared regional cerebral perfusion in healthy, CFS, and major depression groups. They found that CFS and depression were associated with increased blood flow to the right thalamus, whereas only the depressed group had decreased perfusion in the left prefrontal cortex. The researchers speculate that thalamic hyperperfusion may be linked to the similar disturbances of motor and effort perception in depression and CFS (Lawrie, MacHale, Power, & Goodwin, 1997).

As the thalamus plays a crucial role in motor and cognitive coordination, its overactivity may reflect increased need to attend to previously automatic motor and cognitive tasks, thus increasing effort. Yet, Schmaling, Lewis, Fiedelak, Mahurin, and Buchwald (2003) found a pattern of diffuse regional cerebral blood flow among subjects with CFS compared with the more focal pattern among healthy subjects when performing the Paced Auditory Serial Addition Test (PASAT). Although CFS subjects showed less perfusion in the anterior cingulate region, the change in CFS subjects' activation of the left anterior cingulate region during performance of the PASAT was greater than that observed in healthy subjects. In both CFS and depression, fatigue appears to be associated with limbic system dysfunction and white matter abnormalities, although the left prefrontal cortex may be differentially affected in depressed patients.

Functional and structural neuroimaging findings have not been well integrated for either CFS or depression. A recent study (Oda et al., 2003) investigated associations of MRI-defined subcortical hyperintensities with rCBF changes in depressed patients. Depressed patients, with or without subcortical MRI hyperintensities, and healthy volunteers underwent SPECT scanning. Both groups of depressed patients showed decreased rCBF compared with control subjects in the frontal lobe, temporal lobe, and anterior cingulate gyrus; however, only the depressed patients with MRI hyperintensity showed decreased rCBF in the thalamus, basal ganglia, and brainstem in addition to cortical areas. White matter hyperintensity correlated negatively with rCBF in subcortical brain structures, including the thalamus and right basal ganglia. Thus, it appears that depressed patients with white matter hyperintensities are more likely to have subcortical and limbic involvement. Unfortunately, Oda and associates' findings do not replicate those of Machale and coworkers (2000) discussed earlier, which showed *increased* blood flow to the thalamus in both CFS and depressed patients. To clarify current inconsistencies, future studies need to perform alternating SPECT and MRI in CFS patients; such studies should include a depressed group and a CFS with depression group for comparison.

Cytokines in Depression and Fatigue

Cytokines are proteins that mediate between immune cells and brain cells (Kronfol & Remick, 2000). Infusion of cytokines in healthy people produces symptoms of fatigue, depression, myalgia, low-grade fever, and confused thinking (Maier & Watkins, 2000). Recent data indicate that cytokines recruit hypothalamic CRH in a negative feedback loop in which glucocortocoids prevent the immune response from becoming overactivated. Thus, if hypothalamic CRH is insufficient (which may be the case in atypical depression and CFS), restraint of the immune activation could fail (Gold et al., 2002). Immune activation, particularly via the circulating cytokines interleukin-1 (IL-1), interleuken-2, interleukin-6, and tumor necrosis factor levels, has been shown to be greater in depression (Anisman & Merali, 2002). Several studies of CFS have found elevated cytokine levels in some patients (Cannon et al., 1999; Patarca, 2001). Musselman and colleagues (2001) found cancer patients with depression have higher concentrations of IL-6. Wallace and coworkers (2001) found elevated IL-6 and IL-8 levels in fibromylagia patients compared to healthy controls. Cytokines may be a marker for a mind–body connection between distress and fatigue, but because the data are correlational, it is not known whether increased activity of cytokines is secondary to depression, stress, or illness or plays a role in provoking these states. Musselman and associates speculate that IL-6 contributes to "sickness behavior," that is, fatigue, loss of appetite, loss of interest in activity, and poorer self-care—symptoms that clearly overlap with depression. Thus, patients with fatiguing illnesses such as cancer, fibromyalgia, and CFS may be at risk for depression because increased peripheral release of cytokines affects the nervous system. Iversen and Wessely (2003) note significant comorbidity between depression, chronic fatigue, and physical illnesses such as fibromyalgia, lupus, and cancer (see other chapters in this volume).

Studies assessing structural and functional neuroimaging, neuroendocrine, and cytokine abnormalities point to neuropathology in CFS patients. In studies stratified according to psychiatric status, neuropathogical abnormalities appear to be more prominent in CFS subjects without psychiatric disorder. Nonetheless, the neurophysiology of CFS is similar in some ways to that of depression in terms of white matter hyperintensities, HPA axis dysfunction (although in the opposing direction from melancholic depression), elevated cytokines, limbic system abnormalities, and of course, the predominant symptom of fatigue. This data suggest a possible brain model of fatigue in depression. Fatigue symptoms that accompany depression could be modulated through decreased activity in the dorsal AC and its limbic–cortical connections. The prefrontal cortex dysfunction seen in depression could affect its strong NE and 5-HT projections, resulting in reduced NE and 5-HT transmission that may increase somatic sensitivity to fatigue through disinhibiting thalamic, caudate, cerebellum, or even spinal cord inputs. Cortisol dysfunction can increase cytokine release, resulting in fatiguing symptoms as well.

The Genetics of Depression, Anxiety, and Fatigue

Population-based twin studies provide etiological insights into environmental and genetic contributions to anxiety, depression, and fatigue. Multivariate analysis suggests that the liability of female twins to anxiety and depression is influenced by the same genetic factors, so whether a vulnerable woman develops major depression or generalized anxiety disorder depends on her environmental experiences (Kendler et al., 1992; Kendler, 1996). A study of 1004 twin pairs (Hickie et al., 1999) found a common genetic factor for somatic distress, anxiety, and depression; an independent genetic factor that contributes to more severe forms of anxiety and depression; and a third independent genetic factor that contributes to fatigue only. Hickie and colleagues (1999) concluded that 44 percent of genetic variance in chronic fatigue was not shared by anxiety and depression.

Gillespie, Zhu, Heath, Hickie, and Martin (2000) examined 3469 Australian twins, measuring depression, phobic anxiety, somatic distress, and sleep difficulty. They found 33 percent of genetic variance in somatic distress was due to specific gene action unrelated to depression or phobic anxiety; 74 percent of environmental influence on somatic distress was unrelated to depression or anxiety. Although these studies indicate that fatigue symptoms are etiologically distinct from anxiety and depression, Roy-Bryne and colleagues (2002) found no such evidence in a sample of 100 female twin pairs. Their study used more stringent criteria for fatigue, requiring prolonged fatigue of at least 6 months, and they found a strong association between fatigue and psychological distress without evidence of genetic covariation.

Conclusion

Fatigue is both a dominant symptom of and risk factor for depression, and the conditions share several neurobiological abnormalities. A number of studies have isolated fatigue as an independent construct, and others reveal strong associations between the two states. Some evidence supports the idea that fatigue states appear to present subtle variations on depression; other evidence argues for a pure fatigue state, with little overlap with depression. Most likely both exist in the heterogeneous fatigue population. Patients with CF do not present with a depressive cognitive style, they make pervasive physical attributions for symptoms, are generally unresponsive to antidepressant drugs, are more disabled than depressed patients, have increased serotonin levels, and do not exhibit the hyperarousal or hyperactivation of the HPA axis that is seen in most depressed patients. On the other hand, both CF and depression affect women more than men and show similar white matter hyperintensities, HPA axis dysfunction (in atypical depression), elevated cytokines, and limbic system abnormalities.

There may be at least two subtypes of fatigue states, one more psychosocial in origin and one characterized by brain pathology. Both subtypes overlap with chronic fatigue syndromes. As long as the dependent variable remains self-report, however, we are unable to differentiate between the two substypes. Future research needs to examine whether there is evidence for a neurologically based fatigue characterized by psychomotor retardation and profound lethargy. The neurobiology of this fatigue state may include elevated cytokines, MRI hyperintensities, low activation of HPA axis, limbic–prefrontal cortex abnormalities, and serotonin dysfunction. Functional neuroimaging of regions such as the thalamus and anterior cingulate may be particularly fruitful. The psychosocial subtype characterized by a subjective sense of tiredness and a cycle of deconditioning may respond to cognitive behavioral therapy. A more neurologically based fatigue may respond to pharmacological potentiators of CRH secretion and action to activate the HPA axis and increase locus coeruleus–NE responses (Tsigos & Chrousos, 2002).

References

Addington, A. M., Gallo, J. J., Ford, D. E., & Eaton, W. W. (2001). Epidemiology of unexplained fatigue and major depression in the community: the Baltimore ECA follow-up, 1981–1994. *Psychological Medicine, 31*, 1037–1044.

American Psychiatric Association. (1994). *Diagnostic and statistical manual of mental disorders*, 4th ed. Washington, DC: American Psychiatric Association.

Anisman, H., & Merali, Z. (2002). Cytokines, stress, and depressive illness. *Brain, Behavior, and Immunity, 16*, 513–524.

Brody, A. L., Saxena, S., Mandelkern, M., Fairbanks, L. A., Ho, M. L., & Baxter, Jr. L. R. (2001). Brain metabolic changes associated with symptom factor improvement in major depressive disorder. *Biological Psychiatry, 50*, 171–178.

Buchwald, D. P. R., Cheney, D. I., Peterson, B., et al. (1992). A chronic illness characterized by fatigue, neurologic and immunologic disorders, and active human herpesvirus type 6 infection. *Annals of Internal Medicine, 116*, 103–113.

Buchwald, D., Pearlman, T., Umali, J., Schmaling, K., & Katon, W. (1996). Functional status in patients with chronic fatigue syndrome, other fatiguing illnesses, and healthy individuals. *American Medical Journal, 101*, 364–370.

Cannon, J. G., Angel, J. B., Ball, R. W., Abad, L. W., Fagioli, L., & Komaroff, A. L. (1999). Acute phase responses and cytokine secretion in chronic fatigue syndrome. *Journal of Clinical Immunology, 19*, 414–421.

Carroll, B. J., Curtis, G. C., & Mendels, J. (1976). Neuroendocrine regulation in depression. II. Discrimination of depressed from nondepressed patients. *Archives of General Psychiatry, 33(9)*, 1051–1058.

Cook, D. B., Lange, G., DeLuca, J., & Natelson, B. H. (2001). Relationship of brain MRI abnormalities and physical functional status in chronic fatigue syndrome. *International Journal of Neuroscience, 107*, 1–6.

Cope, H., & David, A. S. (1996). Neuroimaging in chronic fatigue syndrome. *Journal of Neurology, Neurosurgery & Psychiatry, 60,* 471–477.

Costa, D. C., Tannock, C., & Brostoff, J. (1995). Brainstem perfusion is impaired in chronic fatigue syndrome. *Quarterly Journal of Medicine, 88,* 767–763.

Dendy, C., Cooper, M., & Sharpe, M. (2001). Interpretation of symptoms in chronic fatigue syndrome. *Behavior Research & Therapy, 39,* 1369–1380.

Drevets, W. C. (2000a). Neuroimaging studies of mood disorders. *Biological Psychiatry, 48,* 813–829.

Drevets, W. C. (2000b). Functional anatomical abnormalities in limbic and prefrontal cortical structures in major depression. *Progress in Brain Research, 126,* 413–431.

Dzurec, L. C. (2000). Fatigue and relatedness experiences of inordinately tired women. *Journal of Nursing Scholarship, 32,* 339–345.

Dzurec, L. C., Hoover, P. M., & Fields, J. (2002). Acknowledging unexplained fatigue of tired women (Clinical Scholarship). *Journal of Nursing Scholarship, 34,* 41.

Gillespie, N. A., Zhu, G., Heath, A. C., Hickie, I. B., & Martin, N. G. (2000). The genetic aetiology of somatic distress. *Psychological Medicine, 30,* 1051–1061.

Gold, P. W., & Chrousos, G. P. (1998). The endocrinology of melancholic and atypical depression: relation to neurocircuitry and somatic consequences. *Proceedings of the Association of American Physicians, 111,* 22–34.

Gold, P. W., Gabry, K. E., Yasuda, M. R., & Chrousos, G. P. (2002). Divergent endocrine abnormalities in melancholic and atypical depression: clinical and pathophysiologic implications. *Endocrinology Metabolic Clinics of North America, 31,* 37–62.

Gold, P. W., Goodwin, F. K., & Chrousos, G. P. (1988). Clinical and biochemical manifestations of depression. *New England Journal of Medicine, 319,* 413–420.

Heim, C., Ehlert, U., Hanker, J. O., & Hellhammer, D. H. (1999). Psychological and endocrine correlates of chronic pelvic pain associated with adhesions. *Journal of Psychosomatic Obstetrics & Gynecology, 20,* 11–20.

Heim, C., Ehlert, U., & Hellhammer, D. H. (2000). The potential role of hypocortisolism in the pathophysiology of stress-related bodily disorders. *Psychoneuroendocrinology, 25,* 1–35.

Hickie, I., Kirk, K., & Martin, N. (1999). Unique genetic and environmental determinants of prolonged fatigue: a twin study. *Psychological Medicine, 29,* 259–268.

Ichise, M., Salit, I. E., Abbey, S. E., Chung, D.-G., Gray, B., Kirsh, J. C., & Freedman, M. (1992). Assessment of regional cerebral perfusion by[99]Tc[m]-HMPAO SPECT in chronic fatigue syndrome. *Nuclear Medicine Communications, 13,* 767–772.

Iversen, A., & Wessely, S. (2003). Chronic fatigue and depression. *Current Opinion in Psychiatry, 16,* 17–21.

Johnson, S. K., DeLuca, J., & Natelson, B. (1996). Depression in fatiguing illness: comparing patients with chronic fatigue syndrome, multiple sclerosis and depression. *Journal of Affective Disorders, 39,* 21–30.

Kalin, N. H., Dawson, G., Tariot, P. Shelton, S., Barksdale, C., Weiler, S., & Thienemann, M. (1987). Function of the adrenal cortex in patients with major depression. *Psychiatry Research, 22(2),* 117–125.

Kathol, R. G. (1985). Persistent elevation of urinary free cortisol and loss of circannual periodicity in recovered depressive patients. A trait finding. *Journal of Affective Disorders, 8(2),* 137–145.

Katon, W., & Russo, J. (1989). Somatic symptoms and depression. *The Journal of Family Practice, 29,* 65–69.

Kendler, K. S. (1996). Major depression and generalized anxiety disorder. Same genes (partly) different environments—revisited. *British Journal of Psychiatry (Suppl 30),* 68–75.

Kendler, K. S., Neale, M. C., Kessler, R. C., Heath, A. C., & Eaves, L. J. (1992). Major depression and generalized anxiety disorder. Same genes (partly) different environments? *Archives of General Psychiatry, 49,* 716–722.

Khan, A. A., Gardner, C. O., Prescott, C. A., & Kendler, K. S. (2002). Gender differences in the symptoms of major depression in opposite-sex dizygotic twin pairs. *American Journal of Psychiatry, 159,* 1427–1429.

Kiecolt-Glaser, J. K., McGuire, L., Robles, T. F., & Glaser, R. (2002). Emotions, morbidity, and mortality: new perspectives from psychoneuroimmunology. *Annual Review of Psychology, 53,* 83–107.

Kirk, K. M., Hickie, I. B., & Martin, N. G. (1999). Fatigue as related to anxiety and depression in a community-based sample of twins aged over 50. *Social Psychiatry Psychiatric Epidemiology, 34,* 85–90.

Kirmayer, L. J., Robbins, J. M., Dworkind, M., & Yaffe, M. J. (1993). Somatization and the recognition of depression and anxiety in primary care. *American Journal of Psychiatry, 150,* 734–741.

Kroenke, K., Spitzer, R. L., Williams, J. B., et al. (1994). Physical symptoms in primary care: predictors of psychiatric disorders and functional impairment. *Archives of Family Medicine, 3,* 774–779.

Kronfol, Z., & Remick, D. G. (2000). Cytokines and the brain: implications for clinical psychiatry. *American Journal of Psychiatry, 157,* 683–694.

Lange, G., DeLuca, J., Maldjian, J. A., Lee, H., Tiersky, L. A., & Natelson, B. H. (1999). Brain MRI abnormalities exist in a subset of patients with chronic fatigue syndrome. *Journal of Neurological Science, 171,* 3–7.

Lawrie, S. M., MacHale, S. M., Power, M. J., & Goodwin, G. M. (1997). Is chronic fatigue syndrome best understood as a primary disturbance of the sense of effort? *Psychological Medicine, 27,* 995–999.

Levitan, R. D., Lesage, A., Parikh, S. V., Goering, P., & Kennedy, S. H. (1997). Reversed neurovegetative symptoms of depression: a community study of Ontario. *American Journal of Psychiatry, 154*, 934–940.

Liotti, M., Mayberg, H. S., Brannan, S. K., McGinnis, S., Jerabek, P., & Fox, P. T. (2000). Differential limbic-cortical correlates of sadness and anxiety in healthy subjects: implications for affective disorders. *Biological Psychiatry, 48*, 30–42.

Machale, S. M., Lawrie, S. M., Cavanagh, J. T. O., Glabus, M. F., Murray, C. L., Goodwin, G. M., & Ebmeier, K. P. (2000). Cerebral perfusion in chronic fatigue syndrome and depression. *British Journal of Psychiatry, 176*, 550–556.

Maier, W., Gansicke, M., Gater, R., Rezaki, M., Tiemens, B., & Urzua, R. F. (1999). Gender differences in the prevalence of depression: a survey in primary care. *Journal of Affective Disorders, 53*, 241–252.

Maier, W., Gansicke, M., Gater, R., Rezaki, M., Tiemens, B., & Urzua, R. F. (1999). Gender differences in the prevalence of depression: a survey in primary care. *Journal of Affective Disorders, 53*, 241–252.

Maier, S. F., & Watkins, L. R. (2000). The immune system as a sensory system: implications for psychology. *Current Directions in Psychological Science, 9*, 98–102.

Maurice-Tison, S., Verdoux, H., Gay, B., Perez, P., Salamon, R., & Bourgeois, M. L. (1998). How to improve recognition and diagnosis of depressive syndromes using international diagnostic criteria. *British Journal of General Practice, 48*, 1245–1246.

Mayberg, H. S., Liotti, M., Brannan, S. K., McGinnis, S., Mahurin, R. K., Jerabek, P. A., Silva, J. A., Tekell, J. L., Martin, C. C., Lancaster, J. L., & Fox, P. T. (1999). Reciprocal limbic-cortical function and negative mood: converging PET findings in depression and normal sadness. *American Journal of Psychiatry, 156*, 675–682.

Moss-Morris, R., & Petrie, K. J. (2001). Discriminating between chronic fatigue syndrome and depression: a cognitive analysis. *Psychological Medicine, 31*, 469–479.

Musselman, D., Miller, A., Porter, M., Manatunga, A., Gao, F., Penna, S., Pearce, B., Landry, J., Glover, S., McDaniel, J., & Nemeroff, C. (2001). Higher than normal plasma interleukin-6 concentrations in cancer patients with depression: preliminary findings. *American Journal of Psychiatry, 158*, 1252–1257.

Natelson, B. H., Cohen, J. M., Brassloff, I., & Lee, H. J. (1993). A controlled study of brain magnetic resonance imaging in patients with fatiguing illnesses. *Journal of the Neurological Sciences, 120*, 213–217.

Natelson, B. H., Johnson, S. K., DeLuca, J., Sisto, S., Ellis, S. P., Hill, N., & Bergen, M. T. (1995). Reducing heterogeneity in chronic fatigue syndrome: a comparison with depression and multiple sclerosis. *Clinical Infectious Diseases, 21*, 1204–1210.

Nemeroff, C. B. (1998). Psychopharmacology of affective disorders in the 21st century. *Biological Psychiatry, 44(7)*, 517–525.

Oda, K., Ishida, R., Murata, Y., et al. (2003). Regional cerebral blood flow in depressed patients with white matter magnetic resonance hyperintensity. *Biological Psychiatry, 53*, 150–156.

Parker, A. J. R., Wessely, S., & Cleare, A. J. (2001). The neuroendocrinology of chronic fatigue and fibromyalgia. *Psychological Medicine, 31*, 1331–1345.

Patarca, R. (2001). Cytokines and chronic fatigue syndrome. *Annals New York Academy of Sciences, 933*, 185–200.

Piccinelli, M., & Wilkinson, G. (2000). Gender differences in depression. *British Journal of Psychiatry, 177*, 486–492.

Posse, M., & Hallstrom, T. (1998). Depressive disorders among somatizing patients in primary health care. *Acta Psychiatric Scandanavia, 98*, 187–192.

Powell, R., Dolan, R., & Wessely, S. (1990). Attributions and self-esteem in depression and chronic fatigue syndrome. *Journal of Psychosomatic Research, 21*, 665–673.

Racciatti, D., Guagnano, M. T., Vecchiet, J., De Remigis, P. L., Pizzigallo, E., Della Vecchia, R., Di Sciascio, T., Merlitti, D., & Sensi, S. (2001). Chronic fatigue syndrome: circadian rhythm and hypothalamic-pituitary-adrenal (HPA) axis impairment. *International Journal Immunopathology and Pharmacology, 14*, 11–15.

Roy-Byrne, P., Afari, N., Ashton, S., Fischer, M., Goldberg, J., & Buchwald, D. (2002). Chronic fatigue and anxiety/depression: a twin study. *British Journal of Psychiatry, 180*, 29–34.

Schmaling, K. B., Lewis, D. H., Fiedelak, J. I., Mahurin, R., & Buchwald, D. S. (2003). Single-photon emission computerized tomography and neurocognitive function in patients with chronic fatigue syndrome. *Psychosomatic Medicine, 65*, 129–136.

Schwartz, R. B., Garada, B. M., Komaroff, A. L., Tice, H. M., Gleit, M., Jolesz, F. A., & Holman, B. L. (1994). Detection of intracranial abnormalities in patients with chronic fatigue syndrome: comparison of MR imaging and SPECT. *American Journal of Radiology, 162*, 935–941.

Schwartz, R. B., Komaroff, A. L., Garada, B. M., Gleit, M., Doolittle, T. H., Bates, D. W., Vasile, R. G., & Holman, B. L. (1994). SPECT imaging of the brain: comparison of findings in patients with chronic fatigue syndrome, AIDS dementia complex, and major unipolar depression. *American Journal of Radiology, 162*, 943–951.

Schweitzer, I., Tuckwell, V., Ames, D., & O'Brien, J. (2001). Structural neuroimaging studies in late-life depression: a review. *World Journal of Biological Psychiatry, 2*, 83–88.

Silverstein, B. (2002). Gender differences in the prevalence of somatic versus pure depression: a replication. *American Journal of Psychiatry, 159*, 1051–1052.

Silverstein, B., & Blumenthal, E. (1997). Depression mixed with anxiety, somatization, and disordered eating: relationship with gender-role-related limitations experienced by females. *Sex Roles, 36*, 709–724.

Silverstein, B., Caceres, J., Perdue, L., & Cimarolli, V. (1995). Gender differences in depressive symptomatology: the role played by "anxious somatic depression" associated with gender-related achievement concerns. *Sex Roles, 33,* 621–636.

Silverstein, B., & Lynch, A. (1998). Gender differences in depression: the role played by paternal attitudes of male superiority and maternal modeling of gender-related limitations. *Sex Roles, 38,* 539–555.

Simon, G. E., VonKorff, M., Piccinelli, M., Fullerton, C., & Ormel, J. (1999). An international study of the relation between somatic symptoms and depression. *New England Journal of Medicine, 341,* 1329–1335.

Stahl, S. (2002). The shared neurobiology of depression and painful physical symptoms. Abstract 15th ECNP Congress, Barcelona, Spain.

Tsigos, C., & Chrousos, G. (2002). Hypothalamic-pituitary-adrenal axis, neuroendocrine factors and stress. *Journal of Psychosomatic Research, 53,* 865–871.

Tylee, A. (2000). Depression in Europe: experience from the DEPRES II survey. *European Neuropsychopharmacology, 10(Suppl 4),* S445–S448.

Tylee, A., Gastpar, M., Lepine, J. P., & Mendlewicz, J. (1999). DEPRES II (Depression Research in European Society II): a patient survey of the symptoms, disability and current management of depression in the community. *International Clinical psychopharmacology, 14,* 139–151.

van der Linden, G., Chalder, T., Hickie, I., Koschera, A., Sham, P., & Wessely, S. (1999). Fatigue and psychiatric disorder: Different or the same? *Psychological Medicine, 29,* 863–868.

Vercoulen, J. H. M. M., Swanink, C. M. A., Zitman, F. G., Vreden, S. G. S., Hoofs, M. P. H., Fennis, J. F. M., Galama, J., van der Meer, J. W. M., & Bleijenberg, G. (1996). Randomized, double-blind, placebo-controlled study of fluoxetine in chronic fatigue syndrome. *Lancet, 347,* 858–861.

Wallace, D. J., Linker-Israeli, M., Hallegua, D., Silverman, S., Silver, D., & Weisman, M. H. (2001). Cytokines play an aetiopathogenetic role in fibromyalgia: a hypothesis and pilot study. *Rheumatology, 40,* 743–749.

Watt, T., Groenvald, M., Bjorner, J. B., Noerholm, V., Rasmussen, N. A., & Bech, P. (2000). Fatigue in the Danish general population. Influence of sociodemographic factors and disease. *Journal of Epidemiology and Community Health, 54,* 827–833.

Weiss, E. L., Longhurst, J. G., & Mazure, C. M. (1999). Childhood sexual abuse as a risk factor for depression in women: psychosocial and neurobiological correlates. *American Journal of Psychiatry, 156,* 816–828.

Wolkowitz, O. M., & Reus, V. I. (1999). Treatment of depression with antiglucocorticoid drugs. *Psychosomatic Medicine, 61,* 698–711.

World Health Organization. (2002). *WHO Collaborative Study on Psychological Problems in General Health Care.* Geneva: World Health Organization.

11 Fatigue and Somatization

Lesley A. Allen and Javier I. Escobar

The presentation of disabling fatigue and multiple medically unexplained physical symptoms creates both diagnostic and management challenges. Typically, the severity of such complaints fails to correspond with objective assessments of symptoms. Further, somatization and fatigue tend to respond poorly to standard treatments. Once these symptoms become chronic, they often result in severe functional impairment and overuse of healthcare services. This chapter aims to synthesize the empirical literature on the assessment of, treatment of, and potential mechanisms involved in somatization and fatigue syndromes.

Definitions

Somatization Disorder

According to the *Diagnostic and Statistical Manual of Mental Disorders* (DSM-IV), somatization disorder is characterized by a lifetime history of multiple medically unexplained physical symptoms, including at least four unexplained pain symptoms, two unexplained nonpain gastrointestinal symptoms, one unexplained sexual symptom, and one pseudoneurological symptom. Although "fatigue" has not been included as a symptom of somatization disorder in any version of the DSM, DSM-III and DSM-III-R include "muscle weakness" as a possible symptom of somatization disorder, and DSM-IV includes "localized weakness" as a possible symptom.

In addition to their numerous somatic complaints, the health status of these patients is a clinical concern. Many somatization disorder patients meet criteria for other psychiatric disorders (Robins et al., 1984; Swartz, Blazer, George, & Landerman, 1986). These patients have been shown to incur nine times the U.S. per capita health care cost (Smith, Monson, & Ray, 1986). Somatization disorder also creates enormous indirect costs to the economy, in the form of lost productivity and time at work. Individuals diagnosed with somatization disorder report spending 2 to 7 days in bed per month (Smith et al., 1986; Katon et al., 1991).

Abridged Somatization

Although DSM-IV classifies somatization disorder as a distinct disorder, it has been argued that this disorder, rarely encountered in primary care clinics, represents the extreme end of a somatization continuum (Escobar, Burnam, Karno, Forsythe, & Golding, 1987; Escobar, Golding, Hough, Karno, Burnam, & Wells, 1987; Escobar, Waitzkin, Silver, Gara, & Holman, 1998; Katon et al., 1991). Patients experiencing multiple unexplained physical symptoms that fail to meet all DSM-IV criteria for somatization disorder have higher rates of healthcare utilization, disability, and emotional distress than do nonsomatizers (Escobar, Burnam, et al., 1987; Escobar, Golding, et al., 1987; Escobar, et al., 1998; Katon et al., 1991).

Escobar introduced the label "abridged somatization" to describe men complaining of at least four unexplained physical symptoms and women complaining of at least six unexplained physical symptoms (Escobar, Burnam, et al., 1987). The diagnosis of abridged somatization requires fewer symptoms than does the diagnosis of somatization disorder and also eliminates the requirement of four different symptom types (i.e., pseudoneurological, pain, gastrointestinal, and sexual). Research suggests that abridged somatization coincides with increased use of medical services as well as with elevated levels of disability and psychopathology (Escobar, Burnam, et al., 1987; Escobar, Golding et al., 1987; Escobar et al., 1998; Katon et al., 1991). Unlike somatization disorder, moderate levels of somatization are widespread in primary care. The prevalence of abridged somatization has been estimated to be 22 percent (Escobar et al., 1998).

Fatigue as a Symptom and Syndrome

"Fatigue" is an elusive symptom. It is defined as a "lassitude or weariness resulting from either bodily or mental exertion" (Weiner & Simpson, 1989). Despite being one of the most frequently reported complaints in primary care, it is rarely associated with clearcut organic pathology (Lane, Matthews, & Manu, 1990; Valdini, Steinhardt, & Feldman, 1989). Semantic ambiguity interferes with our understanding of this symptom. Patients complaining of fatigue may be referring to one or more subjective experiences, such as feeling tired, exhausted, sleepy, listless, slowed down, uninterested, or depressed. Differences between patients' subjective state and objective measures of fatigue add to the vagueness of the fatigue construct. The interval during which the symptom is experienced is also often unclear. *Chronic fatigue* usually refers to fatigue lasting at least 6 months. When chronic fatigue is accompanied by at least four symptoms (e.g., memory impairment, sore throat, tender lymph nodes, muscle pain, joint pain, headache, nonrestorative sleep, or postexertional fatigue) a diagnosis of *chronic fatigue syndrome (CFS)* is applied (Fukuda et al., 1994). With an estimated prevalence of 10 to 20 percent in primary care clinics, chronic fatigue appears to be significantly more common than is full CFS (Bates et al., 1993; Pawlikowska et al., 1994).

Medically unexplained fatigue that interferes with patients' functioning is a public health concern. High rates of disability, use of health care, and psychiatric distress have been associated with chronic fatigue as well as CFS (Bombardier & Buchwald, 1996; Kroenke, Wood, Mangelsdorff, Meier, & Powell, 1988; Sharpe, Hawton, Seagroatt, & Pasvol, 1992). Fatigue experienced concomitantly with psychiatric symptoms such as depression appears to be particularly debilitating (Cathebras, Robbins, Kirmayer, & Hayton, 1992; Hickie, Davenport, Issakidid, & Andrews, 2002; Walker, Katon, & Jemelka, 1993). Patients presenting with chronic fatigue are likely to meet the criteria for comorbid affective, anxiety, and also somatoform disorders (Addington, Gallo, Ford, & Eaton, 2001; Kroenke et al., 1988; Walker et al., 1993). Data from the Epidemiologic Catchment Area Program show the number of somatization symptoms to be the strongest predictor of both new and chronic idiopathic fatigue (Addington et al., 2001).

Nosological Issues

The nosology of unexplained physical symptoms, including fatigue, is controversial. Are somatization and chronic fatigue separate syndromes? Is fatigue a symptom of somatization? Does comorbid fatigue and somatization represent a distinct syndrome that is more severe than either syndrome alone? In the absence of a gold standard, there are no clear answers to these questions.

A review of the literature suggests that patients meeting criteria for abridged somatization, somatization disorder, chronic fatigue, or CFS share many clinical and behavioral characteristics. In fact, many patients meet criteria for all four conditions. This is not to suggest, however, that the same mechanism is producing all unexplained physical symptoms. The pathophysiologies of these syndromes have yet to be defined, and the syndromes have not been carefully differentiated from each other.

Assessment of Somatization and Fatigue

Assessing somatization and idiopathic fatigue is complicated by various factors. Often, discrepancies exist between patients' subjective reports of their symptoms and objective findings. Physicians and patients may not share the same terminology. Patients may present incomplete or inaccurate histories of their complaints. Also, somatization and fatigue are multifaceted conditions.

Structured Clinical Interviews

Capturing the complexities of these patients' conditions requires a comprehensive medical, psychiatric, and psychosocial assessment. Structured clinical interviews, such as the Structured Clinical Interview for DSM-IV (SCID) (First, Spitzer, Gibbon, & Williams, 1997) and the Composite International Diagnostic Schedule (CIDI) (Robins,

Wing, Wittchen, & Helzer, 1988) facilitate eliciting and diagnosing somatoform disorders and other psychiatric disorders.

Self-Administered Instruments

Because diagnostic status may not represent a valid measure of severity of distress or impairment, additional information on the impact of symptoms on personal wellbeing should be explored. Behaviors, cognitions, and emotions associated with medically unexplained symptoms all contribute to impaired functioning (Cathebras, Robbins, Kirmayer, & Hayton, 1992; Katon et al., 1991; Petrie, Moss-Morris, & Weinman, 1995; Sharpe, Hawton, et al., 1992; Smith et al., 1986). Self-report questionnaires used to assess the severity of somatization include the somatization scale of the SCL-90-R (Derogatis, 1977), the SUNYA Psychosomatic Checklist (Attanasio, Andrasik, Blanchard, & Arena, 1984), and the Somatic Symptom Inventory (Barsky & Wyshak, 1990). Despite their usefulness in quantifying patients' level of physical discomfort, self-report scales cannot substitute for diagnostic interviews because these scales fail to assess the nature of the physical symptoms. These self-report measures count medically explained as well as medically unexplained symptoms toward the total somatization score.

Measures of Related Behaviors and Beliefs

Perhaps more important than the number and intensity of symptoms is the quality of patients' lives. Functional impairment may be quantified with questionnaires such as the Medical Outcomes Study (MOS-SF-36) (Ware & Sherbourne, 1992) and the Sickness Impact Scale (Gilson et al., 1975), both of which are behaviorally based measures of health status. The Illness Attitude Scale (Kellner, 1987) and Coping Strategies Questionnaires (Swartzman, Gwadry, Shapiro, Teasell, 1994) can be administered to assess dysfunctional beliefs and coping behaviors.

Assessing Fatigue

Given the frequent co-occurrence of fatigue and somatization, how fatigue is assessed becomes extremely important. As noted earlier, although "fatigue" is not included in the diagnostic criteria for somatization disorder or abridged somatization, "localized weakness" is one of the pseudoneurological symptoms of these disorders. Self-report instruments used to assess somatic symptoms probe "fatigue" along with other common somatic symptoms. Although fatigue is not a key symptom for distinguishing between somatoform and nonsomatoform patients, it is predictive of severity of somatic distress.

Treatment of Fatigue and Somatization

The treatment of persistent fatigue and somatization is in its infancy. Little research supports the use of psychotropic medication for chronic fatigue or for somatization

(Voltz, Moller, Reimann, & Stoll, 2000; Whiting et al., 2001). Some clinicians describe frequent adverse reactions to pharmacological agents, but other clinicians advocate treating comorbid depressive or anxiety disorders with antidepressants and anxiolytics (Sharpe & Wilks, 2002; Wessely, 2001). As an alternative to pharmacological interventions, psychosocial treatments have been proposed and studied. Treatments that help patients change their behaviors and thought processes appear to hold some promise for these conditions.

Exercise treatments have been developed in accordance with evidence suggesting that exercise improves mood, pain thresholds, and sleep (Minor, 1991; Weyerer & Kupfer, 1994). Graded exercise treatments have resulted in reduced pain, fatigue, and disability in somatization and CFS patients (Fulcher & White, 1997; Peters, Stanley, Rose, Kaney, & Salmon, 2002; Wearden et al., 1998). Some investigators have shown exercise to outperform relaxation and stretching comparison interventions (Fulcher & White, 1997); others have found no advantage for exercise over stretching (Peters et al., 2002). Questions also remain regarding the generalizability of these findings. Patients who are unwilling to exercise are unlikely to enroll in exercise studies. And even those patients who do participate in exercise trials may not complete the treatment (Peters et al., 2002; Wearden et al., 1998).

Cognitive behavior therapy (CBT) aims to alter dysfunctional thoughts and behaviors associated with the functional somatic symptoms. When CBT is administered to somatization and CFS patients, gradual increases in activities including exercise is a key component of these interventions. The efficacy of CBT has been examined in six randomized controlled trials (four trials with CFS patients, one with moderate somatization patients, and one with full somatization disorder patients). In one study, CBT was found to be no more effective than the control treatment (Lloyd et al., 1993); however, in all five other studies CBT reduced physical discomfort significantly more than the control treatments did (Allen, Woolfolk, & Gara, 2001; Deale, Chalder, Marks, & Wessely, 1997; Prins et al., 2001; Sharpe et al., 1996; Sumathipala, Hewege, Hanwella, & Mann, 2000). The trials that demonstrated CBT's efficacy employed more intensive treatments than did the one negative trial. Despite the overall support for CBT with these patients, investigators agree that improvement is neither complete nor universal.

Explanatory Models

The mechanisms underlying persistent fatigue and somatization are poorly understood. Although many explanatory theories have been proposed, research examining these theories has either not yet been conducted or produced inconsistent findings. Many investigators have suggested the etiology of these conditions is multifaceted. Thus, biopsychosocial models have been proposed (Sharpe, Peveler, & Mayou, 1992).

Psychosocial factors associated with chronic fatigue and somatization include distorted thinking, such as thinking catastrophically about one's physical sensations or believing one has a serious medical condition (Cathebras et al., 1992; Rief, Hiller, & Margraf, 1998). Such beliefs may prompt heightened awareness of bodily sensations and increased emotional distress, both of which may exacerbate the physical symptoms (Barsky, 1992). Distorted beliefs may also encourage patients to engage in self-defeating behavior, such as avoiding activities and seeking unnecessary medical services (Katon et al., 1991; Kroenke et al., 1988; Smith et al., 1986; 14). In turn, the environment, including family, friends, and physicians, may respond in ways that reinforce the individual's somatic distress.

The most consistent findings on pathophysiological antecedents of somatization and chronic fatigue come from research on the hypothalamic–pituitary–adrenal (HPA) axis. Reduced levels of circulating cortisol have been observed in patients diagnosed with CFS (Cleare et al., 1999; Demitrack et al., 1991), idiopathic pain (Alfven, de la Torre, & Uvnas-Moberg, 1994; Johansson, 1982; Valdes, Garcia, Treserra, de Pablo, & de Flores, 1989; Von Knorring & Almay, 1989), and chronic headache (Elwan, Abdella, el Bayad, Hamdy, 1991). Investigators who have failed to find a glucocorticoid deficiency attribute their results to psychiatric comorbidity in their samples (Rief & Auer, 2000). Because melancholic depression has been associated with excessively high levels of cortisol (Gold, Goodwin, & Chrousos, 1988), comorbid depression and somatization may neutralize each other's effect on the HPA axis, resulting in normal cortisol levels (Rief & Auer, 2000). The fact that fatigue and malaise are key symptoms of primary adrenal insufficiency (i.e., Addison's disease) lends additional support to an association between fatigue/somatization and hypocortisolism.

The cause of hypocortisolism in fatigue and somatization syndromes has yet to be delineated. An enhanced negative feedback of the HPA axis and a diminished release of CRH at the central level have been proposed (Ehlert, Gaab, & Heinrichs, 2001). The morphological bases of these changes have not been determined. Presumably, genetic factors and life experiences set the stage for the dysregulation of the HPA axis.

A separate branch of research has examined the neurophysiological processing of afferent stimuli. This literature suggests that somatization patients may have disturbed sensory regulation, overresponding to high-intensity stimuli. Investigators have found excessive augmentation of sensory evoked potentials in patients diagnosed with somatization disorder, psychogenic pain, chronic pain, and hysterical anesthesia compared with control subjects (James, Gordon, Kraiuhin, Howson, & Meares, 1990; Moldofsky & England, 1975; Mushin & Levy, 1974; von Knorring, Almay, Johansson, & Terenius, 1979). Consistent with these results, Bushbaum found that individuals with high pain tolerances have reduced evoked potentials (Bushbaum, 1975). Possible causes of somatization patients' hypersensitivity include genetic factors and repeated exposure to stress.

The research on the psychological and biological underpinnings of somatization and chronic fatigue must be considered preliminary. Although differences between these patients and controls have been identified, not all patients with somatization or chronic fatigue possess the characteristics described here. What distinguishes patients exhibiting cortisol deficiencies or sensory hypervigilance from others has not yet been determined.

Despite numerous uncertainties, a preliminary synthesis of these findings suggests the following: patients with medically unexplained physical symptoms may be hypersensitive to incoming stimuli. The tendencies of these patients to amplify and think castrophically about somatic sensations may arouse the body's HPA axis. Over time, the stress system may become less reactive and produce less cortisol. Dysregulation of the HPA axis may cause neuroimmune dysfunction.

Conclusion

Etiological questions have hindered the development of precise diagnostic and effective treatment procedures for somatizing and fatigued patients. Currently, our most promising treatments for these patients are designed to provide symptomatic relief. Clearly, more research into the pathophysiological antecedents of somatization and idiopathic fatigue is called for. In the absence of clear pathophysiology, a sharper definition of the syndromes including family studies and laboratory assessments, type of symptoms, and treatment response is called for.

Acknowledgments

This paper was supported by grants from the National Institute of Mental Health (K08 01662 and R01 60265).

References

Addington, A. M., Gallo, J. J., Ford, D. E., & Eaton, W. W. (2001). Epidemiology of unexplained fatigue and major depression in the community: the Baltimore ECA Follow-up, 1981–1984. *Psychological Medicine, 31*, 1037–1044.

Alfven, G., de la Torre, B., & Uvnas-Moberg, K. (1994). Depressed concentrations of oxytocin and cortisol in children with recurrent abdominal pain of non-organic pain. *Acta Paediatrica 83*, 1076–1080.

Allen, L. A., Woolfolk, R. L., & Gara, M. A. (2001). Cognitive behavior therapy for somatization disorder: a controlled study. *Psychosomatic Medicine 63*, 93–94.

Attanasio, V., Andrasik, F., Blanchard, E. B., & Arena, J. G. (1984). Psychometric properties of the SUNYA revision of the Psychosomatic Symptom Checklist. *Journal of Behavior Medicine 7*, 247–258.

Barsky, A. J. (1992). Amplification, somatization, and the somatoform disorders. *Psychosomatics 33*, 28–34.

Barsky, A. J., & Wyshak, G. (1990). Hypochondriasis and somatosensory amplification. *British Journal of Psychiatry 157*, 404–409.

Bates, D. W., Schmitt, W., & Buchwald, D. (1993). Prevalence of fatigue and chronic fatigue syndrome in a primary care practice. *Archives of Internal Medicine 153*, 2759–2765.

Bombardier, C. H., & Buchwald, D. (1996). Chronic fatigue, chronic fatigue syndrome, and fibromyalgia: disability and health care use. *Medical Care 34*, 924–930.

Bushbaum, M. (1975). Averaged evoked response augmenting/reducing in schizophrenia and affective disorders. *Association for Research in Nervous Mental Disease 54*, 29–42.

Cathebras, P. J., Robbins, J. M., Kirmayer, L. J., & Hayton, B. C. (1992). Fatigue in primary care: prevalence, psychiatric comorbidity, illness behavior, and outcome. *Journal of General Internal Medicine 7*, 276–286.

Cleare, A. J., Heap, E., Malhi, G. S., Wessely, S., O'Keane, V., & Miell, J. (1999). Low-dose hydrocortisone in chronic fatigue syndrome: a randomized crossover trail. *Lancet 353*, 455–458.

Deale, A., Chalder, T., Marks, I., & Wessely, S. (1997). Cognitive behavior therapy for chronic fatigue syndrome: a randomized controlled trial. *American Journal of Psychiatry 154*, 408–414.

Demitrack, M. A., Dale, J. K., Straus, S. E., Laue, L., Listwak, S. J., Kruesi, M. J., Chrousos, G. P., & Gold, P. W. (1991). Evidence for impaired activation of the hypothalamic-pituitary-adrenal axis in patients with chronic fatigue syndrome. *Journal of Clinical Endocrinology Metabolism 73*, 1224–1234.

Derogatis, L. R. (1977). *SCL-90-R: Administration, Scoring and Procedures Manual—II for the Revised Version and Other Instruments of the Psychopathology Rating Scale Series*. Towson, MD: Clinical Psychometric Research.

Ehlert, U., Gaab, J., & Heinrichs, M. (2001). Psychoneurological contributions to the etiology of depression, posttraumatic stress disorder, and stress-related bodily disorders: the role of the hypothalamus-pituitary-adrenal axis. *Biological Psychology 57*, 141–152.

Elwan, O., Abdella, M., el Bayad, A. B., & Hamdy, S. (1991). Hormonal changes in headache patients. *Journal of Neurological Science 106*, 75–81.

Escobar, J. I., Burnam, M. A., Karno, M., Forsythe, A., & Golding, J. M. (1987). Somatization in the community. *Archives of General Psychiatry 44*, 713–718.

Escobar, J. I., Golding, J. M., Hough, R. L., Karno, M., Burnam, M. A., & Wells, K. B. (1987). Somatization in the community: relationship to disability and use of services. *American Journal of Public Health 77*, 837–840.

Escobar, J. I., Waitzkin, H., Silver, R. C., Gara, M., & Holman, A. (1998). Abridged somatization: a study in primary care. *Psychosomatic Medicine 60*, 466–472.

First, M. B., Spitzer, R. L., Gibbon, M., & Williams, J. B. W. (1997). *Structured Clinical Interview for DSM-IV Axis I Disorders (SCID-I)*. Washington, DC: American Psychiatric Press.

Fukuda, K., Straus, S. E., Hickie, I. Sharpe, M. C., Dobbins, J. G., & Komaroff, A. (1994). Chronic fatigue syndrome: a comprehensive approach to its definition and study. *Annals of Internal Medicine 121*, 953–959.

Fulcher, K. Y., & White, P. D. (1997). Randomised controlled trial of graded exercise in patients with the chronic fatigue syndrome. *British Medical Journal 341*, 1647–1652.

Gilson, B. S., Gilson, J. S., & Bergner, M. (1975). The Sickness Impact Profile: development of an outcome measure of health care. *American Journal of Public Health 65*, 1304.

Gold, P. W., Goodwin, F. K., & Chrousos, G. P. (1988). Clinical and biochemical manifestations of depression in relation to the neurobiology of stress. *New England Journal of Medicine 319*, 413–420.

Hickie, I. B., Davenport, T., Issakidid, C., & Andrews, G. (2002). Neurasthenia: prevalence, disability, and health care characteristics in the Australian community. *British Journal of Psychiatry 181*, 56–61.

James, L., Gordon, E., Kraiuhin, C., Howson, A., & Meares, R. (1990). Augmentation of auditory evoked potentials in somatization disorder. *Journal of Psychosomatic Research 24*, 155–163.

Johansson, F. (1982). Differences in serum cortisol concentrations in organic and psychogenic chronic pain syndromes. *Journal of Psychosomatic Research 26*, 351–358.

Katon, W., Lin, E., von Korff, M., Russo, J., Lipscomb, P., & Bush, T. (1991). Somatization: a spectrum of severity. *American Journal of Psychiatry 148*, 34–40.

Kellner, R. (1987). Abridged Manual of the Illness Atttitude Scale. Unpublished manual, Department of Psychiatry, School of Medicine, University of New Mexico, Albuquerque.

Kroenke, K., Wood, D. R., Mangelsdorff, A. D., Meier, N. J., & Powell, J. B. (1988). Chronic fatigue in primary care: prevalence, patient characteristics, and outcome. *Journal of the American Medical Association 260*, 929–934.

Lane, T. J., Matthews, D. A., & Manu, P. (1990). The low yield of physical examinations and laboratory investigations of patients with chronic fatigue. *American Journal of Medical Science 299*, 313–318.

Lloyd, A. R., Hickie, I., Brockman, A., Hickie, C., Wilson, A., Dwyer, J., & Wakefield, D. (1993). Immunologic and psychologic therapy for patients with chronic fatigue syndrome: a double-blind, placebo-controlled trial. *American Journal of Medicine 94*, 197–203.

Minor, M. A. (1991). Physical activity and management of arthritis. *Annals of Behavior Medicine 13*, 117–124.

Moldofsky, H., & England, R. S. (1975). Facilitation of somatosensory average-evoked potentials in hysterical anaesthesia and pain. *Archives of General Psychiatry 32*, 193–197.

Mushin, J., & Levy, R. (1974). Averaged evoked responses in patients with psychogenic pain. *Psychological Medicine 4*, 19–27.

Pawlikowska, T., Chalder, T., & Hirsch, S. R. (1994). Population based study of fatigue and psychological distress. *British Medical Journal 308*, 763–766.

Peters, S., Stanley, I., Rose, M., Kaney, S., & Salmon, P. (2002). A randomized controlled trial of group aerobic exercise in primary care patients with persistent unexplained physical symptoms. *Family Practice 19*, 665–674.

Petrie, K., Moss-Morris, R., & Weinman, J. (1995). The impact of catastrophic beliefs on functioning in chronic fatigue syndrome. *Journal of Psychosomatic Research 39*, 31–37.

Prins, J. B., Bleijenberg, G., Bazelmans, E., Elving, L. D., de Boo, T. M., Severens, J. L., van der Wilt, G. J., Spinhoven, P., & van der Meer, J. W. M. (2001). Cognitive behaviour therapy for chronic fatigue syndrome: a multicentre randomized controlled trial. *Lancet 357*, 841–847.

Rief, W., & Auer, C. (2000). Cortisol and somatization. *Biological Psychology 53*, 13–23.

Rief, W., Hiller, W., & Margraf, J. (1998). Cognitive aspects of hypochondriasis and the somatization syndrome. *Journal of Abnormal Psychology 107*, 587–595.

Robins, L. N., Helzer, J. E., Weissman, M. M., Orvaschel, H., Gruenberg, E., Burke, J. D., & Regier, D. A. (1984). Lifetime prevalence of specific psychiatric disorders in three sites. *Archive of General Psychiatry 41*, 949–958.

Robins, L. N., Wing, J., Wittchen, H., & Helzer, J. E. (1988). The Composite International Diagnostic Interview. *Archives of General Psychiatry 45*, 1069–1077.

Sharpe, M., Hawton, K., Seagroatt, V., & Pasvol, G. (1992). Follow up of patients presenting with fatigue to an infectious diseases clinic. *British Medical Journal 305*, 147–152.

Sharpe, M., Hawton, K., Simkin, S., Surawy, C., Hackmann, A., Klimes, I., Peto, T., Warrell, D., & Seagroatt, V. (1996). Cognitive behaviour therapy for the chronic fatigue syndrome: a randomised controlled trial. *British Medical Journal 312*, 22–26.

Sharpe, M., Peveler, R., & Mayou, R. (1992). The psychological treatment of patients with functional somatic symptoms: a practical guide. *Journal of Psychosomatic Research 36*, 515–529.

Sharpe, M., & Wilks, D. (2002). ABC of psychological medicine: fatigue. *British Medical Journal 325*, 480–483.

Smith, G. R., Monson, R. A., & Ray, D. C. (1986). Patients with multiple unexplained symptoms: their characteristics, functional health, and health care utilization. *Archives of Internal Medicine 146*, 69–72.

Sumathipala, A., Hewege, R., Hanwella, R., & Mann, A. H. (2000). Randomized controlled trial of cognitive behaviour therapy for repeated consultations for medically unexplained complaints: a feasibility study in Sri Lanka. *Psychological Medicine 30*, 747–757.

Swartz, M., Blazer, D., George, L., & Landerman, R. (1986). Somatization disorder in a community population. *American Journal of Psychiatry 143*, 1403–1408.

Swartzman, L. C., Gwadry, F. G., Shapiro, A. P., & Teasell, R. W. (1994). The factor structure of the Coping Strategies Questionnaire. *Pain 57*, 311–316.

Valdes, M., Garcia, L., Treserra, J., de Pablo, J., & de Flores, T. (1989). Psychogenic pain and depressive disorders: an empirical study. *Journal of Affective Disorders 16*, 21–25.

Valdini, A., Steinhardt, S., & Feldman, E. (1989). Usefulness of a standard battery of laboratory tests in investigating chronic fatigue in adults. *Family Practice 6*, 286–291.

Voltz, H. P., Moller, H. J., Reimann, I., & Stoll, K. D. (2000). Opipramol for the treatment of somatoform disorders: results from a placebo-controlled trial. *European Neuropsychopharmacology 10*, 211–217.

von Knorring, L., & Almay, B. G. L. (1989). Neuroendocrine responses to fenfluramine in patients with idiopathic pain syndromes. *Nord Psykiatr Tidsskr 43*, 61–65.

von Knorring, L., Almay, B. G. L., Johansson, F., & Terenius, L. (1979). Endorphins in CSF of chronic pain patients, in relation to augmenting-reducing response in visual averaged evoked response. *Neuropsychobiology 5*, 322–326.

Walker, E. A., Katon, W. J., & Jemelka, R. P. (1993). Psychiatric disorders and medical care utilization among people in the general population who report fatigue. *Journal of General Internal Medicine 8*, 436–440.

Ware, J. E., & Sherbourne, C. D. (1992). The MOS-36-item short form health survey (SF-36). *Medical Care 30*, 473–483.

Wearden, A. J., Morris, R. K., Mullis, R., Strickland, P. L., Pearson, D. J., Appleby, L., Campbell, I. T., & Morris, J. A. (1998). Randomized, double-blind, placebo-controlled treatment trial of fluoxetine and graded exercise for chronic fatigue syndrome. *British Journal of Psychiatry 172*, 485–490.

Weiner, E. S., & Simpson, J. A., eds. (1989). *The Oxford English Dictionary.* Oxford: Oxford University Press.

Wessely, S. (2001). Chronic fatigue: symptom and syndrome. *Annals of Internal Medicine, 134 (suppl)*, 838–843.

Weyerer, S., & Kupfer, B. (1994). Physical exercise and psychological health. *Sports Medicine 17*, 108–116.

Whiting, P., Bagnall, A. M., Sowden, A. J., Cornell, J. E., Mulrow, C. D., & Ramirez, G. (2001). Interventions for the treatment and management of chronic fatigue syndrome: a systematic review. *Journal of the American Medical Association 286*, 1378–1379.

IV Fatigue in General Medical and Other Conditions

12 HIV-Related Fatigue

Natasha Dufour, Benoit Dubé, and William Breitbart

According to the Joint United Nations Programme on HIV/AIDS, as of December 2002, 42 million people worldwide were believed to be infected with the human immunodeficiency virus (HIV), the virus believed to cause acquired immunodeficiency syndrome (AIDS). According to the Center for Disease Control, approximately 800,000 to 900,000 Americans are currently infected with HIV. Furthermore, an estimated 40,000 new cases are expected every year. With the advent of antiretroviral therapy, the morbidity and mortality of HIV-infected patients has decreased significantly (O'Dell, 1994; Palella, Delaney, Moorman, Loveless, Fuhrer, Satten, et al., 1998) in the Western world. This advance has increased the attention given to symptom management, especially for those symptoms of greatest concern to patients.

Although the literature has extensively discussed the concept of fatigue, little is known or understood about fatigue in patients with HIV. For example, the presence of fatigue has been associated with impaired overall quality of life and functional limitations in AIDS patients (Vogl et al., 1999; Breitbart, McDonald, Rosenfeld, Sewell, Fishman, & Rabkin, 1998; Ferrando, et al., 1998). However, much of what is known has been extrapolated from findings in other medically ill populations, primarily cancer patients.

Epidemiology of Fatigue in HIV

Fatigue is a common finding even in the general population, where its base rate is almost 20 percent (Pawlikowska, Chalder, Hirsch, Wallace, Wright, & Wessely, 1994). As mentioned previously, fatigue with HIV infection is the most common symptom reported by both the patients and their providers (table 12.1; Fontaine, Larue, & Lassauniere, 1999; Justice, Rabeneck, Hays, & Wu, & Bozette, 1999). The prevalence of fatigue in clinical samples of patients with early stages of asymptomatic HIV illness ranges from 2 to 27 percent (Kaslow et al., 1987; Palenicek, Nelson, Vlahov, Galai, Cohn, & Saah, 1993; Hoover, Saah, Bacellar, Murphy, Visscher, Anderson, et al., 1993; Vlahov, Munoz, Solomon, Amstemborski, Lindsay, Anderson, et al., 1994), and it

Table 12.1
Prevalence of fatigue in HIV/AIDS

Study	Population	Prevalence
Longo et al. (1990)	Homosexual men with AIDS	41%
Darko et al. (1992)	HIV+ homosexual men	57% CDC Stage IV 11% CDC Stage III 10% HIV– controls
Hoover et al. (1993)	HIV+ "asymptomatic" homosexual men	9% HIV+ 6% HIV– controls
Vlahov et al. (1994)	HIV+ male and female intravenous drug users	19.4%–30% depending on CD4 counts
Breitbart et al. (1998)	Ambulatory HIV/AIDS patients	54%
Ferrando et al. (1998)	HIV+ gay/bisexual men	6%–17% depending on CD4 counts
Vogl et al. (1999)	AIDS outpatients	85.1%

increases from 30 to 54 percent among symptomatic HIV-infected and AIDS patients (Palenicek et al., 1993; Vlahov et al., 1994; Darko, McCutchan, Kripke, Gillin, & Golschan, 1992). Of their sample of 14 patients with AIDS, Darko and colleagues found that over 50 percent had fatigue compared to 10 percent of 50 HIV-seronegative controls (Darko et al., 1992). In another study of 34 patients with AIDS, 41 percent described fatigue as a major physical concern (Longo, Spross, & Locke, 1990). A study comparing 916 asymptomatic HIV-infected homosexual men reported a prevalence rate of 9 percent compared to 6 percent of 2161 seronegative control subjects (Hoover et al., 1993). A study of 562 HIV-seropositive injection drug users revealed a prevalence of fatigue ranging from 19 to 30 percent, depending on CD4+ cell count, with higher rates of fatigue being found with lower counts (Vlahov et al., 1994).

Higher prevalence of fatigue in patients with severe immunological compromise has also been reported by other investigators (Darko et al., 1992; Walker, McGown, Jantos, & Anson, 1997; Lee, Portillo, & Miramontes, 1999), but these findings have not been consistent. Many researchers have failed to replicate this association (Vogl et al., 1999; Breitbart et al., 1998; Justice et al., 1999; Vlahov et al., 1994; Barroso, 2001; De Boer, van Dam, Spranger, Frissen, & Lange, 1993; Perkins, Leserman, Stern, Baum, Liao, Golden, et al., 1995; Lyketsos, Hoover, Cuccione, Dew, Wesch, Bing, et al., 1996). Other findings involve HIV viral load: Ferrando and colleagues (Ferrando et al., 1998) found no association between viral load and fatigue, nor did Barroso and colleagues (Barroso, Carlson, & Meynell, 2003). These inconsistencies are likely a result of methodological differences or operational definition caveats, which go beyond the scope of this chapter.

Defining Fatigue: A Clinical Syndrome

Although fatigue is one of the most prominent symptoms affecting people with acute and chronic medical conditions, confusion continues to surround its definition (Ream & Richardson, 1996). Fatigue is a subjective symptom that can be ascertained only through patient reports. Furthermore, individuals use various words to describe fatigue: tired, lethargic, lack of energy, weak, exhausted, bored (Wolfe, 1999). Fatigue often develops slowly and worsens over time; it can be temporary or chronic (Barroso, 1999). Smets and colleagues suggested that fatigue in cancer patients may include physical, mental, and motivational fatigue (Smets, Garssen, Schuster-Uitterhoeve, & de Haes, 1993). Alternatively, Capaldini proposed dividing fatigue into emotional, psychological, and physical components (Capaldini, 1998). Accordingly, emotional fatigue is sometimes associated with frustration and irritability; it can involve decreased motivation as well as anhedonia. Psychological fatigue makes it difficult for people to concentrate, calculate, remember things, or focus on mentally challenging activities. As for physical fatigue, it is often experienced after physical activities and is mostly related to a specific physical malfunction.

Recognizing the need for a standardized definition, a group of investigators developed a set of criteria for the ICD-10 diagnosis of fatigue (Cella, Peterman, Passik, Jacobsen, & Breitbart, 1998). Although the criteria listed in table 12.2 were developed in the context of cancer, they could easily be applied to patients infected with HIV/AIDS. These diagnostic criteria have been submitted for inclusion in the tenth edition of the International Classification of Disease and are undergoing validation.

In the meantime, the Center for Disease Control (CDC) currently defines fatigue as a general and continuous or recurring feeling of sluggishness, lack of concentration ability, aching and tired bones and muscles, and even sleepiness, which progresses with each of the stages of HIV infection.

Measuring Fatigue

If fatigue is difficult to define, it is even harder to quantify (table 12.3). Nevertheless, it is only through repeated assessments that the efficacy of various treatment modalities can be ascertained.

The earliest attempts at quantifying fatigue relied solely on clinician-based observations. Scales were later developed to standardize ratings. Patient-based reports were then used in scales, thus incorporating their subjective reports. However, most scales were developed in the context of cancer or chronic illnesses other than HIV infection.

The earlier scales used a dichotomous approach: fatigue was either present or absent. These scales include, but are not limited to, the Pearson-Byars Fatigue Checklist

Table 12.2

International Classification of Diseases criteria for cancer-related fatigue

---

A. Six (or more) of the following symptoms have been present every day or nearly every day during the same 2-week period in the past month and at least one of the symptoms is significant fatigue.

- Significant fatigue, diminished energy, or increased need to rest, disproportionate to any recent change in activity level
- Complaint of generalized weakness or limb heaviness
- Diminished concentration or attention
- Decreased motivation or interest in usual activities
- Insomnia or hypersomnia
- Experience of sleep as unrefreshing or nonrestorative
- Perceived need to struggle to overcome inactivity
- Marked emotional reactivity (sadness, frustration, or irritability) to feeling fatigued
- Difficulty completing daily tasks attributed to feeling fatigued
- Perceived problems with short-term memory
- Postexertional malaise lasting several hours

B. The symptoms cause clinically significant distress or impairment in social, occupational, or other important areas of functioning.

C. There is evidence from the history, physical examination, or laboratory findings that the symptoms are a consequence of cancer or cancer therapy.

D. The symptoms are not primarily a consequence of comorbid psychiatric disorders such as major depression, somatization disorder, somatoform disorder, or delirium.

(Pearson & Byars, 1956), the Profile of Mood States (POMS) fatigue and vigor subscale (Cella, Jacobsen, Orav, Holland, Silberfard, & Rafla, 1987), the Fatigue Severity Scale (Krupp, LaRocca, Mur-Nash, & Steinberg, 1989), and the European Organization for Research and Treatment of Cancer Quality of Life Questionnaire (EORTC-QLQ-C30) fatigue subscale (Aaronson et al., 1993). Most of these scales use statements endorsed, to various degrees, by Likert scales.

Other scales take a unidimensional approach, probing intensity (e.g., Visual Analogue Scale for Fatigue; Lee, Hicks, & Nino-Murcia, 1991) or measuring consequences such as performance (e.g., Karnofsky Performance Status; Schag, Heinrich, & Ganz, 1984). These instruments are limited by the multiple confounds, such as pain, that can intervene.

Several scales developed primarily for use in cancer populations are multidimensional. The Piper Fatigue Scale (Piper, Lindsey, Dodd, Ferketich, Paul, & Weller, 1989) is perhaps one of the earliest scales to assess multiple dimensions of fatigue. It consists of four subscales: the Affective, Cognitive, Sensory, and Severity subscales. These various subscales reflect the multiple domains of fatigue, which consist of physical, cognitive, and emotional aspects of the fatigue experience. Two recently developed scales are becoming widely used in the study of cancer populations and palliative care populations: the Fatigue Symptom Inventory (FSI; Hann, Jacobsen, Azzarello, Martin,

Table 12.3
Fatigue measures/assessment tools

Scales using a dichotomous approach
Pearson-Byars Fatigue Checklist (Pearson et al., 1956)
Profile of Mood States fatigue and vigor subscale (Cella et al., 1987)
Fatigue severity scale (Krupp et al., 1989)
European Organization for Research and Treatment of Cancer Quality of Life Questionnaire fatigue subscale (Aaronson et al., 1993)

Unidimensional approach
Visual Analogue Scale for Fatigue (Lee et al., 1991)
Karnofsky Performance Status (Schag et al., 1984)
Global Fatigue Index (Bormann et al., 2001)

Multidimensional approach
Piper Fatigue Scale (Piper et al., 1989)
Fatigue Symptom Inventory (Hann et al., 1998)
Brief Fatigue Inventory (Mendoza et al., 1999)
Multidimensional Assessment of Fatigue (Belza et al., 1995)

Specific scales for the HIV population
Sleep and Infection Questionnaire
HIV-Related Fatigue Scale (Barroso et al., 2002)

Curran, Fields, et al., 1998) and the Brief Fatigue Inventory (BFI; Mendoza, Wang, Cleeland, Morrissey, Johnson, Wendt, et al., 1999). The FSI and the BFI both consist of several numerical rating scales that assess the severity of fatigue as well as its impact on various domains of quality of life.

Attempts have been made to validate some of these scales in the HIV patient population, such as the Global Fatigue Index (GFI) (Bormann, Shively, Smith, & Gifford, 2001). It stems from the Multidimensional Assessment of Fatigue (MAF) questionnaire developed for patients with rheumatoid arthritis (Belza, 1995). (The MAF itself is a revision of the Piper Fatigue Scale that had been developed in a cancer-stricken population.) Using 15 of 16 items from the MAF, the GIF yields a 50-point score. The novelty comes from averaging all the scores on the activities of daily living (ADL) items (items 4–14); this was done to appreciate the special ADL restrictions placed on individuals with HIV. Averaging the ADL scores avoids an artificial overinflation of the total score, since HIV-positive subjects may have functional limitations. The easily administered scale takes about 5 minutes to fill out. The resulting score, however, is unidimensional.

Others have attempted to develop scales specifically for patients infected with HIV. One early example is the Sleep and Infection Questionnaire developed by Darko (Darko et al., 1992). Using 11 items, the scale was designed to show how fatigue affects mental agility. Although it targets HIV-infected patients in particular, it does not encompass the full experience of fatigue in HIV-infected patients.

Barroso and her colleagues at the University of North Carolina at Chapel Hill set out to fill this shortcoming by developing an assessment tool specifically for this population (Barroso & Lynn, 2002). The resulting HIV-Related Fatigue Scale (HRFS) is a 56-item scale. It is the amalgam of five preexisting scales with the addition of four items based on the author's preliminary qualitative study of HIV-related fatigue.

The HRFS encompasses all 16 items from the MAF (on which the GIF is based), as well as selected items from the General Fatigue Scale, the Fatigue Impact Scale, the Fatigue Assessment Instrument, and the Sleep and Infection Questionnaire. The 56 items in the resulting instrument probe three domains: intensity (11 items), consequences (14 items), and circumstances (31 items) of fatigue. The consequences of fatigue items relate to the impact of fatigue on activities of daily living, socialization, mental function, and general consequences. Circumstance-related statements probe timing, precipitants, and aggravating and relieving factors of fatigue. Although this assessment tool is relatively young, it shows great promise in that it encompasses the most elements specific to HIV-infected individuals.

As mentioned previously, there is no standardized definition for pathological fatigue in the course of HIV infection. Hence, it is not surprising that no widely recognized gold standard assessment scale exists for HIV-related fatigue. The fatigue intensity, consequences, and circumstance items included in the HRFS nevertheless correspond to three of the five aspects identified by Aaronson in defining the characteristics of fatigue (Aaronson, Teel, Cassmeyer, et al., 1999). These characteristics include the relationship of fatigue to anxiety and depression in HIV/AIDS patients. Fatigue, anxiety, and depression in HIV/AIDS have been assessed with three distinct approaches: the clinical syndrome approach, in which assessment methods focus on the presence of a mood disorder; the symptom-cluster approach, focusing on measuring multiple symptoms of anxiety and depression; and finally, the single-symptom approach that specifically measures anxious or depressed mood. The same assessment methods have also been used to study fatigue.

All three approaches appear to overlap in studies that measure the relationship between fatigue, depression, and anxiety; provide subjective quantification of distress and assessment of impact; and examine correlates and biological parameters of fatigue. This suggests that accessory scales should be used in addition to fatigue assessment tools (e.g., depression scales) and biological markers (e.g., disease progression indicators such as viral load and CD4 count) to obtain the most complete assessment.

Table 12.4
Etiologies of fatigue in HIV/AIDS

Physiological factors
Direct effects of HIV/AIDS
Peripheral and central nervous system
Hepatocyte toxicity
Cytokines
Comorbid medical conditions
Anemia
Hypogonadism
Hypo/hyperthyroidism
Adrenal insufficiency
Opportunistic infections
Nutritional deficiencies
Treatment effects
Medication side effects
Exacerbating factors
Sleep disturbances
Lack of exercise
Inactivity
Pain syndromes

Psychological factors
Depression
Anxiety
Coping with a chronic illness

HIV-Related Fatigue: Etiologies

Fatigue is a multidimensional concept and, as one would expect, has multifactorial causes that coexist and interact (table 12.4). The underlying mechanisms of HIV-related fatigue remain unclear. From a broader theoretical standpoint, several hypotheses have been suggested, but none has been adequately tested specifically in this population. For example, fatigue could be related to a buildup in the muscles of the waste products pyruvic and lactic acids (Simonson, 1971); it may also result in a depletion of adenosine triphosphate (ATP), carbohydrates, fats, or adrenal hormones (Nail & Winningham, 1993). Or it could be a consequence of cytokine activation leading to abnormalities in the hypothalamic-pituitary-adrenal axis (Ur, White, & Grossman, 1992) or neurophysiological changes in the brain.

Piper and colleagues propose diverse mechanisms to comprehend fatigue, including psychological and social patterns, environmental and innate host factors, accumulation of metabolites, activity–rest and sleep–wake patterns, disease, patterns of symptoms and treatment (Piper, Lindsey, & Dodd, 1987). Despite multiple hypotheses, few basic research studies have investigated the biological basis of fatigue (Gutstein, 2001). Treatment options thus become less targeted and more empirically based. Proposed hypotheses for the underlying mechanisms of fatigue in HIV infection explore a variety of factors. In the following sections, we review the most frequently recognized processes.

Anemia

HIV-infected individuals experience a range of hematological complications including thrombocytopenia, lymphopenia, neutropenia, and anemia, anemia being the most prevalent abnormality. Studies have shown anemia to occur in 10 to 20 percent of asymptomatic HIV-seropositive people (Barroso, 1999), and in 66 to 85 percent of individuals with advanced disease (Doweiko & Groopman, 1998). Sullivan and colleagues, in a study examining HIV-infected patients with CD4 cell counts below 200/mm (Vogl et al., 1999) who were not directed to take antiretroviral drugs, found that the 1-year incidence of anemia was higher in women and individuals of African descent (Sullivan, Hanson, Chu, Jones, & Ward, 1998).

Anemia in HIV infection can have multiple etiologies. It may result from opportunistic infections; neoplasia (mostly lymphoma); chronic inflammation (usually leading to erythropoietin-deficient anemia); bone marrow damage or hypoproliferative bone marrow; dietary or iron deficiencies due to poor appetite, oral lesions, difficulty, with digestion, malabsorption, or diarrhea; blood loss; histiocytosis; myelodysplasia, or myelofibrosis (Volberding, 2000).

Anemia could also be iatrogenic, resulting from pharmacotherapeutic interventions that lead to myelosuppression (Zidovadine, or AZT, remains the most widely used myelosuppressive drug in HIV patients; Groopman, 1990).

Alternatively, upregulation of cytokines such as interferons, interleukin-1, tumor necrosis factor, and transforming growth factor in HIV infection may play an important role in impairing erythropoietin response, contributing to ineffective red cell production (Means, 1997).

In a study assessing the prevalence of fatigue in 427 ambulatory patients with HIV/AIDS, Breitbart and colleagues found that fatigue was significantly associated with the number of current AIDS-related physical symptoms, current treatment for HIV-related medical disorders, anemia, and pain (Breitbart et al., 1998). Anemia affects various dimensions of quality of life, especially through fatigue (Ludwig & Strasser, 2001). It is known to be a prognostic marker of disease progression or death in patients with HIV infection, independent of the viral load and CD4 count (Moyle, 2002).

Managing anemia initially requires determination of the need for a transfusion in severely symptomatic patients. However, there are drawbacks to such an intervention in people with HIV. Blood transfusions may directly accelerate disease progression by activating HIV-1 expression (Mudido, Georges, Dorazio, et al., 1996) and trigger transfusion-related immunosuppression. Some studies have reported a transient elevation in the viral load following transfusion (Groopman, 1997). Recombinant human erythropoietin (rHuEPO) is the mainstay of treatment for anemia in patients with a hemoglobin level below 11 g/dl, whether they are being treated with zidovudine or not (Fischl, Galpin, Levine, et al., 1990; Phair, Abels, McNeil, & Sullivan, 1993; Henry, Beall, Benson, et al., 1992). Clinical trials in patients with low endogenous erythropoietin levels have demonstrated that patients who took rHuEPO had higher energy levels and less fatigue. RHuEPO can be administered intravenously or subcutaneously three times a week; it is well tolerated in most patients, with similar rates of adverse events to those with placebo.

Endocrinopathies

Hormonal imbalances are another contributing factor to fatigue in individuals with HIV infection. HIV has a direct effect on immunologic cytokines, some of which are known to affect endocrine processes in animals. However, the clinical correlates of these effects remain unclear (Briggs & Beazlie, 1996).

The most prevalent form of hormonal deficiency in HIV-seropositive people is hypogonadism, defined as impaired testicular or ovarian function resulting in low testosterone levels (Klauke, Falkenbach, Schmidt, Staszewski, Helm, & Althoff, 1990). Testosterone is associated with regulation of energy, sexual drive, nutrient metabolism, and mood. Low testosterone levels, in addition to fatigue, can lead to low libido, impotency, anorexia, weight loss, and depression. An estimated prevalence of 25 percent of asymptomatic untreated HIV-infected men and 45 percent of untreated men diagnosed with AIDS have low testosterone levels (Dobs, 1988).

Many mechanisms have been involved as possible causes of hypogonadism. These include insufficient production due to low stimulation by brain hormones, testicular damage, and medication side effects. Testosterone-deficient patients benefit from treatment with testosterone (or synthetic anabolic steroids), but they are also subjected to its anabolic and androgenic effects (e.g., increased heart rate, blood pressure, and hirsutism). Testosterone can be administered by injection, pill, patch, gel, or cream. Supplementation can have a beneficial effect on fatigue as well as increase sexual interest and appetite and decrease wasting. It can increase energy levels and even concomitant depression. Women can also use these drugs, but careful monitoring is important since androgens can have virilizing effects, some of which might not be reversible when treatment is discontinued.

Adrenal insufficiency is another possible physiological cause of fatigue in seropositive people (Abbott, Khoo, Hammer, & Wilkins, 1995; Norbiato, Galli, Righini, & Moroni, 1994; Piedrola, Casado, Lopez, Moreno, Perez-Elias, & Garcia-Robles, 1996). It may be caused by HIV infection, drugs, cytomegalovirus, tuberculosis, or psychological stress that increases the activity of the hypothalamic-pituitary-adrenal axis. Many studies have reported mean cortisol levels consistently higher in HIV-seropositive individuals than in healthy seronegative controls (Clerici, Trabattoni, Piconi et al., 1997; Enwonwu, Meeks, & Sawiris, 1996; Rondanelli, Solerte, Fioravanti et al., 1997). The cortisol response to ACTH stimulation is reduced in these subjects (Stolarczyk, Rubio, Smolyar, Young, & Poretsky, 1998). Poor adrenal function can be treated with oral hydrocortisone or dexamethasone replacement therapy.

Both hyperthyroidism and hypothyroidism can induce fatigue. The latter can be treated with levothyroxine, which also increases the quality of life and energy levels of HIV-seropositive patients with no evidence of hypothyroidism (Derry, 1995).

Bartlett reported that up to 75 percent of HIV-seropositive patients had abnormal liver function (Bartlett, 1996). As shown by the presence of HIV messenger RNA in hepatocytes and HIV p24 in Kupffer cells and endothelial cells, HIV can involve the liver directly. Whether the liver damage results from primary damage by the virus itself or a secondary mechanism such as hepatitis remains unknown.

Depression as a Cause of Fatigue

According to Perdices and colleagues, anxiety and depression are the most commonly reported disturbances in seropositive individuals, up to 83 percent of whom are diagnosed with a depressive spectrum disturbance (Perdices, Dunbar, Grunseit, Hall, & Cooper, 1992). Major depression is reported in 10 to 20 percent of HIV-infected individuals.

One of the major challenges facing researchers and clinicians who identify, evaluate, and treat individuals with HIV/AIDS is to sort out the relationship between depression and fatigue (Walker et al., 1997). The need to clarify this relationship stems from the fact that, fatigue is not only a symptom of HIV/AIDS and its treatment, but also a symptom of anxiety and mood disorders. Furthermore, anxiety and mood disorders, like fatigue, are also very prevalent in this population. In a previous attempt to clarify the same relationship in cancer patients, Jacobsen and Weitzner proposed four important questions as a theoretical framework. The first question addressed the conceptual similarities and differences between depression and anxiety, on one hand, and fatigue, on the other hand. The second question was to what extent depression and anxiety co-existed with fatigue and how they could be distinguished. Third, what was the possible causal relationships between fatigue and depression and between fatigue and anxiety? The final question was what treatment implications arose from the relationship of fatigue to depression and anxiety (Jacobsen & Weitzner, 2003). These questions have been applied to the fatigue's relationship with anxiety and depression in HIV/AIDS patients.

For example, in a study of fatigue in 438 ambulatory patients with AIDS, Breitbart and colleagues found that patients with fatigue (over 50% of their sample) had higher levels of psychological distress, poorer quality of life, significantly more depressive symptoms (Beck depression Inventory), and higher levels of hopelessness (Beck Hopelessness Scale) than patients without fatigue (Breitbart et al., 1998). They also found that fatigue was associated with severity of anemia, but no significant association was found between fatigue and time of HIV diagnosis, CD4 count, CDC clinical category of HIV infection, or use of antiretroviral medication.

Conversely, in a longitudinal study on changes in depressive symptoms as AIDS develops, Lyketsos and colleagues reported that depressive symptoms and fatigue were closely associated over time across stages of the disease. However, because they found no correlation between fatigue, depression, and measures of the immune status or HIV illness, the researchers concluded that fatigue was most likely a symptom of depression (Lyketsos et al., 1996). In a study of fatigue correlates in 20 HIV-infected men not meeting criteria for AIDS, O'Dell and colleagues found no statistically significant associations between fatigue measurements and physiological parameters (total protein, albumin, hematocrit, hemoglobin, and physical dimension score on the Sickness Impact Profile; O'Dell, Meighen, & Riggs, 1996). The authors concluded that fatigue was more strongly correlated with psychological than physiological parameters among HIV-seropositive men.

On the contrary, Ferrando and colleagues reported that depressed HIV-seropositive men were more likely to experience clinical fatigue. In a 1-year follow-up, they also found an increase in depressive symptoms predicted a small amount of variance in fatigue. Thus, they concluded that although associated with major depression and depressive symptoms, fatigue in advanced HIV illness does not seem to be merely a symptom of depression (Ferrando et al., 1998).

Perkins and colleagues found that depressive symptoms and major depression significantly predicted severity of fatigue, at both the baseline and on 6 month follow-up in HIV-infected asymptomatic men, suggesting that fatigue was a manifestation of depression in the early stages of the disease (Perkins et al., 1995). In trying to predict fatigue and depression in 36 HIV-infected gay men followed longitudinally for 7.5 years, Barroso and colleagues found that fatigue was predicted by both physiological (CDC clinical status) and psychological (anxiety, hopelessness, social conflict, lack of satisfaction with support) risk factors, whereas depression was predicted only by psychological risk factors (Barroso, Preisser, Leserman, Gaynes, Golden, & Evans, 2002). They found that concurrent depression was strongly correlated with previous depression and concurrent fatigue with previous fatigue. Depression at the previous visit was reported to be correlated with fatigue, and fatigue at the previous visit with depression scores. The researchers' results also demonstrate that fatigue and depression are mutually predictive in HIV-infected gay men.

Treatment options for depression are similar to those for other chronic medical illnesses. Once underlying organic causes have been ruled out and treated, for example, hypogonadism or hypothyroidism, treatment options include pharmacological and psychotherapeutic modalities.

Pharmacological interventions for depression include either antidepressants or psychostimulants. Most studies of antidepressants consisted of either randomized, placebo-controlled trials or open-label trials (Jones & Breitbart, 2003). Several studies have suggested that serotonin-specific inhibitors are better tolerated than tricyclic antidepressants (Elliot, Uldall, Bergan, Russo, Claypoole, & Ray-Byrne, 1998; Schwartz & McDaniel, 1999). One notable exception is fluvoxamine, which was less well-tolerated despite its efficacy in treating depression (Grassi, 1995). Because of the frequent concomitant use of antiretrovirals, prescribing clinicians must carefully monitor drugdrug interactions.

Psychiatric Clinics of North America published an excellent review of these psychopharmacological considerations (Robinson & Qaqish, 2002). Psychostimulants such as methylphenidate, pemoline, and dextroamphetamine can be used safely and successfully in HIV-positive patients who present with depression and fatigue (Breitbart, Rosenfeld, Kaim, & Funesti-Esch, 2001; Holmes, Fernandez, & Levy, 1989; Wagner & Rabkin, 2000). Modafinil, a norepinephrine agonist that acts in the human hypothalamus (McClellan & Spencer, 1998), is a new wakefulness-promoting agent that has been used off-label to augment antidepressants in small studies (Menza, Kaufman, & Castellanos, 2000; Schwartz, Leso, Beale, Ahmed, & Naprawa, 2002). It may prove to be a valid treatment option for HIV-positive patients.

Comparatively, much less research has been conducted into the efficacy of psychotherapeutic interventions in HIV-infected individuals who are depressed. Most of the literature supports group cognitive-behavioral approaches to improving mental health-related quality of life indices (Lechner, Antoni, Lydston et al., 2003) as well as depression (Blanch, Rousaud, Hautzinger et al., 2002). Conversely, individual psychotherapy has not been the subject of as much research. It is nevertheless an integral part of the American Psychiatric Association's practice guidelines for the treatment of HIV/AIDS. The paucity of evidence-based research may be attributed to the lack of a widely used manual-driven protocol in this patient population. Studies have shown combined pharmacotherapy and psychotherapy, on the other hand, to be effective (Lee, Cohen, Hadley, & Goodwin, 1999; Lyketsos, Fishman, Hutton et al., 1997).

Miscellaneous Etiologies

As mentioned previously, fatigue is a multifactorial problem. It is often linked to pre-existing conditions in seropositive patients, such as congestive heart failure, or attributed to opportunistic infections or other medical complications encountered throughout the evolution of HIV infection (table 12.5).

Malnutrition states are common and should be identified so that appropriate treatments can be initiated. When severe, they can result in wasting syndrome, which is

Table 12.5
Antiretroviral side effects leading to or contributing to fatigue

Drug Class	Side Effect		
	Fatigue	Nausea, vomiting	Anemia
Nucleoside reverse transcriptase inhibitors	Lamivudine Abacavir	Lamivudine Zalcitabine Zidovudine	Zidovudine
Nucleotide reverse transcriptase inhibitors		Tenofovir	
Nonnucleoside reverse transcriptase inhibitors		Efavirenz	
Protease inhibitors	Amprenavir Saquinavir Lopinavir/ritonavir Ritonavir	Amprenavir Saquinavir Lopinavir/ritonavir Ritonavir Nelfinavir	Indinavir

potentially life-threatening. Medication-induced nausea decreases appetite, and food intake may be reduced because of difficulty in swallowing with painful *Candida albicans* infection. Advanced malnutrition can also result from malabsorption due to gastrointestinal parasitic infections (*Cryptosporidium, Microsporidium*), viral infection (Cytomegalovirus), or neoplasia (Kaposi sarcoma).

The most frequently cause of nutritional deficits is medication side effects, especially in the era of multidrug regimens of highly active antiretroviral therapy (HAART). Antiretrovirals are known to cause nausea and vomiting, which lead to fatigue through decreased food intake. Fatigue is also a significant side effect, and these agents can induce anemia, another confound for fatigue.

Fatigue and Neuropsychological Function

Psychological fatigue is a fatigue component described by Capaldini and defined as difficulty in concentrating, calculating, remembering, or focusing on mentally challenging activities. Perkins and colleagues (Perkins et al., 1995) examined insomnia and fatigue as indicators of a mood disturbance and HIV disease severity. CD4 counts and neuropsychological test performance were chosen as markers of disease severity. More specifically, studies of global neuropsychological functioning focused on measures of attention and information processing, executive function, language, learning and memory, visuospatial function, and motor function. Motor function testing reflects motor speed and dexterity, both thought to be initial indications of central nervous system (CNS) involvement of HIV infection (MMWR, 1987). Severity of depressive symptoms and self-reported dysphoric mood were related to the level of both fatigue and insomnia. According to the researchers, at the start of the study, no significant relationships existed between global and motor neuropsychological function and fatigue or insomnia. At the 6-month follow-up visit, a reduction in motor neuropsychological function was found to be associated with more complaints of fatigue, even after controlling for depression. Perkins and his team argued that this finding suggests a separate relationship between fatigue and HIV effects on the brain. They propose fatigue may be an earlier indicator of HIV CNS involvement.

Fatigue Management Strategies

All successful strategiegies in managing and treating fatigue must start with education. Only when patients and their support network have been taught to recognize signs and symptoms of fatigue can it be detected and treated. Patient education is recommended because most patients do not report fatigue unless directly asked; others do not report it because they assume it is a normal aspect of the disease.

As fatigue is thought to be a multifactorial entity, a multifaceted approach is required to optimize treatment benefits (table 12.6). Cella and colleagues proposed a three-stage hierarchy for the treatment of fatigue: identify and treat the underlying cause(s), treat fatigue directly, then, finally, manage the consequences of fatigue (Cella et al., 1998).

This chapter has explored the underlying causes of fatigue. Once both physiological and psychological causes have been addressed, residual symptoms of fatigue can be targeted directly with either pharmacological or nonpharmacological strategies; the goal is to restore or increase as well as preserve energy to improve fatigue and the level of functioning. Pharmacological approaches include psychostimulants, corticosteroids, anticytokine agents (thalidomide, pentoxifylline), or other agents (amantadine, anabolic steroids, hypnotics) (Portenoy & Itri, 1999). Nonpharmacological interventions include sleep hygiene and exercise.

The last, but certainly not least, step in fatigue management is improving quality of life by addressing the consequences of fatigue. Through counseling and communication, patients learn to reprioritize their activities, adjust to their limitations, and restructure their goals and expectations accordingly. This process also entails sustaining a sense of purpose and meaningfulness (Winningham, Nail, Burke et al., 1994).

What Does the Future Hold?

As death rates from AIDS decline, more and more attention needs to be given to quality-of-life issues. The most prominent of these is undoubtedly fatigue.

Table 12.6
Fatigue intervention strategies in HIV/AIDS

Cause-specific interventions	
Anemia	Transfusions, rHuEPOH
Hypogonadism	Testosterone
Adrenal insufficiency	Corticosteroids
Hypothyroidism	Levothyroxine
Infections	Antibiotics/antiviral, antifungal therapy
Malnutrition	Nutritional supplement, megestrol acetate
Depression	Antidepressants, psychotherapy
Inactivity	Exercise, training
Sleep disturbances	Sleep aids
Nonspecific pharmacological interventions	
Selective serotonin-reuptake inhibitors	
Tricyclic antidepressants	
Psychostimulants	
Methylphenidate	
Dextroamphetamine	
Pemoline	
Modafinil	
Anticytokine agents	
Thalidomide	
Pentoxifyline	
Nonpharmacological interventions	
Good sleep hygiene	
Education	
Meditation, relaxation	
Energy conservation and restoration	
Cognitive-behavioral therapy	

Unfortunately, most of the current knowledge of HIV-related fatigue was inspired by research in cancer and other chronic illnesses. This means that current recommendations are not evidence-based, have not been tested in a randomized, placebo-controlled fashion, and often originated before the era of HAART.

No doubt the qualitative experience of fatigue in HIV-infected patients differs from that of cancer-stricken individuals. We must continue to identify these unique experiential characteristics before we can develop standardized management protocols in this population. The advent of such guidelines will enhance the quality of life of these patients who must struggle daily with a vacillating sense of hope and purpose.

References

Aaronson, L. S., Teel, C. S., Cassmeyer, V., et al.(1999). Defining and measuring fatigue. *Journal of Nursing Scholarship 31*, 45–50.

Aaronson, N. K., Ahmedzai, S., Bergman, B., et al. (1993). The European Organization for Research and Treatment of Cancer QLQ-C30: a quality-of-life instrument for use in international clinical trials in oncology. *Journal of the National Cancer Institute 85*, 365–763.

Abbott, M., Khoo, S. H., Hammer, M. R., & Wilkins, E. G. (1995). Prevalence of cortisol deficiency in late HIV disease. *Journal of Infection 31*, 1–4.

Barroso, J. (2001). "Just worn out:" a qualitative study of HIV-related fatigue. In S. G. Funk, E. M. Tornquist, J. Leeman, M. S. Milles, J. S. Harrell, eds. *Key Aspects of Preventing and Managing Chronic Illness.* pp. 183–194. New York: Springer.

Barroso, J. (1999). A review of fatigue in people with HIV infection. *Journal of the Association of Nurses in AIDS Care 10*, 42–49.

Barroso, J., Carlson, J. R., & Meynell, J. (2003). Physiological and psychological markers associated with HIV-related fatigue. *Clinical Nursing Research 12*, 49–68.

Barroso, J., & Lynn, M. L. (2002). Psychometric properties of the HIV-Related Fatigue Scale. *Journal of the Association of Nurses in AIDS Care 13*, 66–75.

Barroso, J., Preiseer, J. S., Leserman, J., Gaynes, B. N., Golden, R. N., & Evans, D. N. (2002). Predicting fatigue and depression in HIV-positive gay men. *Psychosomatics 43*, 317–325.

Bartlett, J. G. (1996). Medical management of HIV infection. Glenview, IL: Physicians and Scientists Publishing.

Belza, B. L. (1995). Comparison of self-reported fatigue in rheumatoid arthritis and controls. *Journal of Rheumatism 22*, 639–643.

Blanch, J., Rousaud, A., Hautzinger, M., et al. (2002). Assessment of the efficacy of cognitive-behavioral group psychotherapy programme for HIV-infected patients referred to a consultation–liaison psychiatry department. *Psychotherapy and Psychosomatics 71*, 77–84.

Bormann, J., Shively, M., Smith, T. L., & Gifford, A. L. (2001). Measurement of fatigue in HIV-positive adults: reliability and validity of the Global Fatigue Index. *Journal of the Association of Nurses AIDS Care 12*, 75–83.

Breitbart, W., McDonald, M. V., Rosenfeld, B., Sewell, M., Fishman, B., & Rabkin, J. (1998). Fatigue in ambulatory AIDS patients. *Journal of Pain Symptom Management 15*, 159–167.

Breitbart, W., Rosenfeld, B., Kaim, M., & Funesti-Esch, J. (2001). A randomized, double-blind, placebo-controlled trial of psychostimulants for the treatment of fatigue in ambulatory patients with human immunodeficiency virus disease. *Archives of Internal Medicine 161*, 411–420.

Briggs, J. M., & Beazlie, L. H. (1996). Nursing management of symptoms influenced by HIV infection of the endocrine system. *Nursing Clinics of North America 31*, 845–865.

Capaldini, L. (June 1998). Symptom management guidelines. *HIV InSite Knowledge Base* (http://hivinsite.ucsf.edu/InSite.jsp?doc=kb-03-01-06&page=kb-03).

Cella, D., Peterman, A., Passik, S., Jacobsen, P., & Breitbart, W. (1998). Progress toward guidelines for the management of fatigue. *Oncology 12*, 369–377.

Cella, D. F., Jacobsen, P. B., Orav, E. J., Holland, J. C., Silberfard, P. M., & Rafla, S. (1987). A brief POMS measure of distress for cancer patients. *Journal of Chronic Diseases 40*, 939–942.

Clerici, M., Trabattoni, D., Piconi, S., et al. (1997). A possible role for the cortisol/anticortisols imbalance in the progression of human immunodeficiency virus. *Psychoneuroendocrinology 22(1)*, S27–S31.

Darko, D. F., McCutchan, J. A., Kripke, D. F., Gillin, J. C., & Golschan, S. (1992). Fatigue, sleep disturbance, disability, and indices of progression of HIV infection. *American Journal of Psychiatry 149*, 514–520.

De Boer, J. B., van Dam, F. S., Spranger, M. A., Frissen, P. H., & Lange, J. M. (1993). Longitudinal study on quality of life of symptomatic HIV-infected patients in a trial of zidovudine versus zidovudine and interferon-alpha. *AIDS 7*, 947–953.

Derry, D. M. (1995). Thyroid therapy in HIV-infected patients. *Medical Hypotheses 45*, 121–124.

Dobs, A. S. (1988). Endocrine disorders in men infected with HIV. *American Journal of Medicine 84*, 611–616.

Doweiko, J., & Groopman, J. (1998). Hematologic manifestations of HIV infection. In G. Wormser, ed. *AIDS and Other Manifestations of HIV Infection*. Pp. 542–557. Philadelphia: Lippincott-Raven.

Elliot, A. J., Uldall, K. K., Bergam, K., Russo, J., Claypoole, K., & Ray-Byrne, P. P. (1998). Randomized, placebo-controlled trial of paroxetine versus imipramine in depressed HIV-positive outpatients. *American Journal of Psychiatry 155*, 367–372.

Enwonwu, C. O., Meeks, V. I., & Sawiris, P. G. (1996). Elevated cortisol levels in whole saliva in HIV infected individuals. *European Journal of Oral Sciences 104*, 322–324.

Ferrando, S., Evans, S., Goggin, K., et al. (1998). Fatigue in HIV illness: relationship to depression, physical limitations, and disability. *Psychosomatic Medicine 60*, 759–764.

Fischl, M., Galpin, J. E., Levine, J. D., et al. (1990). Recombinant human erythropoietin for patients with AIDS treated with zidovudine. *New England Journal of Medicine 322*, 1488–1492.

Fontaine, A., Larue, F., & Lassauniere, J. M. (1999). Physician's recognition of the symptoms experienced by HIV patients: how reliable? *Journal of Pain Management 18(4)*, 263–270.

Grassi, B. (1995). Notes on the use of fluvoxamine as a treatment of depression in HIV-1 infected subjects. *Pharmacopsychiatry 28*, 93–94.

Groopman, J. (1997). Impact of transfusion on viral load in human immunodeficiency virus infection. *Seminatsin Hematology 34(2)*, 27–33.

Groopman, J. E. (1990). Zidovudine intolerance. *Review of Infectious Disease 12(5)*, S500–S506.

Gutstein, H. B. (2001). The biologic basis of fatigue. *Cancer 92*, 1678–1683.

Hann, D. M., Jacobsen, P. B., Azzarello, L. M., et al. (1998). Measurement of fatigue in cancer patients: development and validation of the Fatigue Symptom Inventory. *Quality of Life Research 7*, 301–310.

Henry, D. H., Beall, G. N., Benson, C. A., et al. (1992). Recombinant human erythropoietin in the treatment of anemia associated with human immunodeficiency virus (HIV) infection and zidovudine therapy. Overview of four clinical trials. *Annals of Internal Medicine 117*, 739–748.

Holmes, V. F., Fernandez, F., & Levy, J. K. (1989). Psychostimulant response in AIDS-related complex patients. *Journal of Clinical Psychiatry 50*, 5–8.

Hoover, D. R., Saah, A. J., Bacellar, H., et al. (1993). Signs and symptoms of "asymptomatic" HIV-1 infection in homosexual men. *Journal of Acquired Immune Deficiency Syndromes 6*, 66–71.

Jacobsen, P. B., & Weitzner, M. A. (2003). Evaluating the relationship of fatigue to depression and anxiety in cancer patients. In *Issues in Palliative Care Research*, R. K. Portenoy & E. Bruera. Pp. 127–149. Oxford University Press.

Jones, K., & Breitbart, W. (2003). Palliative care research in human immunodeficiency virus/acquired immunodeficiency syndrome: clinical trials of symptomatic therapies. In R. K. Portenoy & E. Bruera, eds. pp. 371–401. *Issues in Palliative Care Research*, New York: Oxford University Press.

Justice, A. C., Rabeneck, L., Hays, R. D., Wu, A. W., & Bozette, S. A. (1999). Sensitivity, specificity, reliability, and clinical validity of provider-reported symptoms: a comparison with self-reported symptoms. Outcomes Committee of the AIDS Clinical Trials Group. *Journal of Acquired Immune Deficiency Syndromes 21*, 126–133.

Kaslow, R. A., Phair, J. P., Friedman, H. B., et al. (1987). Infection with the human immunodeficiency virus: clinical manifestations and their relationship to immune deficiency. *Annals of Internal Medicine 107*, 474–480.

Klauke, S., Falkenbach, A., Schmidt, K., Staszewski, S., Helm, E. B., & Althoff, P. H. (1990). Hypogonadism in males with AIDS. (Abstract F. B. 205) *International Confence on AIDS 6*, 209.

Krupp, L. B., LaRocca, N. G., Mur-Nash, J., & Steinberg, A. D. (1989). The fatigue severity scale. *Archives of Neurology 46*, 1121–1123.

Lechner, S. C., Antoni, M. H., Lydston, D., et al. (2003). Cognitive-behavioral interventions improve quality of life in women with AIDS. *Journal of Psychosomatic Research 54*, 253–261.

Lee, K. A., Hicks, G., & Nino-Murcia, G. (1991). Validity and reliability of a scale to assess fatigue. *Psychiatry Research 36*, 291–298.

Lee, K. A., Portillo, C. J., & Miramontes, H. (1999). The fatigue experience for women with human immunodeficiency virus. *Journal of Obstetrics Gynecology and Neonatal Nursing 28*, 193–200.

Lee, M. R., Cohen, L., Hadley, S.W., & Goodwin, F. K. (1999). Cognitive-bahavioral group therapy with medication for depressed gay men with AIDS or symptomatic infection. *Psychiatric Services 50*, 948–952.

Longo, M. B., Spross, J. A., & Locke, A. M. (1990). Identifying major concerns of persons with acquired immunodeficiency syndrome: a replication. *Clinical Nurse Specialist 4*, 21–26.

Ludwig, H., & Strasser, K. (2001). Symptomatology of anemia. *Seminarsin Oncology 28(8)*, 7–14.

Lyketsos, C. G., Fishman, M., Hutton, H., et al. (1997). The effectiveness of psychiatric treatment for HIV-infected patients. *Psychosomatics 38*, 423–432.

Lyketsos, C. G., Hoover, D. R., Cuccione, M., et al. (1996). Changes in depressive symptoms as AIDS develops. *American Journal of Psychiatry 153*, 1430–1437.

McClellan, K. J., & Spencer, C. M. (1998). Modafinil: a review of its pharmacology and clinical efficacy in the management of narcolepsy. *CNS Drugs 9*, 311–324.

Means, R. Jr. (1997). Cytokines and anaemia in HIV infection. *Cytokines Cell Molecular Therapy 3*, 179–186.

Mendoza, T. R., Wang, X. S., Cleeland, C. S., et al. (1999). The rapid assessment of fatigue severity in cancer patients: use of the Brief Fatigue Inventory. *Cancer 85*, 1186–1196.

Menza, M. A., Kaufman, K. R., & Castellanos, A. (2000). Modafinil augmentation of antidepressant in depression. *Journal of Clinical Psychiatry 61*, 378–381.

Moyle, G. (2002). Anaemia in persons with HIV infection: prognostic marker and contributor to morbidity. *AIDS Review 4*, 13–20.

Mudido, P. M., Georges, D., Dorazio, D., et al. (1996). HIV type 1 activation after blood transfusion. *Transfusion 36*, 860–865.

Nail, L., & Winningham, M. (1993). Fatigue. In S. Groenwald, M. Frogge, M. Goodman, & C. Yarboro, eds. *Cancer Nursing: Principles and Practice*, 3rd ed. Pp. 608–619. Boston: Jones et Bartlett.

Norbiato, G., Galli, M., Righini, V., & Moroni, M. (1994). The syndrome of acquired glucocorticoid resistance In HIV infection. *Ballier's Clinical Endocrinology and Metabolism 8*, 777–787.

O'Dell, M. V. (1994). The epidemiology of HIV-related physical disability. In G. J. Stewart, ed. *Could It Be HIV?* North Sydney, Australia: Australasian Medical Publishing Co.

O'Dell, M. W., Meighen, M., & Riggs, R. V. (1996). Correlates of fatigue in HIV prior to AIDS: a pilot study. *Disability and Rehabilitation 18*, 249–254.

Palella, F. J. Jr., Delaney, K. M., Moorman, A. C., et al. (1998). Declining morbidity and mortality in patients with advanced human immunodeficiency virus infection. *New England Journal of Medicine 338*, 853–860.

Palenicek, J., Nelson, K. E., Vlahov, D., Galai, N., Cohn, S, & Saah, A. J. (1993). Comparison of clinical symptoms of human immunodeficiency virus disease between intravenous drug users and homosexual men. *Archives of Internal Medicine 153*, 1806–1812.

Pawlikowska, T., Chalder, T., Hirsch, S. R., Wallace, P., Wright, D. J., & Wessely, S. C. (1994). Population-based study of fatigue and psychological distress. *British Medical Journal 308*, 763–766.

Pearson, P. G., & Byars, G. E. (1956). The development and validation of a checklist measuring subjective fatigue (report no. 56–115). School of Aviation. U.S. Air Force, Randolph Air Force Base, Texas.

Perdices, M., Dunbar, N., Grunseit, A., Hall, W., & Cooper, D. A. (1992). Anxiety, depression, and HIV-related symptomatology across the spectrum of HIV disease. *Australian and New Zealand Journal of Psychiatry 26*, 560–566.

Perkins, D. O., Lesserman, J., Stern, R. A., Baum, S. F., Lia, D., Golden, R. N., & Evans, D. L. (1995). Somatic symptoms and HIV infection: relationship to depressive symptoms and indicators of HIV disease. *American Journal of Phychiatry 152*, 1776–1781.

Phair, J. P., Abels, R. I., McNeil, M. V., & Sullivan, D. J. (1993). Recombinant human erythropoietin treatment: investigational new drug protocol for the anemia of the acquired immunodeficiency syndrome: overall results. *Archives of Internal Medicine 153*, 2669–2675.

Piedrola, G., Casado, J. L., Lopez, E., Moreno, A., Perez-Elias, M. J., & Garcia-Robles, R. (1996). Clinical features of adrenal insufficiency in patients with acquired immunodeficiency syndrome. *Clinical Endocrinology 45*, 97–101.

Piper, B., Lindsey, A., & Dodd, M. (1987). Fatigue mechanisms in cancer patients: developing cancer theory. *Oncology Nursing Forum 14*, 17–23.

Piper, B. F., Lindsey, A. M., Dodd, M. J., Ferketich, S., Paul, S. M., & Weller, S. (1989). The development of an instrument to measure the subjective dimension of fatigue. In S. G. Funk, E. M. Tornquist, M. T. Champagne, L. A. Copp, & R. A. Wiese, eds. *Key Aspects of Comfort: Management of Pain, Fatigue, and Nausea.* Pp. 199–208. New York: Springer Publishing Company.

Portenoy, R. K., & Itri, L. M. (1999). Cancer-related fatigue: guidelines for evaluation and management. *Oncologist 4(1)*, 1–10.

Ream, E., & Richardson, A. (1996). Fatigue: a concept analysis. *International Journal of Nursing Studies 33*, 519–529.

Revision of the CDC surveillance case definition for acquired immunodeficiency syndrome (1987). Council of State and Territorial Epidemiologists, AIDS Program, Center for Infectious Diseases. *MMWR Morbidity & Mortality Weekly Report (1)*, 1S–15S.

Robinson, M. J., & Qaqish, R. B. (2002). Practical psychopharmacology in HIV-1 and acquired immunodeficiency syndrome. *Psychiatric Clinics of North America 25*, 149–175.

Rondanelli, M., Solerte, S. B., Fioravanti, M., et al. (1997). Circadian secretory pattern of growth hormone, insulin-like growth factor type 1, cortisol, adrenocorticotropic hormone, thyroid-stimulating hormone, and prolactin during HIV infection. *AIDS Research and Human Retroviruses 13*, 1243–1249.

Schag, C. C., Heinrich, R. L., & Ganz, P. A. (1984). Karnofsky Performance Status revisited: reliability, validity, and guidelines. *Journal of Clinical Oncology 2*, 187–193.

Schwartz, J. A., & McDaniel, J. S. (1999). Double-blind comparison of fluoxetine and desipramine in the treatment of depressed women in advanced HIV disease: a pilot study. *Depression and Anxiety 9*, 70–74.

Schwartz, T. L., Leso, L., Beale, M., Ahmed, R., & Naprawa, S. (2002). Modafinil in the treatment of depression with severe comorbid medical illness. *Psychosomatics 43*, 336–337.

Simonson, E. (1971). *Physiology of Work Capacity and Fatigue*. Springfield, IL: Thomas.

Smets, E. M., Garssen, B., Schuster-Uitterhoeve, A. L., & de Haes, J. C. (1993). Fatigue in cancer patients. *British Journal of Cancer 68*, 220–224.

Stolarczyk, R., Rubio, S. I., Smolyar, D., Young, I. S., & Poretsky, L. (1998). Twenty-four-hour urinary free cortisol in patients with acquired immunodeficiency syndrome. *Metabolism: Clinical & Experimental 47*, 690–694.

Sullivan, P. S., Hanson, D. L., Chu, S. Y., Jones, J. L., & Ward, J. W. (1998). Epidemiology of anemia in human immunodeficiency virus (HIV)-infected persons: results from the multistate adult and adolescent spectrum of HIV disease surveillance project. *Blood 91*, 301–308.

Ur, E., White, P. D., & Grossman, A. (1992). Hypothesis: cytokines may be activated to cause depressive illness and chronic fatigue syndrome. *European Archives of Psychiatry and Clinical Neuroscience 241*, 317–322.

Vlahov, D., Munoz, A., Solomon, L., et al. (1994). Comparison of clinical manifestations of HIV infection between male and female injecting drug users. *AIDS 8*, 819–823.

Vogl, D., Rosenfeld, B., Breitbart, W., et al. (1999). Symptom prevalence, characteristics, and distress in AIDS outpatients. *Journal of Pain Symptom Management 18*, 253–262.

Volberding, P. (2000). Consensus statement: anemia in HIV infection. Current trends, treatment options, and practice strategies. Anemia in HIV Working Group. *Clinical Therepy 22*, 1004–1020.

Wagner, G. J., & Rabkin, R. (2000). Effects of dextroamphetamine on depression and fatigue in men with HIV: a double-blind, placebo-controlled trial. *Journal of Clinical Psychiatry 61*, 436–440.

Walker, K., McGown, A., Jantos, M., & Anson, J. (1997). Fatigue, depression, and quality of life in HIV-positive men. *Journal of Psychosocial Nursing 35*, 32–40.

Winningham, M. L., Nail, L. M., Burke, M. B., et al. (1994). Fatigue and the cancer experience: the state of the knowledge. *Oncology Nursing Forum 21*, 23–36.

Wolfe, G. (1999). Fatigue in patients with HIV/AIDS. *Journal of Care Management 3*, 8–11.

13 Fatigue and Sleep

Stephen P. Duntley

The restorative power of sleep is a universal experience. A good night's sleep is a requirement for feeling refreshed during the waking hours. Unfortunately, feeling "tired" after a poor night's sleep is also a universal human experience, and persistent tiredness is a key symptom of many sleep disorders. The term "tired" is complex, however, and includes the concepts of fatigue, sleepiness, alertness, and performance capabilities.

Sleepiness and fatigue are often used interchangeably, as if reflecting a unitary neurological response to precipitants such as sleep deprivation. As this chapter shows, increasing evidence is emerging that fatigue and sleepiness arise from distinct neurological mechanisms. The sleep medicine field has emphasized the importance of sleepiness as a sign of sleep disorders such as obstructive sleep apnea syndrome. Recent research indicates that fatigue is a frequent complaint in patients with a variety of sleep disorders and is often considered the most significant and incapacitating symptom. This chapter emphasizes the distinction between excessive sleepiness and fatigue as overlapping but separable manifestations of many sleep disorders, and speculates on the insights into brain function understanding this distinction may give us.

Sleepiness versus Fatigue

Sleep is a basic biological need of most if not all complex organisms. It serves a restorative function, for both body and nervous system, although exactly what is restored and why sleep is necessary to restore it is poorly understood. Nevertheless, sleep is as essential to human well-being as food and water. Sleep deprivation results in increased physiological sleep need, which is expressed as sleepiness, or an increased tendency to fall asleep. Sleepiness is a basic physiological need state, like hunger or thirst, which subsequent sleep reduces. In early stages of sleep deprivation, therefore, it is a gentle reminder that it is time to sleep, allowing the restorative process to occur; when sleep deprivation becomes severe, sleepiness ensures that we obtain sleep as it eventually becomes virtually impossible to maintain wakefulness.

Excessive sleepiness is defined as drowsiness or sleep onset that occurs at inappropriate or undesirable times. While usually associated with a subjective sensation of sleepiness, sleepiness is an objectively definable and measurable phenomenon. Although alertness is sometimes used as an antonym of sleepiness, it is usually defined as the ability to maintain selective attention and vigilance. Decreased alertness is usually seen in sleepy individuals, but the two processes can be separated, and it is possible to have decreased alertness without evident sleepiness.

A sleepy individual is usually easy to identify because of characteristic signs including ptosis, yawning, head bobbing, and decreased attention to the environment. Several standardized questionnaires measure subjective sleepiness. The Stanford Sleepiness Scale (SSS) (Hoddes, Zarcone, Smythe, Phillips, & Dement, 1973) asks individuals to select one of seven statements to best describe their current level of wakefulness. The Epworth Sleepiness scale (ESS) (Johns, 1991) is a widely used questionnaire in which individuals rate their probability of dozing in a variety of situations. The most widely used objective measure of sleepiness is the multiple sleep latency test (MSLT) (Carskadon et al., 1986). In this test, four or five naps are allowed under standardized conditions at 2-hour intervals. Individuals lie in a quiet dark room and are told to allow themselves to fall asleep. Normal individuals have a mean sleep latency greater than 10 minutes. Pathological sleepiness is usually defined as a mean sleep latency of less than 5 minutes (Carskadon & Dement, 1981). Since the ability to stay awake rather than ease of falling asleep is often the clinical question being asked, the multiple sleep latency test has been modified in the maintenance of wakefulness test (MWT) (Mitler, Gujavarty, & Browman, 1982). In this test, the patient is asked to remain awake in a semireclining position in a darkened room. The test is performed at 2-hour intervals as in the MSLT.

Unlike sleepiness, fatigue has a vague biological role, and the medical profession's uncritical use of the term has hindered clear conceptual thinking about fatigue. The Oxford American Dictionary (2002) defines fatigue as "extreme tiredness after exertion" or "a reduction in the efficiency of a muscle, organ, etc., after prolonged activity." Fatigue has been divided into "peripheral" and "central" manifestations. Peripheral fatigue is defined as the inability to sustain a specified force or level of activity because of physical limitations of the muscles, nerves, or cardiovascular system (Chaudhuri & Behan, 2000). Examples include the inability to maintain repetitive physical activity in myasthenia gravis.

Peripheral fatigue is generally easy to quantify, whereas central fatigue is a more difficult concept to define adequately. The Multiple Sclerosis Council for Clinical Practice Guidelines has attempted to define central fatigue in multiple sclerosis research as "the subjective lack of physical and/or mental energy that is perceived to interfere with usual or desired activities" (1998). Chaudhuri and Behan (2000) define central fatigue as "a failure of physical and mental tasks that require self-motivation and internal cues in the absence of demonstrable cognitive failure or motor weakness." Similarly to sleepiness, transient central fatigue is a normal phenomenon after sleep deprivation and is also observed in normal individuals undergoing acute stresses or illnesses. Whether fatigue plays a normal biological role in organisms is less clear than for sleepiness. Although disturbed sleep results in fatigue and a normal night's sleep resolves this fatigue in normal individuals, fatigue does not serve a basic homeostatic role such as sleepiness does. Conceivably, in normal individuals, fatigue indicaties that their resources are near exhaustion and rest is needed.

Although decreased ability to perform on a variety of tasks is undoubtedly a feature of central fatigue, it is often treated as an inherently subjective phenomenon, such as the experience of pain. Because of this, research with widely accepted, standardized measures of fatigue is less common than such research on sleepiness. Often subjects are asked only if they are "fatigued." When quantification is attempted, the most common method of measuring fatigue is patient rating of subjectively perceived fatigue. The Fatigue Severity Scale, Fatigue Impact Scale, and Visual Analog Scale for Fatigue are some scales in current use. The Profile of Mood States (POMS) and Medical Outcomes Study Short-Form 36 also have fatigue subscales as components of larger inventories.

In summary, a sleepy person is on the verge of falling asleep because of an increase in physiological sleep tendency. Excessive sleepiness can result in significant disability from excessive time spent in bed, difficulty awakening in the morning, and unintentional sleep episodes. Sleepiness is typically measured objectively through tests such as the MSLT. Until better definitions are available, the fatigued person is considered to lack the "energy" to initiate or complete necessary or desired tasks. Fatigue, typically measured by subjective assessment, can result in significant disability as an individual fails to participate fully in occupational or social activities.

The sleep medicine field has generally emphasized the importance of excessive daytime sleepiness as a sign of sleep disorders, while giving little attention to fatigue. Sleepiness is seen as an objective, measurable, and inevitable consequence of inadequate sleep that usually resolves with a good night's sleep. Fatigue, on the other hand, is a subjective complaint that can arise from a variety of medical and psychiatric disorders without concomitant sleep disorders, and it may occur without any identifiable precipitant. It often does not improve after a good night's sleep. Fatigue is therefore considered too nonspecific to be useful. The International Classification of Sleep Disorders: Diagnostic and Coding Manual (2000) lists 34 dyssomnias. Excessive sleepiness is included in the diagnostic criteria of 19 of these disorders and fatigue is in only one disorder. As discussed later, however, fatigue may be a more prominent complaint than sleepiness and may occur in sleep disorders in the absence of overt sleepiness.

Fatigue and Sleepiness in Experimental Manipulations of the Sleep–Wake Cycle

Before we discuss how fatigue and sleepiness are related to clinical sleep disorders, it is helpful to understand how experimental manipulation of the sleep–wake cycle may result in the development of fatigue and sleepiness. An extensive experimental literature exists on sleepiness, performance, and mood in the settings of sleep deprivation, sleep fragmentation, and circadian rhythm manipulation. Fatigue is less commonly measured in these experiments. Measurement of sleepiness and performance are typically performed with a well-accepted standardized methodology. In contrast, fatigue is frequently not assessed or may be addressed in a single question or as a minor component of a mood scale.

In normal individuals, increases in sleepiness and fatigue tend to parallel each other. As might be expected from personal experience, total sleep deprivation leads to increases in subjectively and objectively measured sleepiness, increased fatigue, and decreased performance on a variety of measures. These changes are seen after only one night of deprivation, but are also cumulative, increasing in severity over several days of total sleep deprivation. Partial sleep deprivation leads to similar cumulative effects and is extremely common in our society.

In one study the nightly sleep of 16 healthy young adults was restricted to about 5 hours a night for 1 week, while subjective sleepiness was measured with the SSS, mood and fatigue with the POMS, and performance with a brief battery of tests (Dinges et al., 1997). Subjective sleepiness increased over the seven restriction nights, with a similar increase in the fatigue subscale of the POMS. Performance decrements on some tasks such as psychomotor vigilance testing mirrored that of subjective sleepiness and fatigue but tended to lag behind subjective measures by a day. Subjective sleepiness, fatigue, and performance measures all required two nights of recovery sleep for normalization. Although MSLT data in the Dinges's study were limited, Carskadon and Dement (1981) found a similar cumulative lowering of mean MSLT latencies when sleep was restricted to 5 hours a day. In a long-term sleep reduction experiment, subjects reduced their sleep time by 30 minutes every few weeks (Friedmann et al., 1977). Fatigue increased with increasing sleep reduction, leading ultimately to unwillingness to continue the sleep reduction in many subjects. Subjective fatigue appeared at earlier stages of sleep reduction than performance deficits.

To be fully restorative, an adequate quantity and quality of sleep are both necessary. The objective markers of sleep quality are incompletely understood, and experiments manipulating measurable sleep parameters such as quantity of specific sleep stages have yielded inconsistent results. Sleep continuity, however, has been shown to be necessary for restorative sleep in normal individuals. Sleepiness increases and performance decreases with experimentally induced sleep fragmentation, and the magnitude of the deficits predictably follows the frequency of the fragmentation. Bonnett (1986) exposed healthy subjects to either 64 hours of continuous sleep deprivation, or induced brief awakenings throughout the sleep period after 1 minute of accumulated sleep. Subjects awakened every minute experienced performance decrements similar to that experienced after total sleep deprivation. Sleepiness as measured by nap latency was nearly as great in the 1-minute sleep fragmentation group as that in the total sleep deprivation period, as was subjective sleepiness measured by the SSS. Total sleep time was also somewhat reduced in the sleep fragmentation group, but the magnitude of the change in total sleep time is unlikely to result in such marked increases in sleepiness. Fatigue was not directly measured in these experiments, although mood, measured by the Clyde Mood Scale, was impaired.

Similar results were obtained in an experiment by Martin, Engleman, Deary, and Douglas (1996) in which sleep was disrupted after every 2 minutes of sleep for two nights. Brief auditory stimuli were carefully administered to induce an arousal for 3 to 15 seconds. With this protocol, total sleep time remained unchanged, but MSLT and MWT latencies were significantly reduced. Subjective sleepiness measured by the SSS was unchanged. Cognitive function measured by the Trailmaking B task and paced auditory serial addition test was impaired. The energetic arousal score of the UWIST checklist, which includes self-ratings of adjectives such as sluggish and vigorous, was also impaired after sleep fragmentation.

Electroencephalographic (EEG) evidence of arousal or awakening is typically considered to be a marker for poor sleep quality and is used in fragmentation experiments such as those described previously. There is some evidence that stimuli insufficient to cause EEG arousal can also lead to poor sleep quality. In one experiment, subjects exposed to auditory stimuli sufficient to increase their heart rate or arterial blood pressure but not produce visible EEG evidence of arousal resulted in a significant increase in sleepiness as measured by the MSLT and MWT; subjective sleepiness measured by the SSS showed no change (Martin, Wraith, Deary, & Douglas, 1997). Unlike in the EEG fragmentation experiments, energetic tone measured by the UWIST checklist was unchanged.

Circadian rhythms in sleepiness and fatigue have also been consistently demonstrated. In an experiment in which normal individuals had a multiple sleep latency test every 2 hours for a 24-hour period, a clear biphasic pattern of sleep tendency with objective sleepiness peaking in the early morning and midafternoon hours emerged (Richardson, Carskadon, Orav, & Dement, 1982). In a constant routine study, a similar biphasic pattern of unintentional sleep episodes was observed (Carskadon & Dement, 1992). Although Richardson and colleagues did not find a midafternoon increase in self-reported sleepiness, as measured by the Stanford Sleepiness Scale, self-rated fatigue in another group exhibitied a biphasic circadian curve similar to that of objective sleepiness (Monk, 1991). In constant routine experiments with continuous sleep deprivation over several days, the biphasic curves of sleepiness and fatigue are superimposed on the increasing basal levels of sleepiness and fatigue resulting from the sleep deprivation. In has been estimated that in 64-hour sleep deprivation experiments about 39 percent of the variance in psychomotor tests and subjective measures is attributable to the homeostatic processes whereas about 23 percent of the variances is secondary to the circadian time (Bonnet, 2000). Performance measured by a variety of cognitive and psychomotor tests tends to covary with the circadian curve of subjective sleepiness, although it does not consistently show an afternoon dip (Van Dongen & Dinges, 2000).

Experiments such as those discussed here have led to the two-process model of sleep (Borbely, 1982). According to this model, homeostatic and circadian processes interact to account for sleep and waking patterns. During waking, the homeostatic process, termed "process S," results in the accumulation of sleep need. Although the neurological substrates of sleep need remain incompletely understood, it is clear that sleep need accumulates with sustained wakefulness and is dissipated with sustained sleep. This sleep need interacts with a circadian process, termed "process C," which governs an independent circadian distribution of sleep propensity that generally follows the body temperature curve. Normally, these two processes result in a stable sleep–wake cycle. As sleep need accumulates during the day, it is countered by circadian mechanisms until near the habitual bedtime when sleep onset occurs because of high levels of accumulated sleep need and an increasing circadian tendency toward sleep. An individual remains asleep until process S is reduced and circadian rhythms shift to favor waking. In normal individuals, when homeostatic and circadian processes interact properly, the restorative process of sleep helps prevent the development of abnormal sleepiness and fatigue. In pathological conditions, abnormal sleepiness, fatigue, or both may develop from either a disturbance of the homeostatic or circadian process or other factors such as medical or psychiatric illness or drugs.

Clinical Sleep Disorders and Fatigue

An understanding of the two-process model is essential to understanding clinical sleep disorders, because altered homeostatic or circadian processes occur in many disorders and may explain much of the symptomatology. The current classification system—the International Classification of Sleep Disorders (ICSD)—divides sleep disorders into dyssomnias and parasomnias. Parasomnias involve abnormal behavior arising from sleep and not the quality of sleep itself; dyssomnias involve the quality or adequacy of the sleep process itself.

Dyssomnias can result in sleepiness or fatigue from several mechanisms. Homeostasis altered by either insufficient total sleep time or sleep fragmentation plays a role in many sleep disorders. Insufficient sleep time may result from volitional causes, with a progressive tendency for people to overextend themselves, sacrificing sleep. The 2002 national sleep foundation poll found that 30 percent of adults obtained less than 6 hours of sleep a night. Many sleep disorders, however, also result in reduced total sleep time and chronic sleep deprivation. The abnormal sensations of restless legs syndrome interfere with sleep and can result in severe deprivation. Reduced total sleep time is seen in primary insomnia and delayed sleep phase syndrome. In obstructive sleep apnea, sleep fragmentation from repetitive arousals terminating the apneas is believed underlie many of the behavioral symptoms. Frequent awakenings reduce total sleep time and cause excessive sleepiness that is compensated for by increased time in bed and total sleep time. The fragmented sleep obtained, however, is nonrestorative.

Impaired sleep quality may also play a role in the fatigue experienced by patients with medical disorders such as multiple sclerosis, chronic fatigue syndrome, and fibromyalgia. In an actigraphic study of multiple sclerosis patients with and without fatigue, 12 of 15 patients with fatigue had actigraphy patterns suggestive of disturbed sleep whereas only 3 of 15 patients without fatigue had evidence of disturbed sleep (Attarian, Duntley, Brandon, Carter, & Cross (2003). In a small study of chronic fatigue syndrome patients, sleep efficiency was lower in patients than in controls (Morriss et al., 1993). Alpha activity superimposed on non-REM sleep is common in fibromyalgia and has been related to frequent complaints in these patients of shallow sleep (Perlis et al., 1997).

A misalignment between circadian rhythms and desired sleep–wake cycle is responsible for many of the symptoms of shift-work sleep disorder and advanced sleep phase and delayed sleep phase syndromes (Baker & Zee, 2000). This circadian misalignment may also result in reduced total sleep time and sleep fragmentation, which may further contribute to symptomatology. In addition to the mechanisms already noted, sleepiness can result from a dysfunction of the sleep- or wakefulness-generating mechanisms secondary to either exogenous factors such as sedating medications or neurological disease such as narcolepsy.

Since the MSLT, MWT, SSS, and ESS are commonly used in scientific and clinical studies of sleep disorders, we have considerable data on objective and subjective sleepiness in clinical sleep disorders, but relatively little systematic study has been done of fatigue in sleep disorders. When included in studies, fatigue is typically addressed as one question about fatigue as part of larger questionnaires. Mosko and colleagues (1989) reported the fatigue subscale of the POMS on 233 consecutive patients presenting to a sleep disorder center. The POMS fatigue score for all sleep disorder groups was elevated compared to published normal values: sleep apnea with EDS or insomnia, 11.4; PLM/RLS with EDS or insomnia, 13.9; narcolepsy, 10.6; and "all others," 14.0. Women scored higher than men on the fatigue subscale. That the sleep disorder was causal to the elevated fatigue complaint is suggested by the finding of a statistically significant improvement in fatigue after treatment of sleep apnea and periodic limb movement disorder. Narcolepsy patients demonstrated a nonsignificant trend toward improvement after treatment with stimulants. There was no difference in complaints of fatigue in insomnia patients on or off hypnotic medications.

In a systematic study of fatigue and sleepiness in sleep disorders patients, Lichstein, Means, Noe, and Aguillard (1997) studied 206 consecutive patients presenting to a sleep disorders center. Subjects were given the Fatigue Severity Scale, MMPI, polysomnography, and MSLT testing. Patients with sleep disorders averaged 4.8 on the FSS, with 4.8 for sleep apnea patients, 4.5 in narcolepsy patients, 4.3 in periodic limb movement disorder patients, and 6.0 in psychophysiological insomnia patients. The authors noted the values were high compared to control values of 2.3 to 2.8 reported in the literature, and are similar to values of 4.8 for patients with multiple sclerosis and 6.1 for chronic fatigue syndrome. Female gender, MMPI depression scale, and MMPI average score had the highest correlation with fatigue. Objective polysomnogram measures had a weak if any correlation with fatigue, and objective sleepiness, as measured by the MSLT, had no correlation with levels of fatigue.

In some sleep disorders, a dissociation between sleepiness and fatigue has definable mechanisms. Delayed sleep phase syndrome (DSPS) offers the best example. In DSPS the patient's circadian rhythm is phase delayed relative to the patient's desired bedtime and wake time. If patients attempt to adhere to their desired bed and wake times, they experience severe sleep-onset insomnia, despite the complaint of daytime sleepiness and fatigue. Patients often report that the sleepiness is worst in the morning, with improving alertness as the day progresses. Polysomnography reveals prolonged sleep latency and decreased total sleep time. If the patient is allowed to go to bed at a later hour, polysomnography reveals sleep is of normal latency, continuity, and duration and symptoms typically resolve. In DSPS, sleep onset at the desired bedtime is inhibited because the underlying circadian phase at that time is extremely unfavorable to sleep onset. If the patient is able to get up in the morning at the desired wake time, the circadian phase promotes sleepiness and fatigue. Chronic sleep deprivation contributes to the daytime sleepiness and fatigue.

In disorders such as obstructive sleep apnea, the reason for the lack of correlation between severity measures and subsequent sleepiness and fatigue is not clear. Obstructive sleep apnea syndrome (OSA) is characterized by repetitive episodes of pharyngeal obstruction during sleep, resulting in reduced airflow, with transient impairment of oxygen and carbon dioxide exchange that is typically terminated by arousal. OSA, defined as the laboratory finding of an apnea-hypopnea index of greater than 5, is common, occurring in 9 percent of women and 24 percent of men. Even mild sleep apnea has been shown to confer increased risk of hypertension, and cardiovascular and cerebrovascular disease (Newman et al., 2001). Cognitive dysfunction is also common (Beebe, Groesz, Wells, Nichols, & McGee, 2003). Obstructive sleep apnea syndrome, combined with daytime sleepiness is seen in 2 percent of women and 4 percent of men (Young et al., 1993). Although a variety of daytime and nighttime symptoms occur in sleep apnea syndrome, the most prominent complaints are daytime sleepiness and fatigue.

In a systematic study comparing objective sleepiness and subjective complaints in OSA patients, Chervin (2000) studied 190 patients and performed MSLTs and ESSs. Participants were also given a questionnaire that asked if sleepiness, fatigue, tiredness, or lack of energy was a problem for the patient and to rate the problem as occurring never, seldom, occasionally, often, or almost always. Patients were asked to identify which most affected their ability to accomplish what they wanted, which was the worst problem , and if only one of the symptoms could be cured completely, which would they choose. Men had an apnea/hypopnea index (AHI) of 35.1 compared to 27.5 for women. The mean MSLT indicated moderate sleepiness of approximately equal severity for men and women; men, however, reported less subjective sleepiness on the ESS than women. For both men and women, fatigue, tiredness, or lack of energy were the most common complaints, occurring often or almost always in 57, 61, and 62 percent of patients, respectively. Only 47 percent of patients complained of sleepiness. Patients most commonly responded that lack of energy was their worst problem. Among those who reported that sleepiness was never a problem, 27 percent complained that fatigue was often or almost always a problem. The MSLT showed no statistically significant correlation with any of the four subjective complaints. The AHI did not correlate with complaints of sleepiness or lack of energy, but had a slightly negative correlation with fatigue and tiredness. The ESS correlated with the complaints of sleepiness, tiredness, and lack of energy but not fatigue. Female gender was associated with a markedly increased frequency of each subjective complaint.

One potential explanation proposed by Chervin (2000) for the lack of correlation between objective measures of apnea severity and subsequent sleepiness and fatigue is that the measures used are incomplete indicators of the severity and physiological consequences of obstructive sleep apnea syndrome. If there were better measures of "quality" of sleep, perhaps the correlation between apnea severity and fatigue would be better. There are certainly reasons to suspect the adequacy of our current measures. The definitions of apnea and hypopnea contain components that arbitrarily impose a dichotomous definition on a graded phenomenon. Respiratory events that fail to meet scoring criteria are not counted, while severe events resulting in awakening with respiratory distress receive no additional weighting in the AHI. Our measures of arousal are particularly suspect; the inter-scorer reliability remains poor, and the demonstrable physiological significance of common definitions are so uncertain that the presence of an arousal was dropped from Medicare's definition of hypopnea. On the other hand, Chervin (2000) points out that AHI and extent of oxygen desaturations correlate with consequences such as hypertension and cognitive deficits, suggesting that our measures of apnea severity have some validity. An alternative explanation is that apnea has adverse effects on multiple neurological circuits. Individuals exhibit differential susceptibility to impairment of any given network from disturbed sleep. Individuals may therefore respond to the same insult with either sleepiness, fatigue, or some combination of the two depending on incompletely understood predisposing factors.

One factor that consistently adds to the complexity of subjective response to sleep disorders is depression. In two studies of insomniacs with major depression, both nefazodone and fluoxetine alleviated depression to a similar extent (Rush et al., 1998; Gillin, Rapaport, Erman, Winokur, & Albala, 1997). Both groups had objective sleep disturbance before treatment. In the nefazodone group, the subjective complaint of insomnia resolved and was accompanied by objective improvement in sleep architecture. Similarly, in the fluoxetine group, subjective complaints of insomnia resolved with improvement of depression, but sleep architecture deteriorated in this group, demonstrating the primary importance of depression in the perception of sleep disturbance (Gillin, et al., 1997; Rush et al., 1998). Additionally, in a study of patients presenting with obstructive sleep apnea syndrome there was no correlation between objective measures of sleep such as RDI and subjective sleep quality, but there was a strong correlation between perception of sleep quality and the Beck Depression Inventory (Day, Wells, Carney, Freedland, & Duntley, 2003).

Fatigue and depression are both common in a wide range of chronic medical illnesses. Reviewing the literature on this association, Bardwell, Moore, Ancoli-Israel, and Dimsdale (2003) note that most studies have found a significant correlation between depression and fatigue severity in chronic illness; a significant relationship between illness severity and fatigue is less common. These authors studied assessed depression severity in 60 patients with obstructive sleep apnea syndrome, performing polysomnography to determine apnea severity, POMS fatigue subscale scores to assess fatigue, and Center for Epidemiological Studies Depression Scale. The patients presented with a wide range of severity (AHI mean + 48.8; SD + 27.1). Using linear regression analysis, the authors found that apnea severity as measured by the AHI and percentage of time with oxygen saturation less than 90 percent accounted for only 4.2 percent of the variance in the POMS fatigue subscale. The CES-D Scale score accounted for 42.3 percent of the variance.

Despite the lack of correlation between severity of OSA and fatigue, and the strong correlation between depressive symptomatology and fatigue, studies have shown a decrease in fatigue with treatment of OSA. Mosko and colleagues (1989) noted a reduction of the fatigue subscale of the POMS from 13.1 to 7.7 after surgical treatment of obstructive sleep apnea syndrome, while Kribbs and associates (1993) found significant improvement in the fatigue subscale of the POMS after treatment with nasal continuous positive airway pressure (CPAP). There is also evidence that treatment of OSA results in improved mood. In a small study, Derderian, Bridenbaugh, and Rajagopal (1988) found improvement in the depression and fatigue scales of the POMS when sleep apnea was treated with nasal CPAP; Yu, Ancoli-Israel, and Dimsdale (1999) found improved mood in both CPAP-treated and placebo-treated patients with OSA. It is unclear why depressive symptomatology is tightly linked to perception of sleep quality and perception of fatigue resulting from disturbed sleep. The most likely explanation is that neurological substrates critical in the genesis of both depression and fatigue overlap. Sleep disturbance tends to functionally impair both of these neurological substrates to variable degrees in different individuals, resulting in depressive symptomatology and fatigue. The subjective perception of sleep involves the same neurological substrates, or individuals may label their sleep as poor when these substrates are impaired due to fatigue and dysphoria after a poor night's sleep.

The greatest dissociation between sleepiness and fatigue occurs in primary insomnia, a common condition that is estimated to affect 10 to 15 percent of the U.S. population (Ancoli-Israel, & Roth, 1991). In primary insomnia, fatigue is a prominent complaint. Patients may complain of daytime sleepiness, however, with careful questioning they reveal difficulty in falling asleep during the day and at night time. Subjective fatigue and sleepiness, without evidence of objective sleepiness, has been confirmed by polysomnographic studies of primary insomnia patients. In one study, insomnia patients had a sleep efficiency of 64.2 percent and total sleep time of 314.5 minutes compared to 81.9 percent efficiency and 388 minutes for controls. As might be expected with impaired nocturnal sleep, insomnia patients reported more subjective sleepiness in the day than controls, scoring 3.12 on the SSS compared to 2.03 for controls. Despite the increased subjective sleepiness in the insomnia group, objective sleepiness was not found. In a variant of the MSLT used in this study, sleep latency was 20.9 minutes in the control group compared to 24.4 in the insomnia group (Schneider-Helmert, 1987).

Why do patients with demonstrable sleep disturbance and complaints of daytime sleepiness have no demonstrable sleepiness on objective measures? The most likely explanation is that a persistent state of "hyperarousal" in these patients is responsible for both the sleep disturbance and the lack of physiological sleepiness during daytime testing. Hyperarousal is a multidimensional process in primary insomnia, with patients exhibiting increased somatic, cognitive, and cortical arousal. Somatic arousal is evidenced by increased electromyographic activity (Monroe, 1967) and increased 24-hour metabolic rate (Bonnet & Arand, 1995). Cognitive arousal is marked by the racing thoughts and difficulty patients have "turning off" their thought processes. Cortical arousal is characterized by increased high-frequency EEG activity in insomnia (Smith et al., 2002).

In an attempt to experimentally induce the elevated arousal found in primary insomnia, Bonnet and Arand (1992) increased physiological arousal by giving normal subjects 400 milligrams (mg) of caffeine three times a day. The subjects experienced impaired nocturnal sleep approximating that of primary insomnia. In addition, they experienced a variety of disturbances found in primary insomnia including increased metabolic rate, increased body temperature, increased tension, increased personality disturbance as measured by the MMPI, and increased levels of daytime fatigue. Despite the chronic sleep deprivation and fatigue, subjects exhibited prolonged MSLT latencies, and as in primary insomnia patients, overestimated sleep latencies. In an attempt to determine whether the sleep loss of insomniacs was sufficient to cause the symptoms of insomnia, Bonnet and Arand (1996) yoked normal controls to the sleep patterns of insomnia patients for 10 consecutive nights. Simultaneous awakenings were induced in matched controls with auditory stimuli whenever the insomnia patient awakened. Sleep data for the induced insomnia approximately matched that of the insomnia patients on most variables. The secondary symptoms induced by yoked insomnia model were quite different from those induced by the caffeine hyperarousal model. The yoked arousal subjects exhibited increased fatigue, as measured by the POMS. Metabolic rate increased in the evening and decreased in the morning, body temperature decreased, tension decreased, and there was no increase in personality disturbance on the MMPI. Sleepiness, as measured by the MSLT, was increased in the induced insomnia group with no abnormality of sleep latency perception. Findings such as these have led to the hypothesis that chronic sleep deprivation in insomnia patients is a homeostatic mechanism to balance the hyperarousal, which is the underlying etiology of the insomnia. This concept of sleep deprivation countering heightened arousal levels may partially account for the efficacy of sleep restriction therapy in treating chronic insomnia.

Like primary insomnia, many patients with depression are believed to be hyperaroused. Numerous studies have demonstrated that acute total sleep deprivation leads to significant next-day improvement in 30 to 50% of patients with depression (Wu et al., 1999). Sleepiness increases with sleep deprivation in these patients, as would be expected. Unlike normal controls who generally experience worsening mood with sleep deprivation, depressed patients experience a general improvement in a wide variety of measures of mood, psychomotor retardation, and psychomotor testing (Gerner, Post, Gillin, & Bunney, 1979; Pflug, 1976; Hemmeter, Bischof, Hatzinger, Seifritz, & Holsboer-Traschler, 1998). Although the response of subjective fatigue to sleep deprivation in depressed patients has not been systematically studied, patients who are more subjectively "tired" before sleep deprivation are reported to have a better response to sleep deprivation (Bouhuys, van den Burg, & van den Hoofdakker, 1995). Objective sleepiness, as measured by frequency of microsleeps prior to sleep deprivation, does not predict favorable response to sleep deprivation (Hemmeter et al., 1998).

Sleep, Fatigue, and the Brain

In summary, the literature on sleepiness and fatigue in clinical sleep disorders confirms and expands on the findings in experimental manipulations of the sleep–wake cycle in healthy individuals; that is, while sleepiness and fatigue both result from insufficient sleep and tend to overlap in clinical syndromes, they are clearly distinct phenomena that can occur independently. What does this tell us about brain function? The evidence demonstrates that sleepiness and fatigue, on one hand, and alertness, on the other, are not opposite ends of a unitary continuous process, as they are often discussed in literature. Sleepiness and fatigue can be differentially affected by manipulation of the sleep–wake cycle and in various sleep disorders. This implies that they may be mediated by distinct neurophysiological mechanisms. In a trial of modafinil in the treatment of MS fatigue, 200 mg of modafinil resulted in improvement of fatigue and sleepiness as measured by the ESS, while 400 mg resulted in improvement in the ESS similar to the 200-mg dose but without improved fatigue (Rammohan et al., 2002). One implication might be that sleepiness and fatigue are also pharmacologically distinguishable, although other explanations for this finding are possible.

What neurological mechanisms are involved in the expression of fatigue in sleep disorders? Recent evidence, reviewed earlier, indicates that the presence of depressed mood may be the most important single factor determining how we perceive quality of sleep and whether fatigue is experienced in response to at least some sleep disorders. The strength of this link suggests that the responses to disturbed sleep, fatigue, and depressed mood have common neurophysiological mechanisms.

Neuroimaging studies may provide some clues to the nature of this common mechanism. Neuroimaging studies consistently demonstrate hypometabolism of some brain regions in depression and hypermetobalism of others. Depressed patients exhibit decreased metabolic rate in the basal ganglia and elevated metabolic rates in the anterior cingulate gyrus and medial prefrontal cortex (Wu et al., 1999). Consistent with the hypothesis that hyperarousal is responsible for some symptoms of depression and that sleep deprivation dampens this hyperarousal, metabolic rates in these regions of the brain were higher in responders to sleep deprivation than in nonresponders, and sleep reduction is associated with reduced anterior cingulate hypermetabolism (Wu et al., 1999). Sleep deprivation resulted in the greatest reduction in cerebral glucose metabolism in the anterior cingulate cortex, and this reduction in metabolism was associated with symptomatic improvement (Smith et al., 1999). Treatment with sleep deprivation did not affect basal ganglia hypometabolism in depressed patients. The pattern of response to sleep deprivation in control subjects was often the opposite to that of depressed patients, demonstrating decreased metabolism of the basal ganglia and increased metabolism of the anterior cingulate gyrus and medial prefrontal cortex. Symptomatic improvement in fatigue during treatment of depression with antidepressants or psychotherapy is associated with decreases in frontal cortex and increases in right anterior medial temporal metabolism, as demonstrated by position emission tomographic (PET) scanning (Brody et al., 2001).

Neuroimaging data in sleep disorders are limited. Since hyperarousal is a key feature of primary insomnia, as in depression, it would be interesting to know whether the patterns of hypermetabolism and hypometabolism overlap in primary insomnia and depression. Unfortunately, no data are yet available for primary insomnia patients during waking. During non-REM sleep in primary insomnia patients, a single photon emission computed tomography (SPECT) study demonstrated decreased blood flow to the basal ganglia (Smith et al., 2002). No adequate data exist for sleep disorders such as obstructive sleep apnea syndrome. Studies looking specifically at the effect of sleep deprivation on cerebral metabolism produce results similar to those of control subjects in the sleep deprivation and depression studies. In the first study of cerebral glucose metabolism, Wu and colleagues (1991) found that whole brain metabolism was not decreased but there was significant reorganization of regional cerebral metabolism. There were decreases in basal ganglia, thalamus, white matter, and cerebellum. Little change was seen in the limbic system. Benzodiazepines induce sleepiness as a desired effect, but with the longer half-life agents daytime fatigue can be problematic. Administration of the benzodiazepine analogue DD52700, like sleep deprivation, did not result in a global reduction in whole brain metabolism. PET scanning revealed a regional decrease in brain metabolism in the thalamus, cerebellum, and caudate nucleus, which is similar to the pattern seen in sleep deprivation. Performing attentional tasks, the DD5200 group showed increased regional blood flow to the cingulate gyrus and occipitoparietal cortex compared to control subjects. This relative activation was believed to be secondary to increased effort required to maintain attention.

Hypometabolism of the basal ganglia is a prominent finding in neuroimaging studies of several other conditions characterized by fatigue. Patients with multiple sclerosis show a global reduction in cerebral glucose metabolism, but patients with severe fatigue also exhibit distinct regional changes with reduced glucose metabolism in the frontal cortex and basal ganglia. It has been hypothesized that impaired interaction between cortical regions involved in the frontal cortex and basal ganglia may be related to MS-associated fatigue (Roelcke et al., 1997). Fatigue is a prominent symptom of Parkinson's disease. Not surprisingly, hypometabolism of the basal ganglia has been reported in Parkinson's disease (Dethy et al., 1998). The observation that fatigue severity fluctuates with motor function suggests that the basal ganglia may play a role in mediating fatigue in this disease, as has been hypothesized for MS (van Hilten et al., 1993). Recent research indicates that the basal ganglia modulates many processes typically thought of as being cortical phenomena, including "motivation." Impaired motivation may play an important role in the genesis of fatigue. Chaudhuri and Behan (2000) propose that an interruption of the circuits projecting from the cortex to the basal ganglia, and subsequently to the frontal cortex, is an important mediator of fatigue from many sources. The hypothesis that the basal ganglion is involved in mediating fatigue is consistent with the pharmacological data suggesting that dopaminergic mechanisms are important in fatigue and dopaminergic agonists improve fatigue.

Collectively, these data suggest a possible neuroanatomic basis for the dissociation between fatigue and sleepiness in sleep disturbance. Whether sleepiness is present depends on the balance of activity between ascending wakefulness-promoting and sleep-promoting pathways. These pathways are relatively well defined. Wakefulness can be maintained through augmentation of any of several pathways that may not improve function in the circuits underlying fatigue. The pathways underlying the expression of fatigue are less well characterized. Preliminary evidence from the disorders resulting in fatigue reviewed previously suggests that the presence of fatigue may depend on an interruption of the circuits linking the cortex to the basal ganglia. The prominence of hyperarousal in the genesis of sleep disorders resulting in fatigue suggests that cortical hyperarousal of specific regions, such as the cingulate gyrus, with relative hypofunction of subcortical circuits involving the basal ganglia may generate fatigue without marked dysfunction of subcortical circuits. These conclusions about the neuroanatomic substrates of fatigue remain speculative, but are consistent with the current literature on sleep disorders and fatigue and are amenable to empiric testing.

Less speculatively, the data reviewed here also suggest that traditional concepts of homeostasis must be altered to include circadian rhythms when discussing sleepiness and fatigue. Circadian phase directly affects levels of sleepiness and fatigue and can indirectly affect homeostasis, and circadian factors should be considered in any study of fatigue. Finally, a review of the literature on sleep disorders and fatigue definitively argues that the tendency of the sleep field to focus on sleepiness and neglect fatigue is misguided. Sleepiness and fatigue are prominent manifestations of many sleep disorders, and effective treatment of sleep disorders requires an understanding of the neurophysiological mechanisms underlying both symptoms.

Acknowledgment

The author would like to thank Adelaide E. Morrissey for her assistance on this chapter.

References

Ancoli-Israel, S., & Roth, T. (1991). Characteristics of insomnia in the United States: results of the 1991 national sleep foundation survey. *Sleep, 22(supple 2)*, S354–S353.

Attarian, H. P., Duntley, S. P., Brandon, S., Carter, J. D., & Cross, A. (2003). The relationship of abnormal sleep rhythms and fatigue of multiple sclerosis. *Sleep, 26*, A347.

Baker, S. K., & Zee, P. C. (2000). Circadian disorders of the sleep-wake cycle. In M. H. Kryger, T. Roth, & W. C. Dement, eds. *Principles and Practice of Sleep Medicine*. Pp. 606–614. Philadelphia: W. B. Saunders Company.

Bardwell, W. A., Moore, P., Ancoli-Israel, S., & Dimsdale, J. E. (2003). Fatigue in obstructive sleep apnea: driven by depressive symptoms instead of apnea severity? *American Journal of Psychiatry*, *160*, 350–355.

Beebe, D. W., Groesz, L., Wells, C., Nichols, A., & McGee, K. (2003). The neuropsychological effects of obstructive sleep apnea: a meta-analysis of norm-referenced and case-controlled data. *Sleep*, *26*, 298–307.

Bonnett, M. H. (1986). Performance and sleepiness as a function of frequency and placement of sleep disruption. *Psychophysiology*, *23*, 263–271.

Bonnet, M. H. (2000). Sleep deprivation. In M. H. Kryger, T. Roth, & W. C. Dement, eds. *Principles and Practice of Sleep Medicine*. Pp. 53–71. Philadelphia: W. B. Saunders Company.

Bonnett, M. H., & Arand, D. (1995). 24 hour metabolic rate in insomniacs and matched normal sleepers. *Sleep*, *18*, 581–588.

Bonnet, M. H., & Arand, D. L. (1992). Caffeine use as a model of acute and chronic insomnia. *Sleep*, *15*, 526–536.

Bonnet, M. H., and Arand, D. L. (1996). The consequences of a week of insomnia. *Sleep*, *19*, 453–461.

Borbely, A. A. (1982). A two process model of sleep regulation. *Human Neurobiology*, *1*, 147–154.

Bouhuys, A. L., van den Burg, W., & van den Hoofdakker, R. H. (1995). The relationship between tiredness prior to sleep deprivation and the antidepressant response to sleep deprivation in depression. *Biological Psychiatry*, *37*, 457–461.

Brody, A. L., Saxena, S., Mandelkern, M. A., Fairbanks, L. A., Ho, M. L, & Baxter, L. R. (2001). Brain metabolic changes associated with symptom factor improvement in major depressive disorder. *Biological Psychiatry*, *50*, 171–178.

Carskadon, M. A., & Dement, W. C. (1981). Cumulative effects of sleep restriction on daytime sleepiness. *Psychophysiology*, *18*, 107–113.

Carskadon, M. A., & Dement, W. C. (1992). Multiple sleep latency tests during the constant routine. *Sleep*, *15*, 396–399.

Carskadon, M. A., Dement, W. C., Mitler, M. M., Roth, T., Westbrook, P. R., & Keenan S. (1986). Guidelines for the multiple sleep latency test (MSLT): a standard measure of sleepiness. *Sleep*, *9*, 519–524.

Chaudhuri, A., & Behan, P. (2000). Fatigue and basal ganglia. *Journal of the Neurological Sciences*, *179*, 34–42.

Chervin, R. D. (2000). Sleepiness, fatigue, tiredness and lack of energy in obstructive sleep apnea. *Chest, 118*, 372–379.

Day, R. C., Wells, R., Carney, R., Freedland, K., & Duntley, S. (2003). Relationship between subjective sleep quality and depression in patients with obstructive sleep apnea. *Sleep, 23*, A258.

Derderian, S. S., Bridenbaugh, R. H., & Rajagopal, K. (1988). Neuropsychologic symptoms in obstructive sleep apnea improve after treatment with nasal continuous positive airway pressure. *Chest, 94*, 1023–1027.

Dethy, S., Van Blercom, N., Damhaut, P., Wikler, D., Hildebrand, J., & Goldman, S. (1998). Asymmetry of basal ganglia glucose metabolism and dopa responsiveness in parkinsonism. *Movement Disorders, 13*, 275–280.

Dinges, D. F., Pack, F., Williams, K., Gillen, K. A., Powell, J. W., Ott, G. E., Aptowicz, C., & Pack, A. I. (1997). Cumulative sleepiness, mood disturbance, and psychomotor vigilance performance decrements during a week of sleep restricted to 4–5 hours a night. *Sleep, 20*, 267–277.

Friedmann, J., Globus, G., Huntley, A., Mullaney, D., Naitoh, P., & Johnson, L. (1977). Performance and mood during and after gradual sleep reduction. *Psychophysiology, 14*, 245–250.

Gerner, R., Post, R., Gillin, C., & Bunney, W. (1979). Biological and behavioral effects of one night's sleep deprivation in depressed and normals. *Journal of Psychiatric Research, 15*, 21–40.

Gillin, J. C., Rapaport, M., Erman, M. K., Winokur, A., and Albala, B. J. (1997). A comparison of nefazodone and fluoxetine on mood and on objective, subjective and clinician-rated measures of sleep in depressed patients: a double-blind, 8-week clinical trial. *Journal of Clinical Psychiatry, 58*, 185–192.

Hemmeter, U., Bischof, R., Hatzinger, M., Seifritz, E., & Holsboer-Traschler, E. (1998). Microsleep during partial sleep deprivation in depression. *Biological Psychiatry, 43*, 829–839.

Hoddes, E., Zarcone, V., Smythe, H., Phillips, R., & Dement, W. C. (1973). Quantification of sleepiness: a new approach. *Psychophysiology, 10*, 431–436.

The International Classification of Sleep Disorders: Diagnostic and Coding Manual. (2000). Rochester, MN: American Academy of Sleep Medicine.

Johns, M. W. (1991). A new method for measuring daytime sleepiness: the Epworth Sleepiness Scale. *Sleep, 14*, 540–545.

Kribbs, N. B., Pack, A. I., Kline, L. R., Smith, P. L., Schwartz, A. R., Schubert, N. M., Redline, S., Henry, J., Getsy, J. E., & Dinges, D. F. (1993). Objective measurement of patterns of nasal CPAP use by patients with obstructive sleep apnea. *American Review of Respiratory Disease, 147*, 887–895.

Krupp, L. B., Jandorf, L., Coyl, P. K., & Mendelson, W. B. (1993). Sleep disturbance in chronic fatigue syndrome. *Journal of Psychosomatic Research, 37*, 325–331.

Krupp, L. B., Larocca, N. G., Muir-Nash, J., & Steinberg, A. D. (1989). The Fatigue Severity Scale: Application to patients with multiple sclerosis and systemic lupus erythematosus. *Archives of Neurology, 46*, 1121–1123.

Lichstein, K. L., Means, M. K., Noe, S. L., & Aguillard, R. N. (1997). Fatigue and sleep disorders. *Behavior Research Therapy, 35,* 733–740.

Martin, S. E., Engleman, H. M., Deary, I. J., & Douglas, N. J. (1996). The effect of sleep fragmentation on daytime function. *American Journal Respiratory Critical Care Medicine, 153,* 1328–1332.

Martin, S. E., Wraith, P. K., Deary, I. J., & Douglas, N. J. (1997). The effect of nonvisible sleep fragmentation on daytime function. *American Journal Respiratory Critical Care Medicine, 155,* 1596–1601.

Mitler, M. M., Gujavarty, K. S., & Browman, C. P. (1982). Maintenance of wakefulness test: a polysomnographic technique for evaluation of treatment efficacy in patients with excessive daytime somnolence. *Electroencephalography and Clinical Neurophysiology, 53,* 658–661.

Monk T. H, ed. (1991). Sleep, sleepiness and performance. In *Circadian Aspects of Subjective Sleepiness: A Behavioral Messenger?* Pp. 39–63. New York: John Wiley & Sons.

Monroe, L. J. (1967). Psychological and physiological differences between good and poor sleepers. *Journal of Abnormal Psychology, 72,* 255–264.

Morriss, R., Sharpe, M., Sharpley, A. L., Cowen, P. J., Hawton, K., & Morris, J. (1993). Abnormalities of sleep in patients with chronic fatigue syndrome. *British Medical Journal, 306,* 1161–1164.

Mosko, S., Zetin, M., Glen, S., Garber, D., DeAntonio, M., Sassin, J., McAnich, J., & Warren, S. (1989). Self-reported depressive symptomatology, mood ratings and treatment outcome in sleep disorders patients. *Journal of Clinical Psychology, 45,* 51–60.

Multiple Sclerosis Council for Clinical Practice Guidelines. (1998). *Fatigue and Multiple Sclerosis: Evidence based management strategies for fatigue in multiple sclerosis.* Washington, DC: Paralyzed Veterans of America.

Newman, A. M., Nieto, F. J., Guidry, U., Lind, B. K., Redline, S., Pickering, T. G., & Quan, S. F. (2001). Relation of sleep-disordered breathing to cardiovascular disease risk factors: the Sleep Heart Health Study. *American Journal of Epidemiology, 154,* 50–59.

Oxford Dictionary (2002). Oxford, England: Oxford University Press.

Perlis, M. L., Giles, D. E., Bootzin, R. R., Dikman, Z. V., Fleming, G. M., Drummond, S. P., & Rose, M. W. (1997). Alpha sleep and information processing, perception of sleep, pain, and arousability in fibromyalgia. *International Journal of Neuroscience, 89,* 265–280.

Pflug, B. (1976). The effect of sleep deprivation on depressed patients. *Acta Psychiatrica Scandinavica, 53,* 148–158.

Rammohan, K. W., Rosenberg, J. H., Lynn, D. J., Blumenfeld, A. M., Pollak, C. P., & Nagaraja, H. N. (2002). Efficacy and safety of modafinil for the treatment of fatigue in multiple sclerosis: a two center phase 2 study. *Journal of Neurology, Neurosurgery, & Psychiatry, 72,* 179–183.

Richardson, G. S., Carskadon, M. A., Orav, E. J., & Dement W. C. (1982). Circadian variation of sleep tendency in elderly and young adult subjects. *Sleep, 5,* S82–S94.

Roelcke, U., Kappos, L., Lechner-Scott, J., Brunnschweiler, H., Huber, S., Ammann, W., Plohmann, A., Dellas, S., Maguire, R. P., Missimer, J., Radu, E. W., Steck, A., & Leenders, K. L. (1997). Reduced glucose metabolism in the frontal cortex and basal ganglia of multiple sclerosis patients with fatigue: a 18F-fluorodeoxyglucose positron emission tomography study. *Neurology, 48*, 1566–1571.

Rush, A. J., Armitage, R., Gillin, J. C., Younkers, K. A., Winokur, A., Moldofsky, J., Vogel, G. W., Kaplita, S. B., Fleming, J. B., Montplaisir, J., Erman, M. K., Albala, B. J., & McQuade, R. D. (1998). Comparative effects of nefazodone and fluoxetine on sleep in outpatients with major depressive disorder. *Biological Psychiatry, 44*, 3–14.

Schneider-Helmert, D. (1987). Twenty-four-hour sleep-wake function and personality patterns in chronic insomniacs and healthy controls. *Sleep, 10*, 452–462.

Siegel, J. (1999). Narcolepsy: a key role for hypocretins (orexins). *Cell, 98*, 409–412.

Smith, G. S., Reynolds, C. F., Pollock, B., Derbyshire, S., Nofzinger, E., Dew, M. A., Houck, P. R., Milko, D., Meltzer, C. C., & Kupfer, D. J. (1999). Cerebral glucose metabolic response to combined total sleep deprivation and antidepressant treatment in geriatric depression. *American Journal of Psychiatry, 156*, 683–689.

Smith, M. T., Perlis, M. L., Chengazi, V. U., Pennington, J. M., Soeffing, J., Ryan, J. M., & Giles, D. E. (2002). Neuroimaging of NREM sleep in primary insomnia: a Tc-99-HMPAO single photon emission computed tomography study. *Sleep, 25*, 325–335.

Van Dongen, H. P. A., & Dinges, D. F. (2000). Circadian rhythms in fatigue, alertness, and performance. In M. H. Kryger, T. Roth, & W. C. Dement, eds. *Principles and Practice of Sleep Medicine*. Pp. 391–397. Philadelphia: W. B. Saunders Company.

Van Hilten, J. J., Weggeman, M., van der Velde, E. A., Kerkhof, G. A., van Dijk, D. J., & Roos, R. A. (1993). Sleep, excessive daytime sleepiness and fatigue in Parkinson's disease. *Journal of Neural Transmission-Parkinsons Disease & Dementia Section, 5*, 235–244.

Wu, J. C., Gillin, J. C., Buchsbaum, M. S., Hershey, T., Hazlett, E., Sicotte, N., & Bunney, W. E. (1991). The effect of sleep deprivation on cerebral glucose metabolic rate in normal humans assessed with positron emission tomography. *Sleep, 14*, 155–162.

Wu, J., Buchsbaum, M. S., Gillin, J. C., Tang, C., Cadwell, S., Wiegand, M., Najafi, A., Klein, E., Hazen, K., & Bunney, W. (1999). Prediction of antidepressant effects of sleep deprivation by metabolic rates in the ventral anterior cingulate and medial prefrontal cortex. *American Journal of Psychiatry, 156*, 1149–1158.

Young, T., Palta, M., Dempsey, J., Skatrud, J., Weber, S., & Badr, S. (1993). The occurrence of sleep-disordered breathing among middle-aged adults. *New England Journal of Medicine, 328*, 1230–1235.

Yu, B., Ancoli-Israel, S., & Dimsdale, J. (1999). Effect of CPAP treatment on mood states in patients with sleep apnea. *Journal of Psychiatric Research, 33*, 427–432.

14   Heart Disease, Cardiovascular Functioning, and Fatigue

Scott Siegel and Neil Schneiderman

Cardiovascular disease is the leading cause of death, morbidity, and disability in the United States (McGovern, Pankow, Shahar, et al., 1996). Accordingly, identifying new risk factors in addition to the traditional risk factors (e.g., hypertension) is important in classifying those most likely to develop cardiovascular disease. Research in the past decade has demonstrated a consistent relationship between depressive symptomatology and coronary heart disease (CHD) (Rugulies, 2002); specifically, depression predicts both the development of CHD in initially healthy people and survival post-myocardial infarction (MI). These relationships remain even after controlling for traditional risk factors (e.g., hypertension, elevated cholesterol, smoking, age, male sex, etc.) and markers of disease severity. Furthermore, nearly 20 percent of CHD patients meet criteria for major depression (Carney et al., 1987) and an additional 27 percent meet criteria for minor depression (Schleifer et al., 1989). In contrast, the point prevalence of major depression in individuals without CHD of comparable age and gender is only 3 percent (Myers et al., 1984). Depressed CHD patients are at much greater risk of MI (Frasure-Smith, Lespérance, & Talajic, 1995; Lespérance et al., 2002). Therefore, because of its predictive power and elevated prevalence, depression may be an important, independent prognostic indicator of future cardiac events in CHD patients.

Appels (1997) has argued that the depressive symptoms observed in coronary patients may differ from major depression in otherwise healthy individuals. Although symptoms of depression such as depressed affect, hopelessness, and irritability all predict risk of future cardiac events, these variables lose their predictive power when adjusting for fatigue (Appels, Kop, & Schouten, 2000). Furthermore, fatigue remains an independent predictor of MI risk even after controlling for age, cholesterol level, smoking, and systolic blood pressure. Based on these and other findings, Appels and colleagues have advanced the construct of "vital exhaustion" to distinguish between traditional depression and the state of unusual fatigue associated with CHD. Vital exhaustion also includes feelings of demoralization and increased irritability, though these symptoms are considered secondary to the fatigue; that is, CHD patients who experience a sudden, unusual bout of exhaustion may become demoralized and irritable because of their fatigue. Like depression, vital exhaustion is a strong, short-term predictor of MI in initially healthy individuals.

The relationship between depressive symptomatology and poor coronary outcomes has been explained partly in behavioral terms (reviewed in Rozanski, Blumenthal, & Kaplan, 1999). For example, individuals with depression generally have poorer eating habits, are less likely to exercise adequately, and are more likely to smoke; each of these factors is associated with increased risk for future cardiac events and cardiac mortality (e.g., Glassman et al., 1990). Post-MI depressive symptoms may be a reaction to the cardiac event itself. Existential issues and disability are certainly capable of spurring an episode of depression. The relationship between depression and CHD has also been explained in physiological terms. For instance, as reviewed in Rozanski et al. (1999), depression is associated with alterations in the hypothalamic-pituitary-adrenal (HPA) axis resulting in increased production of corticotropin-releasing factor (CRF), dysregulated negative feedback, and an overall increase in cortisol production (e.g., Carroll et al., 1981). There is also evidence of altered platelet reactivity, decreased heart rate variability, and decreased vagal control in patients with depression. Depression may therefore be associated with risk of MI through behavioral or physiological pathways.

Through either behavioral or physiological mechanisms, depression has been historically described as a predisposing, causal risk factor for future MIs. An alternative, more recently developed hypothesis (e.g., Meesters & Appels, 1996) proposes that depression and fatigue are simply symptoms of CHD. As reviewed in the following section, CHD is associated with chronic, low-level inflammation (Ross, 1999). Research in other situations (e.g., influenza) has shown that inflammation can induce a number of behavioral and motivational changes, including fatigue and depressed affect (reviewed in Larson & Dunn, 2001). The mechanisms by which inflammation induces these behavioral and motivation changes involve the central nervous system (CNS). Thus, inflammation associated with the underlying pathophysiology of CHD may be responsible for the fatigue reported by coronary patients (figure 14.1). This is perhaps not the most intuitive hypothesis, because fatigue and depression both precede and predict future cardiac events in initially healthy individuals (Rugulies, 2002). Nevertheless, the classification of "initially healthy" may not be appropriate. CHD develops slowly, often taking several decades to fully manifest (Viikari, Raitakari, & Simell, 2002). In contrast, vital exhaustion is useful only as a short-term predictor, losing its prognostic value beyond 12 to 18 months (Appels, 1997). Patients within 12 to 18 months of an MI are probably not as "healthy" as they initially seem; more likely, they may be exhibiting subclinical markers of CHD that have eluded detection.

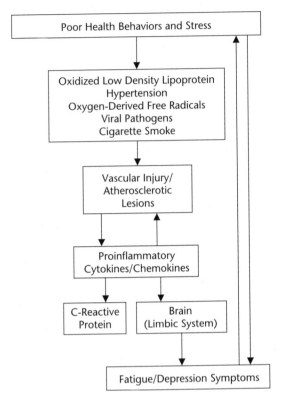

Figure 14.1
Conceptual model delineating the pathway through which poor health behaviors and stress leading to atherosclerotic coronary artery disease produce fatigue and depressive symptoms mediated by the release of proinflammatory cytokines.

Atherosclerosis, Inflammation, and the Acute-Phase Response

Before proceeding, it may be useful to briefly describe the pathophysiology of CHD (for a more thorough review, see Ross, 1999). Only recently has it become generally accepted that CHD contains an inflammatory component. Previously, cardiologists thought infarctions were caused by gradually expanding, yet generally static, accumulations of lipids. Atherosclerotic lesions today are typically understood as dynamic, immunological responses to vascular injury. The exact cause or causes of vascular injury are unknown, but the possibilities include oxidized low-density lipoprotein (e.g., Kaul, 2001), blood flow shear from frequent, sudden shifts in blood pressure (e.g., Leopold & Loscalzo, 2000), oxygen-derived free radicals (e.g., Touyz, 2000), viral pathogens (e.g., Vercellotti, 1998), and cigarette smoke (e.g., McVeigh et al., 1997).

In response to injury, vascular endothelial cells express adhesion molecules that attract platelets, monocytes, and lymphocytes. These leukocytes bind to adhesion molecules and infiltrate the arterial wall. Once within the arterial wall, monocytes mature into macrophages and, together with lymphocytes, produce chemokines and proinflammatory cytokines. Chemokines and cytokines, in turn, promote more inflammation, further enhance expression of adhesion molecules, and lead to greater leukocyte recruitment to the injury (see figure 14.1). Platelets and leukocytes release growth factors that induce smooth muscle to proliferate and migrate to the vessel wall. Thus, the growing plaque is composed of accumulated lipids, smooth muscle, leukocytes, and mediators of inflammation. The plaque is contained by a fibrous cap that can rupture over time, causing a thrombus (i.e., clot). If the thrombus is large enough, it can create a blockage in a coronary artery, leading to cardiac damage (i.e., MI). Additionally, inflammatory mediators contribute to both the instability of the fibrous cap and the formation of the thrombus once the cap has degraded. Inflammatory processes are therefore involved with all stages of atherosclerosis, from initiation of a plaque, to its growth, to the degradation of the cap, and finally to the formation of the thrombus. Occasionally, even without rupturing, plaques can grow large enough to help block blood flow and cause an infarction.

Mediators of inflammation within the vascular lesion also make their way into the circulation, most notably the proinflammatory cytokines (Pollmacher et al., 2002). As described earlier, proinflammatory cytokines are instrumental in the initiation and maintenance of local inflammatory reactions. Proinflammatory cytokines are also important in activating a systemic response, known as acute-phase response. The acute-phase response is characterized by increased white blood cell production (leukocytosis) and increased production of a group of proteins in the liver known as acute-phase proteins. Acute-phase proteins such as serum amyloid A, fibrinogen, and C-reactive protein (CRP) are part of the innate immune system and function to contain microbial infections (see figure 14.1). Interestingly, a history of major depressive episodes has been associated with elevated levels of CRP in men (Danner et al., 2003). Recent reports indicate CRP is an independent risk factor for future cardiac events (Morrow & Ridker, 2000).

Sickness Behavior: A Component of the Acute-Phase Response

Proinflammatory cytokines also initiate behavioral, affective, and motivational changes by binding to receptors in the hypothalamus and other limbic structures of the CNS (Dantzer, 2001; Larson & Dunn, 2001). However, proinflammatory cytokines are large, lipophobic molecules incapable of crossing the blood-brain barrier and are thus forced to take alternative routes (Maier & Watkins, 1998). One interesting alternative pathway proinflammatory cytokines take is the vagus nerve. The proinflammatory cytokine interleukin-1 (IL-1) binds to vagal afferent neurons, which in turn increase afferent vagal activity. The vagus nerve projects to and terminates in the nucleus tractus solitarius (NTS) of the brainstem; the NTS has direct projections to the paraventricular and preoptic nuclei of the hypothalamus (e.g., Watkins et al., 1994). The proinflammatory cytokines IL-1, interleukin-6 (IL-6), and tumor necrosis factor-α (TNF-α) also gain entry into the CNS by diffusing across relatively permeable portions of the blood-brain barrier (i.e., at the circumventricular organs) and engaging active transport mechanisms (for a review, see Rivest, 2001).

As part of a coordinated acute-phase response, central proinflammatory cytokine expression is responsible for inducing fever. By curtailing bacterial replication, fever is an adaptive host response to infection (Blatteis, 1986). Proinflammatory cytokines also produce a set of behavioral changes collectively known as "sickness behavior," a less well understood, purported feature of the acute-phase response. Sickness behavior refers to the subjective feelings of fatigue, weakness, malaise, and listlessness characteristic of sick individuals. Sick individuals also commonly experience changes in appetite and weight, altered sleeping patterns, diminished interest in their surroundings, and difficulty concentrating. These symptoms were once thought to be directly caused by infecting pathogens, but more recently it has become clear that proinflammatory cytokines are both sufficient and necessary (i.e., even without infection) to generate the sickness behavior response (Dantzer, 2001; Larson & Dunn, 2001). For example, cytokine therapy—the therapeutic administration of exogenous cytokines— is sometimes used to treat cancer patients (Capuron & Dantzer, 2003). Exogenous administration of cytokines is thought to activate immune cells in cancer patients capable of curtailing cancerous growth. The efficacy of such therapies aside, physicians have observed that cytokine therapy causes significant side effects, including fatigue, flulike symptoms, and cognitive impairment. Randomized studies substantiate these observations (Capuron et al., 2002; Bonaccorso, Meltzer, & Maes, 2000), and, extensive research with rodents has explicated these findings (reviewed in Larson & Dunn, 2001). For example, peripheral administration of proinflammatory cytokines reduces overall activity levels, decreases food intake, diminishes exploratory behavior, reduces social interactions (including sexual behaviors), and alters sleep patterns. Proinflammatory cytokines also induce anhedonia, the inability to experience and be motivated by pleasurable stimuli. Healthy rodents, for instance, greatly prefer sugary solutions such as sweetened milk to water, whereas animals injected with cytokines show no such preference. Finally, treating infected animals with cytokine antagonists or severing the vagus nerve abrogates sickness behavior (Dantzer, 2001).

In light of these findings, sickness behavior has been advanced as a part of a highly organized strategy of mammals to combat infection. Symptoms of illness, as previously thought, are not inconsequential or even maladaptive. On the contrary, sickness behavior, much like other elements of the acute-phase response (e.g., fever), promotes resistance and facilitates recovery (Dantzer, 2001) For example, an overall decrease in activity allows the sick individual to preserve energy resources that can be redirected toward enhancing immune activity. Similarly, limiting exploration, mating, and foraging further preserves energy resources and reduces the likelihood of risky encounters (e.g., fighting over a mate). Ingesting food, furthermore, increases blood levels of iron, which is essential for bacterial replication; reducing feeding behavior thus hampers bacterial growth. The advantages sickness behavior affords other animals are thought to apply to people as well.

The Role of Proinflammatory Cytokines in the CNS

The immune system can be thought of as a sensory organ capable of perceiving information about an organism's environment (e.g., pathogens) and communicating this information to the brain (Maier & Watkins, 1998). As with other sensory organs (e.g., the eye), the immune system transduces information about the environment perceived by its cells; that is, information from the immune system is encoded into signals the brain can understand. In the eye, transduction occurs when light induces a cascade of biochemical events beginning with photopigments and ultimately leading to a change in the frequency of neural action potentials of the optic nerve. In the immune system, transduction appears to be mediated by the proinflammatory cytokines: peripheral cytokines stimulate the production and release of cytokines in the brain (Laye, Parnet, Boujon, & Dantzer, 1994). Recall that peripheral cytokines can activate the vagus nerve. When activated, the vagus nerve releases glutamate in the NTS of the medulla, which then projects to several limbic structures including the hypothalamus and amygdala (reviewed in Dantzer, 2001). Also recall that peripheral cytokines may enter the brain by diffusing across the most permeable areas of the blood-brain barrier (e.g., area postrema).

Activation of these regions is thought to sensitize target brain areas to centrally produced cytokines, synthesized primarily by microglial cells (Dantzer, 2001; van Dam, Brouns, Louisse, & Berkenbosch, 1992). Cytokine production in these limbic structures is associated with sickness behavior. Fatigue and other symptoms of sickness behavior are attenuated in rodents when the vagus nerve is experimentally severed or when cytokine antagonists are injected centrally. How do central cytokines induce these symptoms? The mechanisms are not yet understood; however, evidence shows that cytokine administration increases norepinephrine, dopamine, and serotonin activity in the hypothalamus. Cytokines also activate the HPA axis and prostaglandin production (for a thorough review on the signal transduction pathways of cytokines in neural circuits, see Rivest, 2001).

Depression, Vital Exhaustion, and Sickness Behavior: Distinct or Identical Constructs?

There is considerable overlap between the symptoms of depression and sickness behavior. The DSM-IV criteria for a major depressive episode require either depressed mood or anhedonia and four other symptoms, including change in appetite or weight, altered sleeping patterns, psychomotor retardation (or agitation), fatigue/loss of energy, feelings of worthlessness/excessive guilt, difficulties concentrating, and recurrent thoughts of death. As reviewed earlier, administration of exogenous proinflammatory cytokines in both animals and humans can induce anhedonia, a change in eating habits, altered sleeping patterns, reduced overall activity levels, fatigue, and cognitive difficulties. Thus, exogenous proinflammatory cytokines are sufficient to produce the symptoms of a major depressive episode. Given the depressive effects of exogenous cytokines and the many known associations between depression and altered immunity (Irwin, 2002), a great deal of interest has been paid to the cytokine hypothesis of depression—that is, endogenously produced proinflammatory cytokines may be necessary and sufficient to induce major depression. Other studies (Capuron & Dantzer, 2003; de Beaurepaire, 2002) indicate that proinflammatory cytokines are probably not necessary but may be sufficient to induce many symptoms of depression. Interestingly, cancer patients undergoing cytokine therapy generally develop symptoms of fatigue, malaise, weakness, and anhedonia before mood symptoms. This raises the possibility that emotions such as sadness are secondary to (i.e., develop in response to) other depressive, cytokine-induced symptoms such as fatigue and anhedonia.

Vital exhaustion, like the depression in cytokine therapy patients, has been conceptualized as a primary fatigue accompanied by a secondary demoralization and irritability (Appels, Kop, & Schouten, 2000). For cytokine therapy patients or patients with an apparent infection (e.g., influenza) who are experiencing sickness behavior symptoms, it is not difficult to attribute feelings of listlessness and malaise to the ongoing treatment or sickness. Nevertheless, cytokine therapy patients frequently meet criteria for depression. In fact, evidence now supports treating cytokine therapy patients prophylactically with antidepressants (Capuron et al., 2002). In contrast, pre-MI patients reporting vital exhaustion may be otherwise symptom-free; unlike someone suffering from influenza, pre-MI individuals with CHD may be completely unaware of their "silent" illness. Because such individuals, who feel especially depleted and uninterested in their world, have no obvious illness or treatment to which they can attribute their symptoms, clinical depression may ensue.

Depressive symptoms in post-MI patients can be easily, and perhaps mistakenly, attributed solely to a reaction to the MI itself. As described previously, fatigue, and not depressed affect or irritability, remains a significant predictor of future MIs, even after controlling for age, cholesterol, smoking, and systolic blood pressure. This finding supports the hypothesis that unusual fatigue is more proximally related to

CHD than other symptoms of depression. The inflammation associated with CHD pathophysiology causes fatigue through cytokine-mediated changes in the brain (see figure 14.1). Inflammation does not necessarily cause other depressive symptoms such as irritability or demoralization. According to our model, fatigue is directly caused by the underlying processes of CHD; other symptoms of depression are secondary and psychosocial in origin. The stress and seemingly unpredictable nature of their unexplained fatigue may be sufficient for individuals to develop negative views of themselves and the world in which they struggle to operate. Without an obvious illness to which patients can attribute their fatigue, demoralization and irritability may be a normal reaction. There is thus some reason to believe that fatigue and depression are not just risk factors, but may be symptoms of heart disease as well.

As sickness behavior is an adaptive response to infection, the inflammatory processes associated with atherosclerosis are adaptive responses to vascular injury. Only with extensive vascular injury, and excessive inflammatory reactions does atherogenesis lead to MI. Likewise, vital exhaustion may be a specific sickness behavior response to the underlying pathophysiology of CHD. In support of this theory, a number of studies have found associations between depression and increased levels of inflammatory molecules, such as IL-6 and CRP (e.g., Maes et al., 1995). One study in particular (Appels, Bar et al., 2000) found that CHD patients with vital exhaustion, compared to nonexhausted CHD controls, had higher levels of the proinflammatory cytokines IL-1β and TNF-α, and a trend toward higher levels of IL-6. These patients also had elevated antibody titers against cytomegalovirus and *C. pneumoniae*, two pathogens purported to induce vascular injury. Another more recent study (van der Ven et al., 2003) reported that, compared to nonexhausted CHD patients, vital exhaustion/CHD patients had greater "pathogen burden," defined as the number of seropositive tests to herpes simplex virus, varicella-zoster virus, Epstein-Barr virus, and cytomegalovirus. Patients with the most vital exhaustion and greatest pathogen burden were also characterized by increased levels of IL-6. The concept of pathogen burden may be significant because viral pathogens such as those investigated in these studies are believed to contribute directly to atherosclerosis through such mechanisms as infection of the arterial wall and induction of cytokines. According to our model, increases in atherosclerosis are accompanied by corresponding increases in systemic inflammation. According to van der Ven and colleagues (2003), increased pathogen burden may be a biological correlate of vital exhaustion.

Future Directions

Because the symptoms of depression, vital exhaustion, and sickness behavior overlap considerably, CHD investigators have yet to address fully two unresolved empirical questions. First, are depression and vital exhaustion different, albeit related constructs, or are these simply different labels for the same underlying phenomenon? The findings reviewed earlier do not yet provide an answer. Many measures to test this question—self-reports, semistructured interview format, and structured interview format—are available to diagnose and rate the severity of depression. To measure vital exhaustion, two measures with adequate psychometric properties have been described: one relies on self-report (Maastricht Questionnaire), the other on a semistructured interview format (Maastricht Interview for Vital Exhaustion; Meesters & Appels, 1996). Though the Maastricht Questionnaire may be more readily administered in research settings, the Maastricht Interview for Vital Exhaustion has a lower false-positive rate. Finally, although behavioral-observation systems have been developed to study sickness behavior in animals, none has yet been developed to characterize sickness behavior in humans.

Wojciechowski and colleagues (2000) examined the associations between several measures of depression and the Maastricht Questionnaire to test the hypothesis that major depression and vital exhaustion are separate entities. The correlations among the measures of depression were nearly identical to those between each of the depression measures and the Maastricht Questionnaire; furthermore, factor analysis findings suggested that all the measures could best be described with a one-factor model. Based on these findings, the authors concluded that major depression and vital exhaustion are not necessarily distinct constructs. However, they did not account for the multiple dimensions of vital exhaustion (i.e., fatigue, irritability, and demoralization), nor did they account for the possibility that participants in their study could have both vital exhaustion and depression. To study a phenomenon, one must be able to define it, label it, and distinguish it from other phenomena. To that end, more research is needed to describe the symptoms that CHD patients experience. One way to better understand the depressive symptom presentations in CHD patients would be to study them longitudinally. Tracking at-risk individuals pre- and post-MI over time would help investigators better ascertain relationships among symptoms. For instance, does fatigue precede irritability? How are patients attributing their symptoms? Finally, research should try to relate symptom reports to biological measures such as CRP, proinflammatory cytokines, and pathogen burden.

The second unresolved empirical question that investigators, and treating physicians, face deals with treatment. Findings from two recent well-conducted studies support treating depressive symptoms in CHD patients with antidepressants. The Sertraline Antidepressant Heart Attack Randomized Trial (SADHART) provides evidence that sertraline, a selective serotonin reuptake inhibitor (SSRI), is both safe and effective for recurrent depression in CHD patients (Glassman et al., 2002). The Enhancing Recovery in Coronary Heart Disease (ENRICHD, 2003) randomized study demonstrated that cognitive behavior therapy (supplemented with sertraline, as indicated) was also effective at reducing symptoms of depression in post-MI patients. However, the treatment had no effect on recurrence of MI or mortality. An interesting and unexpected finding, however, was that antidepressant use, primarily the SSRI sertraline, was associated with a lower risk of recurrent MI and mortality. This latter finding needs to be interpreted with caution; the antidepressant was not assigned to the psychotherapy or control group or randomized, but prescribed as indicated. Taken together, these studies support treating depressed CHD patients with either cognitive behavior therapy or sertraline. Furthermore, preliminary evidence shows that sertraline may improve primary outcomes in CHD patients. If future studies confirm sertraline is effective in reducing risk of MI and mortality, it can be argued that psychotherapy and antidepressants work through different pathways in CHD patients.

Although not common knowledge, SSRIs block platelet aggregation and possess anti-inflammatory properties (de Beaurepaire, 2002). In fact, antidepressants have been shown to block sickness behavior in animal models injected with proinflammatory cytokines (Yirmiya, 1996). Furthermore, vital exhaustion is conceptualized as primary fatigue and secondary depressed affect. Setraline may reduce levels of depression by (1) attenuating the inflammatory response associated with vascular injury, thereby reducing the symptoms of sickness behavior including fatigue and secondary depressed affect; (2) targeting the depressed affect directly via a central mechanism (i.e., modifying central serotonin transmission); or (3) an interaction of these two mechanisms. More work is needed to determine if antidepressants can actually improve survival rates and reduce the risk of future cardiac events; if this effect is demonstrated, then studies in animal models are warranted to delineate the mechanisms through which antidepressants operate. Also, randomizing CHD patients to psychotherapy, antidepressant, psychotherapy plus antidepressant, and control conditions could help sort out the unique relationships among fatigue, other depressive symptoms, and CHD.

Coronary heart disease is the leading cause of death, morbidity, and disability in the United States. Symptoms of depression predict both future cardiac events in initially healthy people and post-MI survival. However, limited research findings indicate that fatigue rather than other symptoms of depression is most strongly related to risk of future cardiac events. Proponents of the vital exhaustion theory argue that fatigue should be the symptom of primary interest in assessing risk factors—depressed affect and irritability are secondary to fatigue, and less important in predicting future cardiac events. Although fatigue and depression can contribute to increased risk of MI through behavioral (e.g., poor lifestyle habits) and physiological (e.g., impaired stress response) mechanisms, others have suggested that fatigue is a symptom of ongoing, subclinical heart disease.

The importance of inflammatory processes in CHD is becoming increasingly apparent to the research community and cardiologists. Furthermore, research from a number of disciplines has demonstrated a direct link between inflammation and behavioral changes such as fatigue and depressed affect. Limited research with coronary patients supports this hypothesis: exhausted patients, compared to their non-exhausted counterparts, had elevated levels of proinflammatory cytokines (e.g., IL-1) and acute-phase proteins (e.g., CRP).

More work is needed to confirm these findings and test for the potential therapeutic benefit of anti-inflammatory pharmaceuticals, antidepressants, and psychotherapy. Finally, work in animal models of coronary disease is warranted to fully delineate the relationships among fatigue, depression, and heart disease.

References

American Psychiatric Association. (1994). *Diagnotic and statistical manual of mental disorders*, 4th ed. Washington, DC: American Psychiatric Association.

Appels, A. (1997). Depression and coronary heart disease: observations and questions. *Journal of Psychosomatic Research, 43*, 443–452.

Appels, A., Bar, F. W., Bar, J., Bruggeman, C., & de Bates, M. (2000). Inflammation, depressive symptomatology, and coronary artery disease. *Psychosomatic Medicine, 62*, 601–605.

Appels, A., Kop, W. J., & Schouten, E (2000). The nature of depressive symptomatology preceding myocardial infarction. *Behavioral Medicine, 26*, 86.

Blatteis, C. M. (1986). Fever: is it beneficial? *Yale Journal of Biology and Medicine, 59*, 107–116.

Bonaccorso, S., Meltzer, H., & Maes, M. (2000). Psychological and behavioural effects of interferons. *Current Opinion in Psychiatry, 13*, 673–677.

Capuron, L., & Dantzer, R. (2003). Cytokines and depression: the need for a new paradigm. *Brain, Behavior, and Immunity, 17*, S119–S124.

Capuron, L., Gumnick, J. F., Musselman, D. L., et al. (2002). Neurobehavioral effects of interferon-alpha in cancer patients: phenomenology and paroxetine responsiveness of symptom dimensions. *Neuropsychopharmacology, 26*, 643–652.

Capuron, L., Hauser, P., Hinze-Selch, D., Miller, A. H., & Neveu, P. J. (2002). Treatment of cytokine-induced depression. *Brain, Behavior, and Immunity, 16*, 575–580.

Carney, R. M., Rich, M. W., Tevelde, A., Saini, J., Clark, K., & Jaffe, A. S. (1987). Major depressive disorder in coronary artery disease. *American Journal of Cardiology, 60*, 1273–1275.

Carroll, B. J., Reinberg, M., Greden, J. F., et al. (1981). A specific laboratory test for the diagnosis of melancholia: standardization, validation, and clinical utility. *Archives of General Psychiatry, 38*, 15–22.

Danner, M., Kasl, S. V., Abramson, J. L., & Vaccarion, V. (2003). Association between depression and elevated C-reactive protein. *Psychosomatic Medicine, 65*, 347–356.

Dantzer, R. (2001). Cytokine-induced sickness behavior: where do we stand? *Brain, Behavior, and Immunity*, *15*, 7–24.

de Beaurepaire, R. (2002). Questions raised by the cytokine hypothesis of depression. *Brain, Behavior, and Immunity*, *16*, 610–617.

Frasure-Smith, N., Lespérance, F., and Talajic, M. (1995). Depression and 18-month prognosis after myocardial infarction. *Circulation*, *91*, 999–1005.

Glassman, A. H., Helzer, J. E., Covey, L. S., et al. (1990). Smoking, smoking cessation, and major depression. *Journal of the American Medical Association*, *264*, 1546–1549.

Glassman, A. H., O'Connor, C. M., Califf, R. M., et al. (2002). Setraline treatment of major depression in patients with acute MI or unstable angina. *Journal of the American Medical Association*, *288*, 701–709.

Irwin, M. (2002). Psychoneuroimmunology of depression: clinical implications. *Brain, Behavior, and Immunity*, *16*, 1–16.

Kaul, D. (2001). Molecular link between cholesterol, cytokines and atherosclerosis. *Mollecular & Cellular Biochemistry*, *219*, 65–71.

Larson, S. J., & Dunn, A. J. (2001). Behavioral effects of cytokines. *Brain, Behavior, and Immunity*, *15*, 371–387.

Laye, S., Parnet, P., Boujon, E., & Dantzer, R. (1994). Peripheral administration of lipopolysaccharide induces the expression of cytokine transcripts in the brain and pituitary of mice. *Brain Research & Molecular Brain Research*, *27*, 157–162.

Leopold, J. A., & Loscalzo, J. (2000). Clinical importance of understanding vascular biology. *Cardiology in Review*, *8*, 115–123.

Lespérance, F., Frasure-Smith, N., Talajic, M., & Bourassa, M. G. (2002). Five-year risk of cardiac mortality in relation to initial severity and one-year change in depression symptoms after myocardial infarction. *Circulation*, *105*, 1049–1053.

Maes, M., Meltzer, H. Y., Bosmans, E., et al. (1995). Increased plasma concentrations of interleukin-6, soluble interleukin-6, soluble interleukin-2, and transferrin receptor in major depression. *Journal of Affective Disorders*, *34*, 301–309.

Maier, S. F., & Watkins, L. R. (1998). Cytokines for psychologists: implications of bidirectional immune-to-brain communication for understanding behavior, mood, and cognition. *Psychological Review*, *105*, 83–107.

McGovern, P. G., Pankow, J. S., Shahar, E., et al. (1996). Recent trends in acute coronary heart disease: mortality, morbidity, medical care, and risk factors. *New England Journal of Medicine*, *334*, 884–890.

McVeigh, G. E., Morgan, D. J., Finkelstein, S. M., Lemay, L. A., & Cohn, J. N. (1997). Vascular abnormalities associated with long-term cigarette smoking identified by arterial waveform analysis. *American Journal of Medicine*, *102*, 227–231.

Meesters, C., & Appels, A. (1996). An interview to measure vital exhaustion. I. Development and comparison with the Maastricht Questionnaire. *Psychology and Health, 11,* 557–571.

Morrow, D. A., & Ridker, P. M. (2000). C-reactive protein, inflammation, and coronary disease. *Medical Clinics of North America, 81,* 149–161.

Myers, J. K., Weissman, M. M., Tischler, G. L., et al. (1984). Six month prevalence of psychiatric disorders in three communities, 1980 to 1982. *Archives of General Psychiatry, 41,* 959–967.

Pollmacher, T., Haack, M., Schuld, A., Reichenberg, A., & Yirmiya, R. (2002). Low levels of circulating cytokines—Do they affect human brain functions? *Brain, Behavior, and Immunity, 16,* 525–532.

Rivest, S. (2001). How circulating cytokines trigger the neural circuits that control the hypothalamic-pituitary-adrenal axis. *Psychoneuroendocrinology, 26,* 761–788.

Ross, R. (1999). Atherosclerosis—an inflammatory disease. *New England Journal of Medicine, 340,* 115–126.

Rozanski, A., Blumenthal, J. A., & Kaplan, J. (1999). Impact of psychological factors on the pathogenesis of cardiovascular disease and implications for therapy. *Circulation, 99,* 2192–2217.

Rugulies, R. (2002). Depression as a predictor for coronary heart disease. *American Journal of Preventive Medicine, 23,* 51–61.

Schleifer, S. J., Macari-Hinson, M. M., Coyle, D. A., et al. (1989). The nature and course of depression following myocardial infarction. *Archives of Internal Medicine, 149,* 1785–1789.

Touyz, R. M. (2000). Oxidative stress and vascular damage in hypertension. *Current Hypertension Reports, 2,* 98–105.

van Dam, A. M., Brouns, M., Louisse, S., & Berkenbosch, F. (1992). Appearance of interleukin-1 in the macrophages and in ramified microglia in the brain of endotoxin-treated rats: a pathway for the induction of non-specific symptoms of sickness? *Brain Research, 588,* 291–296.

Van Der Ven, A., Van Diest, R., Hamulyak, K., Maes, M., Bruggeman, C., & Appels, A. (2003). Herpes viruses, cytokines, and altered hemostatis in vital exhaustion. *Psychosomatic Medicine, 65,* 194–200.

Vercellotti, G. M. (1998). Effects of viral activation of the vessel wall on inflammation and thrombosis. *Blood Coagulation & Fibrinolysis, 9,* S3–S6.

Viikari, J. S., Raitakari, O. T., & Simell, O. (2002). Nutritional influence on lipids and future atherosclerosis beginning prenatally and during childhood. *Current Opinion in Lipidology, 13,* 11–18.

Watkins, L. R., Goehler, L. E., Relton, J. K., Tartaglia, N., Silbert, L., Martin, D., & Maier, S. F. (1994). Blockade of interleukin-1 induced fever by subdiaphragmatic vagotomy: evidence for vagal mediation of immune-brain communication. *Neuroscience Letters, 183,* 1–5.

Wojciechowski, F. L., Strik, J. J. M. H., Falger, P., Lousberg, R., & Honig, A. (2000). The relationship between depressive and vital exhaustion symptomatology post-myocardial infarction. *Acta Psychiatrica Scandinavica, 102*, 359–365.

Writing Committee for the ENRICHD Investigators (2003). Effects of treating depression and low perceived social support on clinical events after myocardial infarction. *Journal of the American Medical Association, 289*, 3106–3116.

Yirmiya, R. (1996). Endotoxin produces a depressive-like episode in rats. *Brain Research, 711*, 163–174.

15 Fatigue in Systemic Lupus Erythematosus and Related Autoimmune Disorders

Elizabeth Kozora

Systemic lupus erythematosus (SLE) is a chronic autoimmune disease characterized by multisystemic involvement and diverse manifestations. Many symptoms of SLE involve significant behavioral changes. In patients with SLE, neuropsychiatric syndromes range from overt disorders such as seizure and stroke, to more subtle changes in cognition and mood. Fatigue is extremely common in patients with SLE as well as other rheumatologic autoimmune disorders such as rheumatoid arthritis (RA) and primary Sjogren's syndrome (PSS). To date, the mechanisms propagating fatigue in these disorders are unknown and, hence, difficult to treat and control.

Fatigue has been described as the most chronic and debilitating symptom SLE patients experience (Krupp et al., 1990; Krupp et al., 1989; Liang et al., 1984; Robb-Nicholson et al., 1989; Shur, 1989). Rates of self-reported complaints of fatigue in SLE patients are extremely high, ranging from 46 to 100 percent (Hall et al., 1981; Hall et al., 1983; Liang et al., 1984; Middleton et al., 1994; Shur, 1989; Taylor et al., 2000; Wysenbeek et al., 1993). Many patients report not having enough energy to perform daily activities (Robb-Nicholson et al., 1989), and fatigue frequently compromises activities, affects physical functioning, reduces quality of life, and interferes with work (Daltroy et al., 1995; Krupp et al., 1990; Krupp et al., 1989). Fatigue has typically been associated with active SLE disease status; however, fatigue has also been described as debilitating for "inactive" patients (Hastings et al., 1986).

The phenomenon of fatigue is difficult to describe, define, and measure as it typically refers to a subjective experience involving feelings of exhaustion and tiredness. Common dictionary definitions emphasize that fatigue is associated with weariness and exhaustion from labor, exertion, or stress. Koike, Kazuma, and Kawamura (2000) define fatigue in rheumatological patients as the "perception of persistent tiredness of the whole body not able to be restored by rest." Krupp and Pollina (1996) indicate that the mechanisms that bring about subjective feelings of fatigue differ across various neurological disorders. They suggest that the most likely pathogenic processes involve "immunologic etiologies, neuroendocrine disturbances, impaired psychophysiologic responses, and dysfunction in central and peripheral motor pathways."

This chapter explores the possible links between self-reported fatigue and a variety of biomedical, psychological, and psychosocial factors in SLE and other autoimmune disorders. First, the measurement and prevalence of fatigue in published SLE studies are reviewed. Next, we describe the research on physiological and psychosocial mechanisms that may underlie fatigue in SLE, then the importance of biopsychosocial models in understanding fatigue in SLE. A brief review of fatigue in other autoimmune disease such as RA and PSS is presented, followed by treatment applications for reduction of fatigue in SLE and other related autoimmune disorders. Finally, the chapter is completed with a summary and recommendations for future clinical and empirical directions.

Prevalence and Measurement of Fatigue in SLE

The measurement of fatigue varies across studies in SLE and autoimmune patients. However, several select measures have been consistently used. The type of "fatigue scale" used influences the reported prevalence of fatigue in SLE and requires careful examination and evaluation. To date, all of the measures of fatigue in SLE have relied on subjective self-report measures such as visual analogue scales, Likert scales, or empirically derived fatigue questionnaires.

The Fatigue Severity Scale

The most widely used measure in SLE appears to be the Fatigue Severity Scale (FSS), first derived by Krupp and colleagues (1990; 1989) via factor analysis and validated through statistical procedures. In the original studies, the FSS score was significantly higher in patients with multiple sclerosis (MS) and SLE (mean of 4.6) compared to controls (mean of 2.3). In another study, sedentary controls had a mean FSS score of 3.3 (Tench et al., 2000). Several studies have used the FSS to analyze SLE patients. The mean FSS score has ranged from 4.6 to 6.08 (Bruce et al., 1999; Omdal, 2002; Tayer et al., 2001; Tench et al., 2000; Wang et al., 1998; Zonana-Nacach et al., 2000) in SLE patients with a mean age ranging from 42.6 to 47.2, and years of diagnosis ranging from 11.9 to 14.7. Most studies describe FSS scores at or above 3 as a cutoff index designating fatigue in SLE patients. Tench and colleagues (2000) reported that 81 percent of SLE patients had elevated fatigue, and Zonana-Nacach and coworkers (2000) report that 85.3 percent of their SLE patients have elevated FSS scores, with rates in Hispanic, African-American, and Caucasian SLE subjects ranging from 82 to 86 percent. Recent studies have confirmed these high rates of fatigue. Omdal and colleagues (2002) reported 79 percent of the SLE patients were elevated on the FSS, and in our recent data, 92 percent of SLE patients without neuropsychiatric symptoms (non-NP-SLE), 94 percent of SLE patients with overt neuropsychiatric symptoms (NP-SLE), and 16 percent of healthy controls had elevated FSS scores (Kozora et al., 2005).

Visual Analogue Scales (VAS) and Ranking Systems

VAS and Likert type scales have also been used to measure fatigue in patients with SLE. Using a VAS scale, Krupp and colleagues (1990) reported that SLE patients had a score of 0.6 compared to 0.16 in healthy controls. Wysenbeek and associates (1993) used a patient rating from 0 to 3 (with 0 representing no fatigue, and 1–3 representing fatigue after strenuous, regular, or mild activity). Patients with a 0 or 1 were categorized as "not fatigued," and patients with a 2 or 3 were categorized as "fatigued." Results indicated that 76 percent of the SLE patients were reporting fatigue. Taylor and coworkers (2000) found greater fatigue in SLE patients using a "yes or no" question asking whether the patients had experienced fatigue in the last 3 months. Robb-Nicholson and colleagues (1989) and Daltroy and colleagues (1995) used several VAS scales to assess stamina in the last 7 days (0–10), having less energy in the last 7 days (0–10), and total energy level in the last 7 days (0–10). Tench and colleagues (2000) used four VAS scales, noting greater fatigue in SLE across total fatigue, mental fatigue, and physical fatigue.

Other Scales of Fatigue

Several studies have used scales rarely replicated in other SLE groups. McKinley and coworkers (1995) reported that SLE patients had greater overall fatigue than controls on the Piper Fatigue Scale (Piper, 1989), a scale designed to measure subjective tiredness, decreased energy, and ability to perform activities. SLE patients scored higher on the temporal scale (chronic, continuous) and affective scale (emotional meaning of fatigue as negative, abnormal, agreeable, destructive). Godaert and colleagues (2002) reported that SLE and PSS patients had greater general fatigue and physical fatigue and reduced activity, but they did not differ on measures of motivational or mental fatigue than controls on the 20-point Multidimensional Fatigue Scale (Smets et al., 1995). This was interpreted to mean that physical aspects of the disease may be most important (e.g., sleep, neuroendocrine functions, and physical conditioning). They also indicated that fatigue varies throughout the day and may need to be assessed at various times. Tench and associates (2002) used the 14-item Chalder Fatigue Scale (Chalder et al., 1993) and the SLE patients had significantly higher fatigue (23.5) compared to controls (15.0).

Several studies use subscales of fatigue derived from broader measures of mood and quality of life. The Fatigue subscale from the Profile of Mood States (POMS) (McNair et al., 1980) has been used in SLE patients (Robb-Nicholson et al., 1989) and was found to be in the normal range. In contrast, Daltroy and colleagues (1995) reported a mean score of 10.8, suggesting relatively high fatigue in SLE patients. In our study using the POMS Fatigue subscale (Kozora et al., 2005), our non-NP-SLE patients had a mean score of 12.6 compared to 4.5 in healthy controls. Finally, the SF-36 subscale of Vitality/Fatigue (Ware & Sherbourne, 1992) has been used in prior SLE studies (Dobkin et al., 2001). This subscale includes four questions (feeling pep, lots of energy, worn out, and tired), and SLE patients scored significantly lower (showing greater fatigue) compared to controls (Gilboe et al., 1999; Lwin et al., 2003).

Mechanisms of Fatigue in SLE

The mechanisms underlying fatigue in patients with SLE are most likely multifactorial. Thirty-eight percent of SLE patients reported that inadequate rest, overactivity, stress, and depression were the causes of their fatigue (Hastings et al., 1986). Evidence to date suggests that physiological as well as psychosocial and behavioral factors underlie this phenomenon. This section first examines studies that support these specific approaches, and then the recent evolution of a multidisciplinary biopsychosocial perspective.

Physiological Processes of Fatigue in SLE

Abnormal physiological processes directly related to lupus activity may be responsible for fatigue in SLE patients. These processes can be categorized into the following subsections: clinical disease activity, inflammatory processes, medication side effects, and concomitant medical disorders (fibromyalgia, physical deconditioning, pulmonary problems, sleep disturbance, and central nervous system dysfunction).

Overall Disease Activity   In earlier studies, clinical disease activity (defined by physician rating of SLE disease manifestations) of SLE was thought to be associated with fatigue. Rothfield (1989) reported an association between fatigue and disease activity, and Liang and colleagues (1984) proposed that disease activity was the primary cause of fatigue in SLE. Krupp and others (1990; 1989) reported that fatigue (FSS) was related to physician ratings of disease activity but not to other laboratory measures. Interestingly, 56 percent of the SLE patients reported that the onset of fatigue predated their disease manifestations. Rothfield (1989) reported a similar phenomenon wherein the SLE patients indicated that fatigue predated their actual diagnosis and onset of SLE. Both authors suggested that a biological mechanism, possibly systemic inflammation, may be responsible for the association between fatigue and early symptoms of the disease.

Several studies have investigated the relationship of fatigue to SLE disease activity with standardized measures such as the Systemic Lupus Erythematosus Disease Activity Index (SLEDAI) (Bombardier et al., 1992), the Systemic Lupus Activity Measure (SLAM) (Liang et al., 1989), and the European Consensus of Lupus Activity Measure

(ECLAM) (Vitali et al., 1991). Tench and coworkers (2000) found significant correlations between fatigue and measures of standardized disease activity (i.e. SLAM and ECLAM). Because fatigue items were embedded within SLAM, clinical items related to fatigue were removed and a significant relationship between fatigue and disease activity remained. Fatigue scores were up to 33 percent higher in patients with active SLE disease versus those with inactive disease.

Wysenbeek and colleagues (1993) reported that SLE patients with greater fatigue had higher overall disease activity (based on rankings of physical and history information) as well as significant declines in lymphocyte counts and increased ratings of physical distress (headache, nervousness, and musculoskeletal symptoms, muscle pain, abdominal pain, fever, and weight loss). Patients also had a greater history of nephritis and higher creatine levels. In correlational analysis, the relationship between fatigue and disease activity was quite high ($r = 0.49$; $p < 0.001$). Correlations were also found with nervousness, lymphopenia, muscle pain, and headache. Taylor and colleagues (2000) reported a relationship between fatigue and disease activity including mucutaneous and hematological conditions. The investigation by Zanona-Nacach and coworkers (2000) supported a relationship between fatigue and disease activity using the SLAM, with fatigue-related items removed. Additionally, the FSS was associated with neurological manifestations, headache, pain, and elevated lymphocyte count. Finally, Tayer and associates (2001) reported that, out of multiple variables, only disease status predicted fatigue in SLE patients over time.

In contrast, one author found no strong correlation between disease activity and fatigue measures in SLE (Wang et al., 1998). This study used the SLEDAI, a scale that does not have any clinical items identifying fatigue, and this may account for the lack of correlations. Additionally, those patients had mild disease, which may have weakened possible associations. Overall, studies would suggest a relationship between fatigue and lupus disease activity, and methodological differences may contribute to the discrepancies in those studies with negative findings.

Inflammatory Mechanisms of Fatigue Given the inflammatory nature of SLE and other autoimmune disorders, there has been considerable interest and speculation regarding the inflammation process as it relates to fatigue. Substances called interleukins (IL), or cytokines, are released during inflammation and signal cells to perform certain actions. In fact, some cytokines have been known to cause fatigue and sleepiness (Kelley et al., 2003). The inflammatory response activates a variety of immune cells (macrophages and neutrophils) that contribute to tissue damage and may be partly related to symptoms of fatigue. The inflammatory process also triggers a general or systemic response. The systemic reaction is mediated by the action of proinflammatory cytokines on distant target cells and is characterized by leukocytosis, an increased sedimentation rate, activation of complement and clotting cascades, and synthesis and release of acute-phase proteins (including C-reactive protein).

In addition to regulating and coordinating responses between different types of immune cells, cytokines can also affect distant organs including the central nervous system (CNS). Evidence has been growing that nerve, endocrine, and immune cells share communication molecules and receptors and are functionally linked to form a brain-endocrine-immune axis that integrates the physiological responses in the organism (DeSouza, 1993; Maier et al., 1998). Cytokines act directly within the CNS to alter growth and differentiation, to modulate neuronal and neuroendocrine activities, and to produce pyrogenic, somnogenic, thermogenic, anorexigenic and behavioral effects (DeSouza, 1993). Proinflammatory cytokines such as IL-2r, IL-2, IL-6, IL-10, interferon (INF), and tumor necrosis factor (TNF) are elevated in acute inflammatory responses in both animal models and patient studies of RA and SLE (al-Janadi et al., 1993; Boswell et al., 1988; Elliott & Maini, 1995; Feldman et al., 1993; Linker-Israeli et al., 1991; Maury & Teppo, 1989; Singh, 1992).

In patients with SLE, relationships between fatigue and measures of inflammation such as cytokine and complement activity have been suggested. Complement C3 and C4 (indirect measures of inflammation that are likely related to interleukin changes) have been associated with fatigue. Taylor and colleagues (2000) found higher levels of C3 associated with greater fatigue, but all other studies show that lower complement in SLE is related to fatigue. Rothfield (1989) first described a decline in complement C3 associated with fatigue in SLE patients. Wysenbeek and associates (1993) also reported a significant decline in complement C3 in patients with SLE reporting high levels of fatigue. Omdal and others (2002) also found a relationship between lower C4 and higher fatigue levels, and they reported abnormal levels of C3 in 28 percent of their SLE patients. However, they found no relationship between fatigue and C3 or other cytokines (INF-α, TNF-α, IL-2, IL-6, and IL-10). The researchers indicated that the cytokine and complement levels were low in their patient sample, and a stronger relationship to fatigue may be found in SLE patients with higher overall levels of these immune factors. They also indicate that measuring cytokine in serum may have been problematic, and "paracrine effects of neuronal cells of intrathecally produced cytokines may be a more relevant target for research." In general, declines in C3 and C4 may be related to decreased production, thus a sign of active disease. Overall, studies to date suggest that complement activity in SLE is lower, and typically associated with fatigue.

Medication-Induced Fatigue   In early descriptive studies of SLE, corticosteroids were thought to reduce fatigue (Rothfield, 1989). In studies to date, prednisone, hydroxychloroquine, and psychotropics appear to contribute to fatigue changes in SLE. However, little or no consistent evidence supports the suggestion that medication is primarily or even secondarily responsible for the improvement or worsening of fatigue in SLE patients. Wysenbeek and colleagues (1993) reported that SLE patients with the highest levels of fatigue were also taking higher levels of prednisone (33.9 mg per day versus 19.5 mg per day). Tench and coworkers (2000) reported higher fatigue scores in patients taking hydroxychloroquine. Both studies suggest that medication use may be mediated by and indirectly affected by disease activity. Zonana-Nacach and colleagues (2000) report that self-reported fatigue in SLE was associated with psychotropic medications only. They further suggest that depression and mood disorders, not the medication, mediate this relationship. Several studies have not found any correlation between medication use and fatigue in SLE. Krupp and colleagues (1990) found no correlations between fatigue and various medications. In another study (Omdal et al., 2002), 25 percent of the SLE patients were on prednisone (and another 37 percent on prednisone plus cytotoxins), yet no relationship was found between prednisone and fatigue. Finally, in a hierarchical analysis (Tayer et al., 2001), neither demographics nor presence of any medication use contributed to fatigue. Overall, the studies to date are not conclusive regarding the effect of medications, although it is unlikely that they are the primary contributor of fatigue in SLE.

Concurrent Medical Conditions   Investigations to date indicate that medical disorders concurrent with, but not exclusively related to, SLE may contribute to fatigue in lupus patients. For example, SLE patients with subclinical hypothyroidism have reported higher levels of fatigue (Tench et al., 2000), which suggest that disorders of the endocrine system may contribute to fatigue. Four major processes appear to predominate: (1) fibromyalgia, (2) pulmonary difficulties and deconditioning, (3) sleep disorders, and (4) CNS alterations.

Presence of Fibromyalgia   Early studies indicated that 20 to 30 percent of patients with SLE have a diagnosis of fibromyalgia (Akkasilpa et al., 1997; Gladman et al., 1996; Middleton et al., 1994; Wallace, 1995). Bruce and colleagues (1999) reported a significant correlation between fatigue and the number of tender points (a common objective measure of fibromyalgia) in SLE patients. Wang and associates (1998) also reported that fatigue correlated with the number of tender points in SLE patients. Their results implied that factors associated with pain in fibromyalgia contributed to fatigue in SLE. However, Morand and colleagues (1994) found no difference in self-reported fatigue in SLE patients with or without fibromyalgia. Taylor and others (2000) found that SLE patients reporting fatigue in the past 3 months had more tender points; however, only 11 percent of the patients in this group were actually diagnosed with fibromyalgia (and only 5 percent of the total SLE sample had a diagnosis of fibromyalgia). Middleton and colleagues (1994) reported that 89 percent of SLE patients without fibromyalgia, 100 percent of the SLE patients with probable fibromyalgia, and 95 percent of the SLE patients with fibromyalgia reported symptoms of fatigue. In addition, 35 percent of the SLE patients without fibromyalgia and 81 percent of the SLE patients with fibromyalgia reported having fatigue most or all of the time. Overall, some patients with SLE may have concurrent fibromyalgia, which may contribute to their overall fatigue.

Physical Endurance and Poor Lung Function   A number of studies suggest that physical deconditioning and pulmonary difficulties may contribute to fatigue in SLE patients. Robb-Nicholson and colleagues (1989) reported that SLE patients were at 45 percent of their maximal aerobic activity using age- and gender-matched norms. In addition, fatigue was inversely related with exercise duration but not with maximal aerobic capacity. Fatigue in select SLE patients has also declined following exercise training. For example, Liang and colleagues (1984) reported that following an 8-month exercise program, SLE patients showed reduced fatigue. Robb-Nicholson and coworkers (1989) randomized SLE patients into a treatment group that received 30 minutes of exercise three times per week for 8 weeks and a control group of select SLE patients who participated in nonaerobic exercise and stretching at the same frequency. At baseline, the patients were "very deconditioned" and performed at 45 percent of expected aerobic capacity. Higher fatigue was associated with decreased duration of exercise. Following 8 weeks, the SLE patients in aerobic exercise showed significant improvement in terms of fatigue, exercise duration tolerance, and aerobic capacity compared to the controls. A significant relationship between change in fatigue and change in pulmonary function was also noted.

Finally, 70 percent of the patients in the aerobic treatment group reported feeling more energy and increased psychological wellbeing, though they experienced no change in their disease activity or joint pain after exercising. Daltroy and colleagues (1995) reported that following 3 months of exercise on a stationary bike, SLE patients reported lowered fatigue, depression, and helplessness. In both studies of exercise in SLE patients with stable disease, aerobic activity was likely to reduce fatigue and not worsen physical disease. The studies further suggest that seeking "more rest" may not be the best treatment strategy.

Several studies have suggested that pulmonary dysfunction occurs in SLE patients, and this may be associated in part with other symptoms of the disease such as fatigue and deconditioning. Silberstein and colleagues (1980) report that 88 percent of SLE patients had pulmonary dysfunction. Specifically, 72.5 percent of the patients had abnormal diffusing capacity, 49 percent had reduction in lung volumes, 44.5 percent had hypoxemia, and 9 percent had airways obstruction. Tench and colleagues (2002) reported that SLE patients were significantly different from controls on most physiological measures (lower VO_2 peak, lower maximum minute ventilation, and a lower respiratory exchange ratio). Resting lung function was also significantly reduced across this population. Sakauchi and associates (1995) reported impaired oxygen diffusion in inflamed peripheral muscles in SLE patients with active disease. Forte and coworkers

(1999) found decreased exercise capacity in SLE patients, which they suggested was due to peripheral muscle deconditioning. The etiology of the pulmonary dysfunction and general deconditioning across studies is unclear. However, results thus far suggest that both poor lung function and low exercise capacity contribute to fatigue in SLE patients.

Sleep Disturbance   Another proposed biological mechanism associated with fatigue in SLE patients may be related to sleep disturbance. Liang and coworkers (1984) reported that 61 percent of SLE patients were reporting sleep problems. Robb-Nicholson and colleagues (1989) reported that 61 percent of SLE patients report that they do not feel refreshed from sleep. In addition, they noted that 74 percent of SLE patients indicated that fatigue is worse between 1 and 5 pm, and they typically feel better later in the day. McKinley and associates (1995) suggested that sleep problems are one of several factors mediating fatigue. In their study, SLE patients reported more total sleep time and had a greater sleep latency. They suggested that patients were "too protective of their sleep time" as a strategy to reduce fatigue. Tench and colleagues (2000) reported that almost two-thirds (59%) of their SLE patients had poor sleep quality based on a structured sleep questionnaire, and the degree of sleep difficulties were highly correlated with increased fatigue. They suggested that multiple comediators such as physical pain, depression, and anxiety likely contribute to sleep problems as well as fatigue. Similarly, Dobkin and colleagues (2001) reported that sleep was related to fatigue but was mediated by depression. Overall, studies to date suggest that sleep problems contribute to fatigue in SLE patients. Sleep difficulties are likely mediated by several factors, including pain and depression and possibly deconditioning.

Central Nervous System Alterations   Neuropsychiatric (NP) symptoms are common in SLE and may be associated with fatigue. NP symptoms have been reported in more than half of SLE patients, and in addition to overt disorders such as stroke and seizure, behavioral changes such as psychosis, depression, anxiety, and cognitive dysfunction have been included in the recent nomenclature for NP-SLE (Liang & Committee, 1999). Unfortunately, few studies have directly investigated CNS alterations as a potential pathway for fatigue in SLE. One study reported that changes in fatigue in SLE patients following exercise may represent a mechanism associated with pyramidal CNS deficits (Iriarte & Castro, 1998). Two studies have reported an association between fatigue and neurological manifestations (Wysenbeek et al., 1993; Zonana-Nacach et al., 2000). Gilboe and colleagues (1999) reported that fatigue was more strongly associated with NP symptoms than musculoskeletal and pulmonary symptoms. One study found fatigue was not correlated with overt CNS symptoms. Omdal and associates (2002) completed a standard neurological exam and cranial MRI scans on SLE patients. Neurological exams showed that 9 percent had stroke activity and 17 percent had cerebral infarcts. Fatigue did not differ between SLE patients with and without infarcts or stroke. These findings suggest that structural brain damage does not influence fatigue in SLE.

Studies using neuropsychological assessment of brain function may, however, be a more sensitive approach to understanding fatigue in SLE. For example, in one of our early pilot studies, declines in sustained attention were strongly associated with fatigue versus depression in SLE patients (Kozora et al., 2001). As indicated previously, we have found higher levels of fatigue for SLE patients with and without overt histories of neurological or psychiatric symptoms (NP-SLE; SLE only) (Kozora et al., 2005). However, only the NP-SLE group demonstrated significant correlations between the fatigue and specific cognitive measures including measures of verbal learning and verbal recall (Delis et al., 1987), immediate and delayed recall of nonverbal material (Meyers & Meyers, 1995), and complex visuomotor attention (Reitan & Wolfson, 1988).

Findings also suggested that only the NP-SLE group had significant associations between an overall cognitive index, fatigue, pain, and depression. These preliminary findings might suggest that fatigue is highly related to other NP aspects of SLE. Bruce and colleagues (1999) had also suggested fatigue may reflect "subtle changes in CNS structure and physiology" that require functional testing such as neuropsychological evaluations. Although neuroimaging studies (structural, functional, and neurometabolite) of the brain are frequently abnormal in SLE patients (West, 2002), these methods to date have not been incorporated into fatigue research designs. Thus, including neuroimaging and continuing neuropsychological studies may be useful in expanding our understanding of relationships between fatigue and the brain in SLE.

Psychological and Psychosocial Contributions to Fatigue in SLE
Some studies also suggest that depression and psychosocial factors are the main mechanism underlying fatigue in SLE. Depression is a commonly reported syndrome in SLE patients and appears to be their most common major psychiatric complaint (Magner, 1991; Omdal et al., 1995; Wekking, 1993). The prevalence of depression varies across studies, but in one study using formal psychiatric interviews, the range was between 31 and 52 percent (Giang, 1991). Studies with self-report questionnaires typically report higher levels of depressive symptoms (Kozora et al., 2001). The role of depression in lupus remains controversial, and depression is most likely associated with the effects of chronic illness as well as a mechanism of CNS involvement in this population.

Depression/Helplessness and Stress   A number of studies have suggested that psychosocial factors such as depression, helplessness, and stress are the main mechanisms of self-reported fatigue in patients with SLE. There is considerable debate regarding the prevalence and diagnosis of depression in SLE (Iverson, 1993). In our own studies, clinical impressions from physicians, structured psychiatric interviews, and standardized self-report measures have not provided consistent convergent information (Kozora & West, 2002). Robb-Nicholson and colleagues (1989) reported that 39 percent of their sample of SLE patients met clinical diagnostic criteria for depression, which is lower than the frequency expected from psychiatric outpatients but higher than that expected from healthy controls. The Center for Epidemiological Studies–Depression (CES–D) measure is a common self-report instrument of depression for SLE patients, and scores at or above 16 have been suggested as evidence of mild symptoms (Radloff, 1977). In SLE patients, 39 to 85 percent appear to be elevated on this scale (Daltroy et al., 1995; Kozora & West, 2002; Krupp et al., 1990; Krupp et al., 1989).

Although many findings imply that depression is psychosocially produced, some studies outside the fatigue literature suggest that depression in SLE may have a biological pathophysiology. In the recent classifications of neuropsychiatric disease by the American College of Rheumatology, mood disorders (depression and anxiety) are listed as one of the 19 specific neuropsychiatric symptoms and presentations in SLE (Liang & Committee, 1999). Early studies (Cardenas & Kutner, 1982) suggested that depression in SLE patients was related to fatigue, and some subsequent studies using self-report measures have corroborated these early impressions. However, many of the depression questionnaires have fatigue-related items that tend to falsely inflate these correlations. Iverson (2002) reported that 90.2 percent of SLE patients endorsed the fatigue item on the British Columbia Major Depression Inventory. Tayer and colleagues (2001), removed two items assessing fatigue from the CES–D and continued to report a relationship between depression and fatigue.

Krupp and associates (1989) used the CES–D and reported a significant relationship between depressive symptoms and fatigue ($r + 0.46$, $p < 0.05$). As indicated previously, they also found a relationship between fatigue and disease severity. They suggest that fatigue is separate but overlaps with depression. In their subsequent study, Krupp and colleagues (1990) found that 43 percent of SLE patients were categorized as depressed with the CES–D cutoff. Their SLE patients had neuropsychiatric manifestations, which suggests the depression may be related to adjustment to a variable course of illness. Tayer and colleagues (2001) reported overall high scores on the CES–D in SLE patients at two time points, and these scores correlated highly with fatigue at the same two time points. Wang and associates (1998) found a strong correlation between fatigue and the CES–D, and reported that fatigue correlated with tender points as well as depression and some psychosocial factors from quality of life subscales. In addition to depression, anxiety may also be related to fatigue. Tench and colleagues (2002) indicated that 60 percent of their SLE patients had elevated anxiety and 37 percent had elevated depression measured by the Hospital Anxiety and Depression Scale (HADS) (Zigmond & Smith, 1983). Anxiety and depression were also associated with increased fatigue. Tench et al. (2002) reported that SLE patients had significantly more depression on the HADS than sedentary controls, and fatigue correlated with depression.

Specific aspects of depression, such as helplessness, have also been studied in association with fatigue in SLE. Zonana-Nacach and coworkers (2000) reported a relationship between fatigue and helplessness. Tayer and colleagues (2001) reported fatigue was associated with depression ($r + 0.59$) as well as helplessness, and they concluded that helplessness and depression mediate the relationship between disease status and fatigue. Their findings also indicated that helplessness itself likely mediates the relationship between disease activity and depression. Stress is another factor that has recently been investigated in relation to fatigue. Dobkin and associates (2001) found that decreased stress and depression at 15 months predicted reduced fatigue in SLE patients, whereas additional analysis showed that depression was related to sleep problems.

In summary, measures of depression, anxiety, and helplessness tend to be associated with fatigue in patients with SLE. Results to date suggest these factors all interact. In fact, depression is likely a complex phenomenon that represents a CNS manifestation of SLE and may also be exacerbated by psychosocial factors such as chronic disease, inadequate coping styles, and financial problems. Although multiple psychological factors appear to be associated with self-reported fatigue, the true mechanism underlying the relationships remains unclear.

Quality of Life   Several studies to date indicate that increased perceived fatigue is associated with a decline in quality of life. Wang and others (1998) reported that fatigue was related to decline in overall health status on a formal quality of life scale (SF-20) for physical, role, social, mental, health, and pain subscales. Bruce and colleagues (1999) had similar findings for SLE patients in that the FSS was correlated with all aspects of decline in quality of life on the SF-36. Tench and colleagues (2002) reported that fatigue was associated with overall deceased ability to perform daily tasks as well as all of the SF-36 subscales. In a later study, they reported that a combination of factors influence scores on the SF-36 physical disability subscale, including aerobic fitness, fatigue, high BMI, and depression (Tench et al., 2002). Overall, these studies indicate that fatigue is associated with poor perception of health status and could be associated with psychosocial factors not yet studied. Zanona-Nacach and coworkers (2000) found increased fatigue associated with decreased physical and mental functioning on the SF-36 subscales.

Conclusions: Toward a Biopsychosocial Model of Fatigue in SLE
Early studies suggested that both biological and psychological factors were likely contributors to fatigue in SLE (Krupp et al., 1990; Shur, 1989). Shur (1989) first proposed a multifactorial approach to fatigue in SLE including lupus activity, lack of sleep, depression, unhealthy habits (i.e., smoking, drinking, sedentary living, drug abuse) internal conflicts (inaccurate role perception), deconditioning, anemia medications,

and increased family demands and employment workload. Recent studies have taken advanced multivariate statistical approaches to more clearly identify and understand factors associated with fatigue in SLE. McKinley and colleagues (1995) used multivariate analyses to combine several factors, and results indicated that depression and sleep were the primary moderators of fatigue in their sample of SLE patients. The researchers conclude that fatigue is "precipitated or exacerbated by disease activity, depression and sleep problems and can act as mediators of mechanisms that produce or worsen fatigue. Sleep problems, including both sleep disruption and anxiety about one's sleep are the most proximal link to fatigue in this process." They also suggest that the "affective" component of depression and anxiety may perpetuate sleep disturbance and depression.

Tench and associates (2002) showed that aerobic fitness, fatigue, high body mass index, and depression influenced physical disability in select SLE patients. Depression and poor sleep were related to fatigue, and fatigue was related to depression and exercise capacity. Zonona-Nacach and others (2000) also suggested that the perception of fatigue was multifactorial, including psychosocial and biological realms. Using a stepwise multivariate regression, they reported that fatigue was associated with abnormal ill behavior, older age, higher pain, increased helplessness, increased disease activity, Caucasian race, and lack of health insurance. Overall, these multivariate designs tend to suggest that fatigue may be initiated by the disease process and sustained by a host of biopsychosocial variables. Tayer and colleagues (2001) suggested that depression and helplessness may "exacerbate or maintain fatigue that initially was generated from the physiological process of SLE." Alternatively, there may be separate and distinct forms of fatigue in SLE, one associated with biological mechanisms such as systemic and neurological abnormalities, and another specific to psychosocial factors.

Fatigue in Other Autoimmune Disorders

Fatigue is also a debilitating symptom in other rheumatological disorders such as rheumatoid arthritis (RA) and primary Sjogren's syndrome (PSS). Barendregt and colleagues (1998) and Lwin and others (2003) both report that RA and PSS patients had more self-reported fatigue than healthy controls. RA is a chronic inflammatory disease, and fatigue is frequently the most distressing symptom (Katz, 1998; Tack, 1990). Barendregt and colleagues (1998) reported that fatigue was greater in RA patients than controls and general fatigue and physical fatigue remained greater in RA after controlling for depression. The mechanisms of fatigue in RA are similar to those in SLE, and physical as well as psychosocial factors have been implicated. Physical relationships between fatigue and disease activity, inflammation, and sleep have been reported. In addition, the experience of pain appears to be a specific contributor to fatigue that is not found among SLE patients. Fatigue in RA has been related to disease activity

(Huyser et al., 1998), and in one study fatigue was noted in 88 percent of active disease and 40 percent of nonactive disease states (Pinals et al., 1981).

Koike and colleagues (2000) reported that fatigue was greater in the inflammatory RA patients than in the noninflammatory RA patients and controls. Dekkers et al. (2000) found that increased fatigue was associated with an early morning increase in cortisol. Sleep and pain have been strongly associated with fatigue in a variety of studies (Belza, 1995; Crosby, 1991; Huyser et al., 1998; Mahowald et al., 1989). Neuberger and colleagues (1997) also indicated that fatigue in RA can be improved with appropriate exercise. Several studies further suggest that psychosocial factors such as depression and poor social support may contribute to fatigue (Belza, 1995; Huyser et al., 1998). Fifield and others (2001) reported that RA patients with an affective disorder had more fatigue and higher levels of fatigue over time than RA patients without affective disorders. Fatigue has also been noted to worsen overall quality of life in RA (Belza, 1994; Pincus et al., 1989). Self-reported fatigue appears to be somewhat lower in RA than SLE patients. In patients with relatively mild disease, 27 percent of the SLE and 9 percent of the RA reported that fatigue was their biggest problem (Liang et al., 1984). Fatigue was also elevated in non-NP-SLE patients compared to RA patients in our study (Kozora et al., 2005). In contrast, Gilboe and colleagues (1999) indicated that fatigue was equally elevated in SLE and RA patients compared to controls.

PSS is another rheumatologic/autoimmune disorder with high levels of self- reported fatigue. Sjogren's syndrome is a symptom complex associated with the presence of a connective tissue disease marked by conjunctivitis. Fatigue has ranged from 52.5 to 83 percent across studies (Gudbjornsson et al., 1993; Jacobsson et al., 1995; Manthorpe et al., 1995; Tensing et al., 2001). Barendregt and colleagues (1998) report fatigue in 55 percent of the PSS patients, and decreased motivation and mental fatigue were specifically associated with depression. Additionally, significant levels of general and physical fatigue and decreased activity remained in the PSS patients after controlling for depression.

Treating Fatigue in SLE

The treatment of fatigue in patients with SLE and other autoimmune disorders has not received extensive empirical attention to date, and the published studies primarily involve activities aimed to decrease depression and improve exercise tolerance. In a survey of SLE patients, approximately 70 percent of the patients report seeking rest to cope with fatigue, 21 percent exercise, and 9 percent report that they do nothing. Interestingly, in a survey, the patients' physicians reported that 32 percent of their patients rest, 32 percent exercise, and 32 percent accept their fatigue (Robb-Nicholson et al., 1989).

The rational approach to treatment of fatigue in SLE and other autoimmune groups corresponds with the actual mechanism underlying fatigue. As reviewed previously, there are many possible contributing factors with as many potential treatment approaches. McKinley and colleagues (1995) propose that treatment should address sleep, depression, and disease activity simultaneously. Specifically, getting less sleep and increasing physical activity may improve sleep. Tench and others (2002) suggested that treatment for fatigue should consider managing depression and improving aerobic fitness. Other studies (Robb-Nicholson et al., 1989; Daltroy et al., 1999) have found that increased exercise reduces fatigue in SLE. Understanding the individual nature of the fatigue is likely the key to managing fatigue for patients. Based on the data so far, attempting to obtain both optimal physical and psychological functioning may improve fatigue. Clearly, managing the disease activity itself with appropriate medications is the first step. Other behavioral health factors such as good sleep hygiene, exercise, and healthy living guidelines (no excessive alcohol, smoking, caffeine, etc.) will likely decrease fatigue levels. Additional recommendations are maintaining healthy psychological functioning (use of adaptive coping skills and increased social support) and interventions (such as counseling and psychotropic treatment Nicassio et al., 1997).

Conclusion

Based on the review of literature to date, levels of self-reported fatigue in SLE are extremely high and associated with a variety of biological and psychosocial parameters. The main factors associated with fatigue in SLE and other autoimmune disorders include disease activity, inflammation (cytokine and complement activity), lung dysfunction and deconditioning, sleep, pain, and depression. Clearly, continued studies integrating biopsychosocial variables are necessary to sort through and more clearly identify factors that mediate and improve fatigue.

Addressing some methodological problems in current SLE studies may facilitate the development of more effective research designs in this area. Discrepancies in the research reviewed in this chapter may represent primary design issues such as procedures, patient populations, and instruments used. For example "objective measures" of fatigue have not yet been included in SLE studies. Iriarte and Castro (1998) raised similar issues in patients with multiple sclerosis and suggest that measurement of fatigue must include objective and subjective ratings and signs of fatigue (such as objective signs of speed, strength, and potency) that likely differ from symptoms of fatigue (including subjective feelings of tiredness). Measuring fatigue at only one time point may also be problematic, and measurement at various time points has been recommended. In addition to sampling various time points during the day, cross-sectional studies need to be extended into longitudinal studies to investigate the "causal" relationships between various mediators of fatigue.

Studies to date suggest that symptoms of fatigue are related to multiple processes in SLE and other autoimmune diseases. Fatigue is generally a subjective phenomenon and may be difficult to quantify over time on many biological, psychological, and social levels. As indicated by the literature review, no clear model of fatigue in SLE exists at this time. However, some strong findings suggest changes in complement activity and cytokine changes are common in SLE and are associated with fatigue. In addition, studies demonstrate that lung dysfunction is common and related to fatigue in SLE. Based on current literature, immune dysregulation and lung dysfunction activated by autoimmune processes appear to be the most relevant physiological mechanisms underlying fatigue in SLE. The cascade of psychosocial changes, particularly depression, could be triggered in part by the immune and respiratory changes, and then exacerbate fatigue.

Conversely, psychosocial and biological factors (immune and respiratory mechanisms) may represent a completely different form of fatigue in SLE. For individual SLE patients, one or the other or both mechanisms may underlie the phenomenon. Overall, these multivariate designs suggest that the disease process may initiate fatigue, and fatigue may be sustained by a host of biopsychosocial variables. It is likely that disease activity has a direct effect on the brain, causing fatigue that is modulated by psychosocial factors.

References

Akkasilpa, S., Minor, M., Goldman, D., Petri, M., & Magder, L. (1997). Association of health status with fibromyalgia tender points in systemic lupus erythematosus. *Arthritis & Rheumatism, 40*, S209.

al-Janadi, M., al-Balla, S., al-Dalaan, A., & Raziuddin, S. (1993). Cytokine profile in systemic lupus erythematosus, rheumatoid arthritis, and other rheumatic diseases. *Journal of Clinical Immunology, 13*(1), 58–67.

Barendregt, P. J., Visser, M. R., Smets, E. M., et al. (1998). Fatigue in primary Sjogren's syndrome. *Annals of the Rheumatic Diseases, 57*(5), 291–295.

Belza, B. (1994). The impact of fatigue on exercise performance. *Arthritis Care and Research, 7*(4), 176–180.

Belza, B. L. (1995). Comparison of self-reported fatigue in rheumatoid arthritis and controls. *Journal of Rheumatology, 22*(4), 639–643.

Bombardier, C., Gladman, D. D., Urowitz, M. B., Caron, D., & Chang, C. H. (1992). Derivation of the SLEDAI. A disease activity index for lupus patients. The Committee on Prognosis Studies in SLE. *Arthritis and Rheumatism, 35*(6), 630–640.

Boswell, J. M., Yui, M. A., Endres, S., Burt, D. W., & Kelley, V. E. (1988). Novel and enhanced IL-1 gene expression in autoimmune mice with lupus. *Journal of Immunology, 141(1)*, 118–124.

Bruce, I. N., Mak, V. C., Hallett, D. C., Gladman, D. D., & Urowitz, M. B. (1999). Factors associated with fatigue in patients with systemic lupus erythematosus. *Annals of the Rheumatic Diseases, 58(6)*, 379–381.

Cardenas, D. D., & Kutner, N. G. (1982). The problem of fatigue in dialysis patients. *Nephron, 30(4)*, 336–340.

Chalder, T., Berelowitz, G., Pawlikowska, T., et al. (1993). Development of a fatigue scale. *Journal of Psychosomatic Research, 37(2)*, 147–153.

Crosby, L. J. (1991). Factors which contribute to fatigue associated with rheumatoid arthritis. *Journal of Advanced Nursing, 16(8)*, 974–981.

Daltroy, L. H., Robb-Nicholson, C., Iversen, M. D., Wright, E. A., & Liang, M. H. (1995). Effectiveness of minimally supervised home aerobic training in patients with systemic rheumatic disease. *British Journal of Rheumatology, 34(11)*, 1064–1069.

Dekkers, J. C., Greenen, R., Godaert, G. L., Van Doornen, L. J. P., & Bijlsma, J. W. (2000). Diurnal courses of cortisol, pain, fatigue, negative mood, and stiffness in patients with recently diagnosed RA. *International Journal of Behavioral Medicine, 7(4)*, 353–371.

Delis, D. C., Kramer, J. H., Kaplan, E., et al. (1987). *The California Verbal Learning Test Manual*. San Antonio: The Psychological Corporation.

DeSouza, E. B. (1993). *Neurobiology of Cytokines*, San Diego: Academic Press.

Dobkin, P. L., Da Costa, D., Fortin, P. R., et al. (2001). Living with lupus: a prospective pan-Canadian study. *Journal of Rheumatology, 28(11)*, 2442–2448.

Elliott, M. J., & Maini, R. N. (1995). Anti-cytokine therapy in rheumatoid arthritis. *Baillieres Clinical Rheumatology, 9(4)*, 633–652.

Feldman, J., Brennan, F. M., Chu, C. Q., et al. (1993). Does TNF-alpha have a pivotal role in the cytokine network in rheumatoid arthritis? In W. Fiers & W. A. Buurman, eds. *Tumor Necrosis Factor: Molecular and Cellular Biology and Clinical Relevance*. New York: Karger.

Fifield, J., McQuillan, J., Tennen, H., et al. (2001). History of affective disorder and the temporal trajectory of fatigue in rheumatoid arthritis. *Annals of Behavioral Medicine, 23(1)*, 34–41.

Forte, S., Carlone, S., Vaccaro, F., et al. (1999). Pulmonary gas exchange and exercise capacity in patients with systemic lupus erythematosus. *Journal of Rheumatology, 26(12)*, 2591–2594.

Giang, D. W. (1991). Systemic lupus erythematosus and depression. *Neuropsychiatry, Neuropsychology, and Behavioral Neurology, 4*, 78–82.

Gilboe, I. M., Kvien, T. K., & Husby, G. (1999). Health status in systemic lupus erythematosus compared to rheumatoid arthritis and healthy controls. *Journal of Rheumatology, 26(8)*, 1694–1700.

Gladman, D. D., Urowitz, M. B., Ong, A., Gough, J., & MacKinnon, A. (1996). A comparison of five health status instruments in patients with systemic lupus erythematosus (SLE). *Lupus, 5(3)*, 190–195.

Godaert, G. L., Hartkamp, A., Geenen, R., et al. (2002). Fatigue in daily life in patients with primary Sjogren's syndrome and systemic lupus erythematosus. *Annals of the New York Academy of Sciences, 966*, 320–326.

Gudbjornsson, B., Broman, J. E., Hetta, J., & Hallgren, R. (1993). Sleep disturbances in patients with primary Sjogren's syndrome. *British Journal of Rheumatology, 32(12)*, 1072–1076.

Hall, R. C. W., & Stickney, S. K. (1983). Medical and psychiatric features of systemic lupus erythematosus. *Psychiatric Medicine, 1*, 287–301.

Hall, R. C., Stickney, S. K., & Gardner, E. R. (1981). Psychiatric symptoms in patients with systemic lupus erythematosus. *Psychosomatics, 22(1)*, 15–19, 23–14.

Hastings, C., Joyce, C., Yarbarac, et al. (1986). Factors affecting fatigue in SLE (Abstract). *Arthritis & Rheumatism, 29(Suppl)*, 51.

Huyser, B. A., Parker, J. C., Thoreson, R., Smarr, K. L., Johnson, J. C., & Hoffman, R. (1998). Predictors of subjective fatigue among individuals with rheumatoid arthritis. *Arthritis & Rheumatism, 41(12)*, 2230–2237.

Iriarte, J., & Castro, P. (1998). Correlation between symptom of fatigue and muscular fatigue in MS. *European Journal of Neurology, 5*, 1–7.

Iverson, G. L. (1993). Psychopathology associated with systemic lupus erythematosus: a methodological review. *Seminars in Arthritis and Rheumatism, 22(4)*, 242–251.

Iverson, G. L. (2002). Screening for depression in systemic lupus erythematosus with the British Columbia Major Depression Inventory. *Psychological Reports, 90(3 Pt 2)*, 1091–1096.

Jacobsson, L., Kirtava, Z., Olsson, G., Axell, T., & Manthorpe, R. (1995). Tiredness in patients with primary Sjogren's syndrome. *Clinical Rheumatology, 14(Suppl)*, 51.

Katz, P. P. (1998). The stresses of rheumatoid arthritis: appraisals of perceived impact and coping efficacy. *Arthritis Care and Research, 11(1)*, 9–22.

Kelley, K. W., Bluthe, R. M., Dantzer, R., et al. (2003). Cytokine-induced sickness behavior. *Brain, Behavior & Immunity, 17(Suppl)*, S112–S118.

Koike, T., Kazuma, K., & Kawamura, S. (2000). The relationship between fatigue, coping behavior, and inflammation in patients with RA. *Modern Rheumatology, 10(3)*, 141–149.

Kozora, E., Ellison, M. C., & West, S. G. (2005). Association of depression, pain, fatigue, and perceived functioning to the ACR SLE neuropsychological battery. Paper presented at the 43rd annual meeting of American Psychosomatic Society, Vancouver, B.C., Canada.

Kozora, E., & West, S. (2002). Diagnostic dilemmas: measurement of mood disorders and depression in systemic lupus erythematosus. *Psychosomatic Medicine, 64*, 126.

Kozora, E., West, S. G., Forrest, S., & Young, L. (2001). Attention and depression in systemic lupus erythematosus. Paper presented at the 59th annual meeting of American Psychosomatic Society, Monterey, CA.

Krupp, L. B., LaRocca, N. G., Muir, J., & Steinberg, A. D. (1990). A study of fatigue in systemic lupus erythematosus. *Journal of Rheumatology, 17(11)*, 1450–1452.

Krupp, L. B., LaRocca, N. G., Muir-Nash, J., & Steinberg, A. D. (1989). The fatigue severity scale. Application to patients with multiple sclerosis and systemic lupus erythematosus. *Archives of Neurology, 46(10)*, 1121–1123.

Krupp, L. B., & Pollina, D. A. (1996). Mechanisms and management of fatigue in progressive neurological disorders. *Current Opinion in Neurology, 9(6)*, 456–460.

Liang, M. H., & Ad Hoc Committee on Neuropsychiatric Lupus Nomenclature (1999). The American College of Rheumatology nomenclature and case definitions for neuropsychiatric lupus syndromes. *Arthritis and Rheumatism, 42(4)*, 599–608.

Liang, M. H., Rogers, M., Larson, M., et al. (1984). The psychosocial impact of systemic lupus erythematosus and rheumatoid arthritis. *Arthritis and Rheumatism, 27(1)*, 13–19.

Liang, M. H., Socher, S. A., Larson, M. G., & Schur, P. H. (1989). Reliability and validity of six systems for the clinical assessment of disease activity in systemic lupus erythematosus. *Arthritis and Rheumatism, 32(9)*, 1107–1118.

Linker-Israeli, M., Deans, R. J., Wallace, D. J., Prehn, J., Ozeri-Chen, T., & Klinenberg, J. R. (1991). Elevated levels of endogenous IL-6 in systemic lupus erythematosus. A putative role in pathogenesis. *Journal of Immunology, 147(1)*, 117–123.

Lwin, C. T., Bishay, M., Platts, R. G., Booth, D. A., & Bowman, S. J. (2003). The assessment of fatigue in primary Sjogren's syndrome. *Scandinavian Journal of Rheumatology, 32(1)*, 22–27.

Magner, M. B. (1991). Psychiatric morbidity in outpatients with systemic lupus erythematosus. *South African Medical Journal, 80(6)*, 291–293.

Mahowald, M. W., Mahowald, M. L., Bundlie, S. R., & Ytterberg, S. R. (1989). Sleep fragmentation in rheumatoid arthritis. *Arthritis and Rheumatism, 32(8)*, 974–983.

Maier, S. F., Goehler, L. E., Fleshner, M., & Watkins, L. R. (1998). The role of the vagus nerve in cytokine-to-brain communication. *Annals of the New York Academy of Sciences, 840*, 289–300.

Manthorpe, R., Kirtava, Z., Jacobsson, L., Tabery, H., Hendricsson, V., & Axell, T. (1995). Main subjective symptoms in 217 patients with primary Sjogren's syndrome. *Clinical Rheumatology, 14(Suppl)*, 50.

Maury, C. P., & Teppo, A. M. (1989). Tumor necrosis factor in the serum of patients with systemic lupus erythematosus. *Arthritis and Rheumatism, 32(2)*, 146–150.

McKinley, P. S., Ouellette, S. C., & Winkel, G. H. (1995). The contributions of disease activity, sleep patterns, and depression to fatigue in systemic lupus erythematosus. A proposed model. *Arthritis and Rheumatism, 38(6)*, 826–834.

McNair, D. M., Lorr, M., & Droppleman, L. F. (1980). *Profile of Mood States (POMS) Manual*. San Diego: Education and Industrial Testing Services.

Meyers, J. E., & Meyers, K. R. (1995). *Rey Complex Figure Test and Recognition Trial: Professional Manual*. Odessa, Psychological Assessment Resources, Inc.

Middleton, G. D., McFarlin, J. E., & Lipsky, P. E. (1994). The prevalence and clinical impact of fibromyalgia in systemic lupus erythematosus. *Arthritis and Rheumatism, 37(8)*, 1181–1188.

Morand, E. F., Miller, M. H., Whittingham, S., & Littlejohn, G. O. (1994). Fibromyalgia syndrome and disease activity in systemic lupus erythematosus. *Lupus, 3(3)*, 187–191.

Neuberger, G. B., Press, A. N., Lindsley, H. B., et al. (1997). Effects of exercise on fatigue, aerobic fitness, and disease activity measures in persons with rheumatoid arthritis. *Research in Nursing and Health, 20(3)*, 195–204.

Nicassio, P. M., Radojevic, V., Weisman, M. H., et al. (1997). A comparison of behavioral and educational interventions for fibromyalgia. *Journal of Rheumatology, 24(10)*, 2000–2007.

Omdal, R. (2002). Some controversies of neuropsychiatric systemic lupus erythematosus. *Scandinavian Journal Rheumatology, 31(4)*, 192–197.

Omdal, R., Husby, G., & Mellgren, S. I. (1995). Mental health status in systemic lupus erythematosus. *Scandinavian Journal Rheumatology, 24(3)*, 142–145.

Omdal, R., Mellgren, S. I., Koldingsnes, W., Jacobsen, E. A., & Husby, G. (2002). Fatigue in patients with systemic lupus erythematosus: lack of associations to serum cytokines, antiphospholipid antibodies, or other disease characteristics. *Journal of Rheumatology, 29(3)*, 482–486.

Pinals, R. S., Masi, A. T., & Larsen, R. A. (1981). Preliminary criteria for clinical remission in rheumatoid arthritis. *Arthritis and Rheumatism, 24(10)*, 1308–1315.

Pincus, T., Callahan, L. F., Brooks, R. H., Fuchs, H. A., Olsen, N. J., & Kaye, J. J. (1989). Self-report questionnaire scores in rheumatoid arthritis compared with traditional physical, radiographic, and laboratory measures. *Annals of Internal Medicine, 110(4)*, 259–266.

Piper, B. F. (1989). *Fatigue, Current Basis for Practice: The Development of an Instrument*. New York: Spring.

Radloff, L. S. (1977). The CES-D Scale: a self-report depression scale for research in the general population. *Applied Psychology Measures, 1*, 385–401.

Reitan, R. M., & Wolfson, D. (1988). *The Halstead-Reitan Neuropsychology Test Battery*. Tucson: Neuropsychological Press.

Robb-Nicholson, L. C., Daltroy, L., Eaton, H., et al. (1989). Effects of aerobic conditioning in lupus fatigue: a pilot study. *British Journal of Rheumatology, 28(6)*, 500–505.

Rothfield, N. (1989). *Clinical Features of Systemic Lupus Erythematosus*. Philadelphia: W.B. Saunders.

Sakauchi, M., Matsumura, T., Yamaoka, T., et al. (1995). Reduced muscle uptake of oxygen during exercise in patients with systemic lupus erythematosus. *Journal of Rheumatology, 22(8)*, 1483–1487.

Shur, P. H. (1989). *Clinical Features of Systemic Lupus Erythematosus*. Philadelphia: W.B. Saunders.

Silberstein, S. L., Barland, P., Grayzel, A. I., & Koerner, S. K. (1980). Pulmonary dysfunction in systemic lupus erythematosus: prevalence classification and correlation with other organ involvement. *Journal of Rheumatology, 7(2)*, 187–195.

Singh, A. K. (1992). Cytokines play a central role in the pathogenesis of systemic lupus erythematosus. *Medical Hypotheses, 39(4)*, 356–359.

Smets, E. M., Garssen, B., Bonke, B., & De Haes, J. C. (1995). The Multidimensional Fatigue Inventory (MFI) psychometric qualities of an instrument to assess fatigue. *Journal of Psychosomatic Research, 39(3)*, 315–325.

Tack, B. B. (1990). Fatigue in rheumatoid arthritis. Conditions, strategies, and consequences. *Arthritis Care and Research, 3(2)*, 65–70.

Tayer, W. G., Nicassio, P. M., Weisman, M. H., Schuman, C., & Daly, J. (2001). Disease status predicts fatigue in systemic lupus erythematosus. *Journal of Rheumatology, 28(9)*, 1999–2007.

Taylor, J., Skan, J., Erb, N., et al. (2000). Lupus patients with fatigue—is there a link with fibromyalgia syndrome? *Rheumatology, 39(6)*, 620–623.

Tench, C., Bentley, D., Vleck, V., McCurdie, I., White, P., & D'Cruz, D. (2002). Aerobic fitness, fatigue, and physical disability in systemic lupus erythematosus. *Journal of Rheumatology, 29(3)*, 474–481.

Tench, C. M., McCurdie, I., White, P. D., & D'Cruz, D. P. (2000). The prevalence and associations of fatigue in systemic lupus erythematosus. *Rheumatology, 39(11)*, 1249–1254.

Tensing, E. K., Solovieva, S. A., Tervahartiala, T., et al. (2001). Fatigue and health profile in sicca syndrome of Sjogren's and non-Sjogren's syndrome origin. *Clinical and Experimental Rheumatology, 19(3)*, 313–316.

Vitali, C., Bencivell, W., Isenberg, D., et al. (1991). Disease activity in systemic lupus erythematosus: report for the Consensus Study Group of the European Workshop for Rheumatology Research. II. Identification of the variables indicative of disease activity and their use in the development of an activity score. *Clinical and Experimental Rheumatology, 10*, 541–547.

Wallace, D. J. (1995). *The Lupus Book: A Guide for Patients and Their Families*. New York: Oxford University Press.

Wang, B., Gladman, D. D., & Urowitz, M. B. (1998). Fatigue in lupus is not correlated with disease activity. *Journal of Rheumatology, 25(5)*, 892–895.

Ware, J. E., Jr., & Sherbourne C. D. (1992). The MOS 36-item short-form health survey (SF-36). I. Conceptual framework and item selection. *Medical Care, 30(6)*, 473–483.

Wekking, E. M. (1993). Psychiatric symptoms in systemic lupus erythematosus: an update. *Psychosomatic Medicine, 55(2)*, 219–228.

West, S. G. (2002). Systemic lupus erythematosus and the nervous system. In D. J. W. B. H. Hann, ed. *Dubois' Lupus Erythematosus*, 6th ed. Pp. 693–738. Philadelphia: Lippincott Williams & Wilkins.

Wysenbeek, A. J., Leibovici, L., Weinberger, A., & Guedj, D. (1993). Fatigue in systemic lupus erythematosus. Prevalence and relation to disease expression. *British Journal of Rheumatology, 32(7)*, 633–635.

Zigmond, A. S., & Smith R. P. (1983). The hospital anxiety and depression scale. *Acta psychiatrica Scandinavica, 67(6)*, 361–370.

Zonana-Nacach, A., Roseman, J. M., McGwin, G., Jr., et al. (2000). Systemic lupus erythematosus in three ethnic groups. VI: factors associated with fatigue within 5 years of criteria diagnosis. LUMINA Study Group. Lupus in minority populations: nature vs nurture. *Lupus, 9(2)*, 101–109.

16 Cancer and Fatigue: Insights from Studies of Women Treated for Breast Cancer

Paul B. Jacobsen and Kristine A. Donovan

Interest in the problem of fatigue in cancer patients is growing among clinicians and researchers alike (de Jong, Courtens, Abu-Saad, & Schouten, 2002; Groopman, 1998; Morrow, Andrews, Hickok, Roscoe, & Matteson, 2002), and is consistent with an increasing awareness of the importance of quality of life as an outcome in oncology. Although fatigue has been studied in several populations of cancer patients, much of the research has focused on women previously treated for breast cancer. In addition to descriptive studies, research in this area includes several studies examining the relationship of fatigue to cognitive and immune functioning. The latter studies represent the most relevant attempts yet within oncology to examine fatigue as a window to the brain. For these reasons, this chapter focuses on fatigue in this patient population. Before reviewing the research, however, we first need to identify several important methodological issues in the study of fatigue in cancer patients.

Methodological Issues in the Study of Fatigue

Research on fatigue in cancer patients has been characterized by a number of methodological limitations. One issue is the manner in which fatigue is measured. At present, there is no consensus regarding the optimal means of assessing fatigue in cancer patients. As a result, a variety of self-report techniques are used. Much of the time, fatigue is measured by a single item embedded in a symptom checklist such as the Symptom Distress Scale (McCorkle & Quit-Benoliel, 1983) or the Rotterdam Symptom Checklist (deHaes, van Knippenberg, & Neijt, 1990). Visual analogue scales and the single-item Rhoten Fatigue Scale (Rhoten, 1982) are also used. Because of their format, these single-item measures have limited reliability and provide only the most perfunctory information about patients' experience of fatigue. Fatigue is also frequently assessed with multi-item measures such as the Fatigue Scale of the Profile of Mood States (POMS) (McNair, Lorr, & Droppleman, 1992). Although multi-item measures have better psychometric properties than single-item measures, they are limited in that they provide information only about patients' general level of fatigue severity.

In a more comprehensive approach to the assessment of fatigue, several investigators have developed multidimensional measures (Piper, Dibble, Dodd, Weiss, Slaughter, & Paul, 1998; Smets, Garssen, Bonke, & deHaes, 1995). Two measures our research group has developed illustrate this approach. The Fatigue Symptom Inventory (FSI) (Hann et al., 1998) is a 14-item measure consisting of separate subscales that assess the intensity and duration of fatigue, as well as its perceived interference with quality of life. The FSI is designed to be used in conjunction with the 30-item Multidimensional Fatigue Symptom Inventory-Short Form (MFSI-SF) (Stein, Martin, Hann, & Jacobsen, 1998), which provides information about the patient's experience of behavioral, cognitive, physical, and affective manifestations of fatigue.

A second methodological limitation involves the frequent use of cross-sectional research designs to study changes in fatigue over time. In using cross-sectional designs, researchers attempt to draw conclusions about the persistence or resolution of fatigue by comparing individuals who vary in when they completed cancer treatment. The problem is that the observed changes across time also reflect individual differences in patients' experience of fatigue. Longitudinal designs provide a more methodologically sound approach, assessing the same patients on multiple occasions following completion of treatment. Although longitudinal studies are costly in terms of both time and resources, their data could greatly clarify the natural history of fatigue in cancer survivors.

A third methodological limitation of previous research is the absence of comparison groups. Since fatigue is a common symptom in the general population, some frame of reference is necessary to evaluate reports of fatigue obtained from cancer patients. Ideally, researchers should also obtain fatigue data from samples of individuals without cancer whose sociodemographic characteristics (e.g., age, gender, and education) are similar to those of the patients under study. In addition to providing useful reference values, data from comparison groups may also help us evaluate the sensitivity of different fatigue measures and identify the symptoms of fatigue that distinguish different patient and nonpatient populations.

A fourth methodological limitation is the tendency to recruit samples of breast cancer survivors that are heterogeneous regarding their previous treatment. That is, the samples include women treated with varying combinations of surgery, chemotherapy, and radiotherapy. Typically, these samples do not include enough women who received the same forms of therapy to make meaningful comparisons based on treatment type. A more useful strategy, illustrated in the studies reviewed in the following sections, is to recruit a sufficient numbers of patients who received the same therapy to be able to examine important treatment-specific differences in fatigue.

With these considerations in mind, we now turn to a review of research examining fatigue in women with breast cancer treated with adjuvant radiotherapy, adjuvant chemotherapy, or autologous bone marrow transplantation.

Fatigue after Adjuvant Radiotherapy

Previous research has consistently shown that women with breast cancer generally experience heightened fatigue during the course of adjuvant radiotherapy (Blesch et al., 1991; Greenberg, Sawicka, Eisenthal, & Ross, 1992; Irvine, Vincent, Graydon, & Bubela, 1998; Irvine, Vincent, Graydon, Bubela, & Thompson, 1994; Kobashi-Schoot, Hanewald, van Dam, & Bruning, 1985). Evidence of persistent fatigue following the completion of adjuvant radiotherapy comes primarily from a study conducted by Berglund and colleagues (Berglund, Bolund, Fornander, Rutqvist, & Sjoden, 1991). In this study, fatigue was assessed in women with breast cancer who had been treated with adjuvant radiotherapy between 2 and 10 years previously and were recurrence free at the time of follow-up. Data obtained with a symptom checklist indicated that fatigue was the most commonly reported symptom and was present in 76 percent of patients. Additional results indicated that fatigue severity was unrelated to either patient age or time since completion of radiotherapy.

In contrast to these findings, results from four other studies suggest that fatigue does not persist following completion of adjuvant radiotherapy. In one of the first studies to address this issue, Greenberg and colleagues (Greenberg et al., 1992) assessed fatigue in women with breast cancer during the course of adjuvant radiotherapy and at 3 and 11 to 14 weeks posttreatment. Fatigue was assessed using the average score from three separate fatigue scales: the Profile of Mood States Fatigue Scale (McNair et al., 1992), the Pearson-Byars Fatigue Feeling Checklist (Irvine et al., 1994), and a visual analogue scale. Results indicated that fatigue decreased from baseline during the first 2 weeks of treatment, then increased steadily before reaching a plateau by the fourth week of treatment. Levels of fatigue thereafter diminished significantly, reaching pretreatment levels by the third week following treatment completion. No further changes in fatigue severity were noted.

Irvine and colleagues (Irvine et al., 1998) obtained similar results in a study that assessed fatigue in women with breast cancer during adjuvant radiotherapy and at 3 and 6 months following treatment completion by means of the Pearson Byars Feeling Checklist (Irvine et al., 1994). Consistent with findings of prior research, their results indicated that levels of fatigue during radiotherapy were significantly higher than the pretreatment level. However, by the 3-month follow-up, the severity of fatigue had returned to the pretreatment level. Fatigue severity remained at this level at the 6-month follow-up.

Hann and colleagues (Hann, Jacobsen, Martin, et al., 1998) also obtained results indicating that fatigue does not persist following completion of adjuvant radiotherapy. In this study, the Profile of Mood States Fatigue Scale (McNair et al., 1992), the Fatigue Symptom Inventory (Hann, Jacobsen, Azzarello, et al., 1998), and the Multidimensional Fatigue Symptom Inventory (Stein et al., 1998) were used to assess fatigue in breast cancer patients who had completed treatment with adjuvant radiotherapy an average of 22 months previously and were recurrence free at the time of follow-up. Fatigue was also assessed in an age-matched comparison sample of women with no history of cancer. The two groups did not differ in terms of the duration or disruptiveness of fatigue or in their levels of global, somatic, cognitive, affective, or behavioral symptoms of fatigue. Differences in fatigue severity were also nonsignificant, with the exception of ratings of the most fatigue experienced in the past week. Compared to the age-matched comparison group, the former radiotherapy patients reported higher levels of fatigue on the day they felt most fatigued in the past week.

A study by Geinitz and colleagues (Geinitz et al., 2001) assessing patients 2 months following completion of adjuvant radiotherapy yielded similar results. As measured by a visual analogue scale, levels of fatigue at the follow-up assessment were significantly below pretreatment levels.

Taken together, these findings fail to provide clear evidence that fatigue following adjuvant radiotherapy is a clinically significant phenomenon. Although heightened fatigue does appear to be common during the course of radiotherapy, the studies reviewed indicate that recovery to a pretreatment level typically occurs within several weeks of completing treatment (Greenberg et al., 1992; Irvine et al., 1998; Geinitz et al., 2001). Moreover, one study demonstrated that the level of fatigue experienced by women previously treated with adjuvant radiotherapy could not be distinguished from the level experienced by women of similar age with no history of cancer (Hann, Jacobsen, Martin, et al., 1998). Although one study reviewed did report a relatively high prevalence of fatigue among women previously treated with radiotherapy (Berglund et al., 1991), the significance of this finding remains unclear in the absence of comparison or normative data. To the extent that fatigue is common in the general population, relatively high prevalence rates may not be clinically significant. It should be noted that findings suggesting the absence of heightened fatigue following adjuvant radiotherapy refer to the experience of the "average" patient. In each of the studies reviewed, there was evidence of considerable variability in patient reports of fatigue. Accordingly, fatigue may be an important clinical problem in a subgroup of former radiotherapy patients. Identifying these patients and determining why they experience heightened fatigue should be a focus of future research.

Fatigue after Adjuvant Chemotherapy

Previous research has shown that fatigue is one of the most common symptoms experienced during the course of adjuvant chemotherapy for breast cancer. For example, Greene and colleagues (Greene, Nail, Fieler, Dudgeon, & Jones, 1994) reported that, among women receiving adjuvant chemotherapy, 82 percent reported fatigue after the first treatment cycle and 77 percent reported fatigue after the second treatment cycle.

In one of the first studies to examine fatigue after completion of adjuvant chemotherapy, Knobf (Knobf, 1986) surveyed women who had finished treatment an average of 28 months previously. Using the Symptom Distress Scale (McCorkle & Quit-Benoliel, 1983) to assess seven common symptoms, the investigator found that fatigue and insomnia were perceived as causing the greatest distress.

Three subsequent studies provide more specific information regarding the prevalence of fatigue among women treated with adjuvant chemotherapy. Berglund and colleagues (Berglund et al., 1991) assessed fatigue in a sample of women who had received adjuvant chemotherapy between 2 and 10 years previously. Patients were treated for a minimum of 6 months and a maximum of 18 months and were recurrence free at the time of assessment. Using a 16-item self-report symptom measure, the authors found that 68 percent of patients were currently experiencing fatigue. Additional findings indicated that the presence of fatigue was associated with more time elapsed since treatment completion. It should be noted, however, that the length of chemotherapy and the number of treatment cycles also tended to be greater in patients for whom more time had elapsed. In another study examining prevalence, Beisecker and colleagues (Beisecker, Cook, & Ashworth, 1997) surveyed a sample of women with node-negative disease in which the median time since treatment completion was 7.5 months. Using a semistructured interview to assess common treatment side effects, the investigators found that 83 percent of patients reported the current presence of fatigue and 60 percent reported that fatigue interfered with their functioning.

A study by Broeckel and colleagues (Broeckel, Jacobsen, Horton, Balducci, & Lyman, 1998) provides additional information about the characteristics and correlates of fatigue following adjuvant chemotherapy. Participants in this study were recurrence-free breast cancer patients who had completed adjuvant chemotherapy an average of 471 days previously and an age-matched comparison group of women with no history of cancer. Fatigue was assessed in both groups with the Profile of Mood States Fatigue Scale (McNair et al., 1992), the Fatigue Symptom Inventory (Hann, Jacobsen, Azzarello, et al., 1998), and the Multidimensional Fatigue Symptom Inventory (Stein et al., 1998). Compared to women with no history of cancer, former adjuvant chemotherapy patients reported more severe fatigue, worse quality of life due to fatigue, and more physical and mental symptoms of fatigue. Among the former chemotherapy patients, more severe fatigue was related to poorer sleep quality, more menopausal symptoms, and greater use of catastrophizing as a coping strategy. In contrast, fatigue severity was unrelated to age, time since treatment completion, additional treatment with radiotherapy, or current use of tamoxifen.

Several preliminary conclusions can be drawn from these studies. First, the data suggest that fatigue is an extremely common and distressing symptom following adjuvant chemotherapy (Beisecker et al., 1997; Berglund et al., 1991; Knobf, 1986). Second, fatigue following adjuvant chemotherapy appears to be a clinically significant phenomenon. Levels of fatigue among former adjuvant chemotherapy patients have been shown to be 50 percent greater than those reported by women with no history of cancer (Broeckel et al., 1998). Third, evidence indicates that the presence of menopausal symptoms may exacerbate the degree of fatigue former adjuvant chemotherapy patients experience (Broeckel et al., 1998). One possible explanation for this relationship is that the occurrence of vasomotor symptoms of menopause (e.g., night sweats) may disrupt sleep, resulting in heightened fatigue (Kronenberg, 1994). Fourth, preliminary evidence shows that the strategies patients use to cope with fatigue may also have an impact on the severity of their symptoms. In particular, the tendency to catastrophize (i.e., to engage in overly negative thoughts about oneself and the future) appears to be associated with a worse experience of fatigue (Broeckel et al., 1998). Fifth, at least one study (Broeckel et al., 1998) provides evidence that mental symptoms (e.g., perceived problems with attention and concentration) are part of the fatigue experience among women previously treated with chemotherapy.

Fatigue after Autologous Bone Marrow Transplantation

Autologous bone marrow transplantation or, more precisely, high-dose chemotherapy with autologous stem cell support, is one of the newest and more controversial forms of breast cancer treatment. The controversy relates to recently published findings suggesting that this form of therapy does not significantly improve breast cancer survival over more established treatments (Dicato, 2002). Accordingly, this therapy is now less commonly used than it was a few years ago.

In one of the first studies to examine fatigue following this form of treatment, Hann and colleagues (Hann, Jacobsen, Martin, Kronish, Azzarello, & Fields, 1997) surveyed women who had completed autologous bone marrow transplantation for metastatic or nonmetastatic breast cancer an average of 20 months previously and an age-matched comparison group of women with no history of cancer. Eligibility was limited to women with no clinical evidence of disease at follow-up. Fatigue was assessed in both groups using the Profile of Mood States Fatigue Scale (McNair et al., 1992), the Fatigue Symptom Inventory (Hann, Jacobsen, Azzarello, et al., 1998), and the Multidimensional Fatigue Symptom Inventory (Stein et al., 1998). Versus an age-matched comparison group of women with no history of cancer, former transplant patients reported more severe fatigue, greater duration of fatigue, worse quality of life due to fatigue, and more behavioral, mental, and global symptoms of fatigue. Among former transplant patients, more severe fatigue was related to poorer sleep quality, higher levels of anxiety and depression, and more time elapsed since transplant. In contrast, fatigue severity was unrelated to patient age, disease stage at transplant, length of hospitalization for transplant, or current use of tamoxifen.

Winer and colleagues (Winer et al., 1999) examined quality of life, including fatigue in women who had undergone autologous bone marrow transplantation for metastatic or nonmetastatic breast cancer at least 1 year previously (median, 30.6 months). Based on responses to the Symptom Distress Scale (McCorkle & Quit-Benoliel, 1983), the authors determined that fatigue was one of the most commonly reported symptoms. At the time of assessment, 60 percent of patients were characterized as experiencing mild to moderate fatigue and 8 percent experienced severe fatigue.

Taken together, the results of these studies provide preliminary evidence that fatigue following autologous transplantation for breast cancer is a clinically significant phenomenon. Among women with breast cancer an average of more than 1 year posttransplant, fatigue was common (Winer et al., 1999) and more severe than in women with no history of cancer (Hann et al., 1997). Preliminary evidence also suggests that fatigue in former transplant patients is accompanied by sleep disturbance and heightened emotional distress and includes mental symptoms, such as perceived problems with attention and concentration (Hann et al., 1997).

Comparisons of Fatigue Across Different Types of Treatment

The studies reviewed suggest that the degree of fatigue experienced following breast cancer treatment may vary according to the specific type of treatment received. Specifically, evidence indicates that fatigue is a significant clinical problem in patients treated previously with adjuvant chemotherapy and autologous bone marrow transplantation but not in patients treated previously with adjuvant radiotherapy. To directly address the issue of differences in fatigue related to type of treatment, it would be useful to compare patients who received different type treatments and were assessed with the same measures of fatigue at comparable time points following treatment completion. At least two studies meet these criteria (van Dam et al., 1998; Schagen, van Dam, Muller, Boogerd, Lindeboom, & Bruning, 1999), and both included assessments of cognitive functioning as well as fatigue.

In the study by van Dam and colleagues (van Dam et al., 1998), participants were breast cancer patients with nonmetastatic disease who had been randomly assigned to receive either standard-dose adjuvant chemotherapy or high-dose chemotherapy with stem cell rescue (i.e., autologous bone marrow transplantation). Patients were assessed an average of 1.6 years (transplant group) or 1.9 years (chemotherapy group) following treatment completion. Data were also obtained from a sample of breast cancer patients treated with surgery and radiotherapy alone an average of 2.4 years previously. As part of a larger investigation of quality of life, fatigue and perceived cognitive functioning were assessed in all three groups with the scales from the EORTC QLQ-C30 (Aaronson et al., 1993). In addition, all three groups completed a battery of neuropsychological tests that included measures of attention/concentration (e.g.,

WAIS Digit Span), mental flexibility (e.g., Trailmaking B), memory (e.g., Rey Auditory Verbal Learning), motor function (e.g., Fepsy Finger Tapping), and processing speed (e.g., Fepsy Visual Searching). Results indicated that patients who underwent transplant reported significantly greater fatigue and more perceived problems with cognitive functioning than patients treated with surgery and radiotherapy alone. Differences between transplant patients and standard-dose chemotherapy patients were in the same direction for both fatigue and perceived cognitive functioning but did not reach statistical significance. The same study also found that transplant patients performed significantly poorer than patients treated with surgery and radiotherapy on measures of attention/concentration, processing speed, visual memory, and motor functioning. The only analysis to directly examine the relationship of fatigue to cognitive functioning consisted of a multivariate analysis designed to identify factors associated with classification of patients as impaired or not impaired regarding neuropsychological test performance. Findings indicated that fatigue was not a significant predictor of cognitive impairment.

In the study by Schagen and colleagues (Schagen et al., 1999), participants were breast cancer patients with axillary node involvement who received standard-dose adjuvant chemotherapy and breast cancer patients without axillary node involvement who did not receive adjuvant chemotherapy. Patients were assessed an average of 1.9 years (chemotherapy group) or 2.4 years (no chemotherapy group) following completion of treatment. Fatigue, perceived cognitive functioning, and neuropsychological test performance were assessed with the same methods used in the study by van Dam and colleagues (van Dam et al., 1998). Results indicated that patients who underwent chemotherapy reported greater fatigue than patients not treated with chemotherapy, however, this difference was not statistically significant ($p = 0.16$). The chemotherapy group did report significantly more problems with cognitive functioning than the no chemotherapy group and also performed significantly poorer on tests assessing attention/concentration, mental flexibility, speed of information processing, memory, verbal function, and motor function. As in the study by van Dam and colleagues (van Dam et al., 1998), fatigue did not predict the classification of patients as impaired or not impaired based on neuropsychological test performance.

Recently, Schagen and colleagues (Schagen, Hamburger, Muller, Boogerd, & van Dam, 2001) reported neurophysiological findings for a subset of patients from the study by van Dam and colleagues (van Dam et al., 1998). Analyses based on event-related potentials indicated a significant correlation between P300 latencies and the total number of deviant scores, with longer P300 latencies corresponding to more deviant test results. However, no significant relations were observed between fatigue and neurophysiological functioning as measured by either event-related potentials or quantitative electroencephalography.

The pattern of results observed in these two studies is consistent with the view that, among breast cancer survivors, treatment with high-dose chemotherapy (autologous bone marrow transplantation) is associated with greater fatigue than treatment with standard-dose chemotherapy, which, in turn, is associated with greater fatigue than treatment with nonsystemic therapy (surgery with or without radiotherapy). The evidence of trends, but not statistically significant differences for several of these comparisons, may reflect the limited statistical power the generally small sample sizes provide (ranging from 19 to 36 patients). Regarding the relationship of fatigue to cognitive functioning, the findings are equivocal. Although the pattern of differences among groups in cognitive performance and cognitive complaints tended to mirror the pattern of differences among groups in fatigue, analyses directly comparing fatigue with cognitive performance and neurophysiological functioning yielded no evidence of relationships.

Comparisons of Fatigue with Cognitive Functioning

One additional study (Servaes, Verhagen, & Bleijenberg, 2002) merits discussion since it focused specifically on the relationship of fatigue to cognitive functioning in women previously treated for breast cancer. Participants in this study were women under age 50 who completed various combinations of treatments for breast cancer (i.e., surgery with or without chemotherapy and/or radiotherapy) between 6 and 60 months previously and an age-matched comparison group of women with no history of breast cancer. Fatigue and perceived cognitive functioning were assessed with the Checklist of Individual Strength (Vercoulen, Swanink, Fennis, Galama, Van-der-Meer, & Bleijenberg, 1994) and the Sickness Impact Profile (Bergner, Bobbitt, Carter, & Gilson, 1981), as well as diaries completed over a 12-day period. Participants were also administered neuropsychological measures of information processing speed (Complex Reaction Time Test) and concentration (WAIS Symbol Digit). Based on responses to the Fatigue Severity subscale of the Checklist of Individual Strength, the breast cancer sample was divided into severely and nonseverely fatigued subgroups. Findings indicated that severely fatigued patients reported more problems with concentration and alertness behavior than nonseverely fatigued patients and women with no history of breast cancer. The latter two groups did not differ significantly on these measures. Performance on neuropsychological measures was not entirely consistent with self-reported cognitive functioning. Severely fatigued patients evidenced significantly slower speed of information processing than women with no history of cancer but not patients who were nonseverely fatigued. Moreover, the three groups did not differ significantly on a standardized concentration task.

Findings from this study suggest that reports of fatigue among breast cancer survivors correspond more closely with reports of cognitive complaints than with performance on cognitive tasks. Research with other populations of cancer patients has yielded similar results. For example, reports of memory and concentration problems by lymphoma patients were found to be significantly associated with self-reports of fatigue but not with performance on neuropsychological measures of memory and concentration (Cull, Hay, Love, Mackie, Smets, & Stewart, 1996).

Unanswered Questions

Although considerable progress has been made in identifying the characteristics and correlates of fatigue in breast cancer survivors, two major questions remain unanswered. First, what mechanisms can explain why women with breast cancer continue to experience fatigue months or even years after systemic therapy? In particular, what role might brain functioning play in patients' reports of fatigue? And second, what interventions may be effective in preventing or reducing this fatigue?

There is general agreement that fatigue in cancer patients has a multifactorial origin (Winningham, Nail, Burke, et al., 1994). Fatigue in breast cancer patients may be the direct result of treatment-related physiological changes (e.g., occurrence of anemia and accumulation of toxic metabolites) (Glaspy, Bukowski, Steinberg, Taylor, Tchekmedyian, & Vadhan-Raj, 1997) as well as the indirect result of other treatment-related side effects, such as pain and fever (Blesch et al., 1991). These mechanisms can explain the occurrence of fatigue during treatment, however, they cannot account for its persistence once treatment is completed (i.e., when most patients are no longer experiencing direct physiological effects of treatment or acute side effects).

One possible explanation is that heightened fatigue following treatment completion is a consequence of longer-term changes in physiological functioning or the occurrence of longer-term side effects. Among women who are premenopausal prior to cancer diagnosis, heightened fatigue may be due to the sudden and often irreversible onset of treatment-induced menopause and its accompanying vasomotor symptoms (e.g., hot flashes). Among women who are postmenopausal before breast cancer diagnosis, discontinuation of estrogen replacement therapy may contribute to heightened fatigue if vasomotor symptoms of menopause are not well controlled by other means. If so, this would suggest that nonhormonal interventions effective in relieving vasomotor symptoms of menopause might also be effective in relieving fatigue in breast cancer survivors. Along these lines, we recently reported on the benefits of paroxetine in relieving hot flashes and fatigue in women with breast cancer (Weitzner, Moncello, Jacobsen, & Minton, 2002). In addition to this indirect effect on fatigue, reduced estrogen levels due to treatment-induced menopause or discontinuation of estrogen replacement therapy may also have a direct effect on fatigue. A growing body of evidence suggests that estrogen regulates functioning in brain regions important to mood, memory, and learning (McEwen, 2002), and treatment of estrogen deficiency results in selective improvements in cognitive functioning (LeBlanc, Janowsky, Chan, & Nelson, 2001). These same findings suggest that lack of estrogen may contribute to fatigue because mood and cognitive functioning problems are often subjectively experienced as fatigue. To clarify this potential mechanism, it would be useful to determine whether changes in levels of estrogen and its metabolites in women undergoing breast cancer treatment are related to changes in fatigue and cognitive functioning.

A second possible physiological explanation for persistent fatigue following treatment completion is immune function changes. Basic research in neuroimmune signaling has shown that inflammatory stimuli can signal the central nervous system to generate a variety of illness symptoms, including fatigue (Kent, Bluthe, Kelley, & Dantzer, 1992). Based on this research, Bower and colleagues (Bower, Ganz, Aziz, & Fahey, 2002; Bower, Ganz, Aziz, Fahey, & Cole, 2003) investigated whether fatigue in women previously treated for breast cancer was associated with proinflammatory cytokine activity. Findings indicated that, compared to nonfatigued patients, fatigued patients had higher serum levels of interleukin-1 receptor antagonist (IL-1ra), soluble tumor necrosis factor, and neopterin. Additional analyses indicated that alterations in circulating T-cell levels (CD3$^+$ and CD3$^+$/CD4$^+$) accounted for the relationship between IL-1ra and fatigue. The authors speculate that the observed alternations could be due to changes in immune regulatory systems, such as the autonomic nervous system and the hypothalamic–pituitary–adrenal axis. To better understand the contribution of proinflammatory cytokines to fatigue, prospective studies are needed to examine associations between changes in cytokines and fatigue over the course of cancer treatment. The role of proinflammatory cytokines might also be clarified by examining whether pharmacological agents known to be effective in reducing proinflammatory cytokines levels have a beneficial impact on fatigue in cancer patients.

A third possible physiological explanation for persistent fatigue following treatment completion is neurotoxicity. Evidence supporting this explanation comes from findings reviewed in this chapter that indicate patients receiving systemic therapies (i.e., high-dose or standard-dose chemotherapy) generally report greater fatigue and exhibit poorer cognitive functioning than patients treated with local or regional therapies (i.e., surgery or radiotherapy) (van Dam et al., 1998; Schagen et al., 1999). This pattern of results is consistent with the fact that, unlike local or regional therapies for breast cancer, several commonly used chemotherapy agents have been documented to be neurotoxic (Keime-Guibert, Napolitano, & Delattre, 1998; Tuxen & Hansen, 1994). Clearly, more studies are needed to clarify whether the fatigue and cognitive problems observed in breast cancer patients are manifestations of chemotherapy-induced neurotoxicity. One such approach is to conduct longitudinal studies to determine whether changes in fatigue and cognitive functioning with initiation of chemotherapy are associated with functional or structural changes in the brain. Another approach is to determine whether efforts to limit neurotoxicity, such as by reducing drug doses or developing neuroprotective agents, have beneficial effects on fatigue and cognitive functioning.

A fourth, and not mutually exclusive, explanation is that cognitive and behavioral responses to fatigue during the active phase of treatment contribute to the perpetuation of fatigue following treatment completion. Evidence from other patient populations indicates that patients who respond to fatigue cognitively by catastrophizing and focusing on their symptoms and behaviorally by avoiding activity and accommodating their lifestyles to illness are more likely to develop chronic forms of fatigue (Wessely, Hotopf, & Sharpe, 1998). Two pieces of evidence suggest that this explanation is applicable to breast cancer patients. First, greater use of catastrophizing has been shown to be related to greater fatigue in breast cancer patients previously treated with adjuvant chemotherapy (Broeckel et al., 1998). Second, restrictions in physical activity have been shown to be related to greater fatigue in breast cancer patients currently receiving adjuvant chemotherapy (Berger, 1998). Evidence in support of this explanation suggests the use of a psychosocial intervention designed to change maladaptive cognitive and behavioral responses to treatment-related fatigue. Consistent with this view, we recently demonstrated the effectiveness of a stress management training intervention in relieving fatigue and improving quality of life in cancer patients undergoing chemotherapy (Jacobsen, Meade, Stein, Chirikos, Small, & Ruckdeschel, 2002). In addition, a growing body of evidence suggests that interventions designed to increase physical activity are effective in relieving fatigue in cancer patients (Courneya & Friedenreich, 1999).

Conclusion

A growing body of evidence demonstrates that fatigue is a long-term side effect of certain forms of breast cancer treatment. The studies conducted to date generally show that breast cancer patients treated with systemic therapies (i.e., high-dose or standard-dose chemotherapy) are more likely to experience heightened fatigue in the post-treatment period than breast cancer patients treated with local or regional therapies (i.e., surgery or radiotherapy). Differences in fatigue among treatment groups are accompanied by similar differences in cognitive complaints and, to a lesser extent, cognitive performance. At least four mechanisms mediated by or originating in the central nervous system may account for heightened fatigue following treatment completion in this patient population: (1) changes in hormonal functioning including changes in estrogen levels attributable to chemotherapy-induced menopause or discontinuation of estrogen replacement therapy; (2) changes in immune functioning, particularly changes in production of proinflammatory cytokines; (3) neurotoxic effects of chemotherapeutic agents; and (4) maladaptive cognitive and behavioral responses to treatment-related fatigue. The challenge for the future is to learn more about these and other potential causes of fatigue among cancer survivors and develop effective interventions to prevent or reduce fatigue following completion of cancer treatment.

References

Aaronson, N. K., Ahmedzi, S., Bergman, B., et al. (1993). The European Organization for Research and Treatment of Cancer QLQ-C30: a quality-of-life instrument for use in international clinical trials in oncology. *Journal of the National Cancer Institute, 85,* 365–376.

Beisecker, A. E., Cook, M. R., & Ashworth, J. (1997). Side effects of adjuvant chemotherapy: perceptions of node-negative breast cancer patients. *Psycho-Oncology, 6,* 85–93.

Berger, A. M. (1998). Patterns of fatigue and activity and rest during adjuvant breast cancer chemotherapy. *Oncology Nursing Forum, 25,* 51–62.

Berglund, G., Bolund, C., Fornander, T., Rutqvist, L. E., & Sjoden, P. O. (1991). Late effects of adjuvant chemotherapy and postoperative radiotherapy on quality of life among breast cancer patients. *European Journal of Cancer, 27,* 1075–1081.

Bergner, M., Bobbitt, R. A., Carter, W. B., & Gilson, B. S. (1981). The Sickness Impact Profile: development and final revision of a health status measure. *Medical Care, 19,* 787–805.

Blesch, K., Paice, J. A., Wickham, R., et. al. (1991). Correlates of fatigue in people with breast or lung cancer. *Oncology Nursing Forum, 18,* 81–87.

Bower, J. E., Ganz, P. A., Aziz, N., & Fahey, J. L. (2002). Fatigue and proinflammatory cytokine activity in breast cancer survivors. *Psychosomatic Medicine, 64,* 604–611.

Bower, J. E., Ganz, P. A., Aziz, N., Fahey, J. L., & Cole, S. W. (2003). T-cell homeostatis in breast cancer survivors with persistent fatigue. *Journal of the National Cancer Institute, 95,* 1165–1168.

Broeckel, J. A., Jacobsen, P. B., Horton, J., Balducci, L., & Lyman, G. H. (1998). Characteristics and correlates of fatigue following adjuvant chemotherapy for breast cancer. *Journal of Clinical Oncology, 16,* 1689–1696.

Courneya, K. S., & Friedenreich, C. M. (1999). Physical exercise and quality of life following cancer diagnosis: a literature review. *Annals of Behavioral Medicine, 21,* 171–179.

Cull, A., Hay, C., Love, S. B., Mackie, M., Smets, E., & Stewart, M. (1996). What do cancer patients mean when they complain of concentration and memory problems? *British Journal of Cancer, 74,* 1674–1679.

deHaes, J. C., van Knippenberg, F. C., & Neijt, J. P. (1990). Measuring psychological and physical distress in cancer patients: structure and application of the Rotterdam Symptom Checklist. *British Journal of Cancer, 62,* 1034–1038.

de Jong, N., Courtens, A. M., Abu-Saad, H., & Schouten, H. C. (2002). Fatigue in patients with breast cancer receiving adjuvant chemotherapy: a review of the literature. *Cancer Nursing, 25,* 283–297.

Dicato, M. (2002). High-dose chemotherapy in breast cancer: Where are we now? *Seminars in Oncology, 29*, 16–20.

Geinitz, H., Zimmerman, F. B., Stoll, P., et al. (2001). Fatigue, serum cytokine levels, and blood cell counts during radiotherapy of patients with breast cancer. *International Journal of Radiation Oncology, Biology, and Physics, 51*, 691–698.

Glaspy, J., Bukowski, R., Steinberg, D., Taylor, C., Tchekmedyian, S., & Vadhan-Raj, S. (1997). Impact of therapy with epoetin alfa on clinical outcomes in patients with nonmyeloid malignancies during cancer chemotherapy in community oncology practice. *Journal of Clinical Oncology, 15*, 1218–1234.

Greenberg, D. B., Sawicka, J., Eisenthal, S., & Ross, D. (1992). Fatigue syndrome due to localized radiation. *Journal of Pain & Symptom Management, 7*, 38–45.

Greene, D., Nail, L. M., Fieler, V. K., Dudgeon, D., & Jones, L. S. (1994). A comparison of patient-reported side effects among three chemotherapy regimens for breast cancer. *Cancer Practice, 2*, 57–62.

Groopman J. E. (1998). Fatigue in cancer and HIV/AIDS. *Oncology, 12*, 335–344.

Hann, D. M., Jacobsen, P. B., Azzarello, L. M., et al. (1998). Measurement of fatigue in cancer patients: development and validation of the Fatigue Symptom Inventory. *Quality of Life Research, 7*, 301–310.

Hann, D. M., Jacobsen, P. B., Martin, S. C., Azzarello, L. M., & Greenberg, H. (1998). Fatigue and quality of life following radiotherapy for breast cancer: a comparative study. *Journal of Clinical Psychology in Medical Settings, 5*, 19–33.

Hann, D. M., Jacobsen, P. B., Martin, S. C., Kronish, L. E., Azzarello, L. M., & Fields, K. K. (1997). Fatigue in women treated with bone marrow transplantation for breast cancer: a comparison with women with no history of cancer. *Supportive Care in Cancer, 5*, 44–52.

Irvine, D., Vincent, L., Graydon, J. E., & Bubela, N. (1998). Fatigue in women with breast cancer receiving radiation therapy. *Cancer Nursing, 21*, 127–135.

Irvine, D., Vincent, L., Graydon, J. E., Bubela, N., & Thompson, L. (1994). The prevalence and correlates of fatigue in patients receiving treatment with chemotherapy and radiotherapy: a comparison with the fatigue experienced by healthy individuals. *Cancer Nursing, 17*, 367–378.

Jacobsen, P. B., Meade, C. D., Stein, K. D., Chirikos, T. N., Small, B. J., & Ruckdeschel, J. C. (2002). Efficacy and costs of two forms of stress management training for cancer patients undergoing chemotherapy. *Journal of Clinical Oncology, 20*, 2851–2862.

Keime-Guibert, F., Napolitano, M., & Delattre, J. Y. (1998). Neurological complications of radiotherapy and chemotherapy. *Journal of Neurology, 245*, 695–708.

Kent, S., Bluthe, R. M., Kelley, K. W., & Dantzer, R. (1992). Sickness behavior as a new target for drug development. *Trends in Pharmacological Sciences, 13*, 24–28.

Knobf, M. T. (1986). Physical and psychologic distress associated with adjuvant chemotherapy in women with breast cancer. *Journal of Clinical Oncology, 4,* 678–684.

Kobashi-Schoot, J. A., Hanewald, G. J., van Dam, F. S., & Bruning, P. F. (1985). Assessment of malaise in cancer treated with radiotherapy. *Cancer Nursing, 8,* 306–314.

Kronenberg, F. (1994). Hot flashes: phenomenology, quality of life, and search for treatment options. *Experimental Gerontology, 29,* 319–336.

LeBlanc, E. S., Janowsky, J., Chan, B. K., & Nelson, H. D. (2001). Hormone replacement therapy and cognition: systematic review and meta-analysis. *Journal of the American Medical Association, 285,* 1489–1499.

McCorkle, R., & Quit-Benoliel, J. (1983). Symptom distress, current concerns and mood disturbance after diagnosis of life threatening disease. *Social Science in Medicine, 17,* 431–438.

McEwen, B. (2002). Estrogen actions throughout the brain. *Recent Progress in Hormone Research, 57,* 357–384.

McNair, D. M., Lorr, M., & Droppleman, L. (1992). *Profile of Mood States,* 2nd ed. San Diego: Educational and Industrial Testing Service.

Morrow, G. R., Andrews, P. L., Hickok, J. T., Roscoe, J. A., & Matteson, S. (2002). Fatigue associated with cancer treatment. *Supportive Care in Cancer, 10,* 389–398.

Piper, B. F., Dibble, S. L., Dodd, M. J., Weiss, M. C., Slaughter, R. E., & Paul, S. M. (1998). The Revised Piper Fatigue Scale: psychometric evaluation in women with breast cancer. *Oncology Nursing Forum, 25,* 677–684.

Rhoten, D. (1982). Fatigue and the post surgical patient. In C. Norris, ed. *Concept Clarification in Nursing.* Rockville, Md.: Aspen Systems Corporation.

Schagen, S. B., Hamburger, H. L., Muller, M. J., Boogerd, W., & van Dam, F. S. (2001). Neurophysiological evaluation of late effects of adjuvant high-dose chemotherapy on cognitive function. *Journal of Neuro-Oncology, 51,* 159–165.

Schagen, S. B., van Dam, F. S., Muller, M. J., Boogerd, W., Lindeboom, J., & Bruning, P. F. (1999). Cognitive deficits after postoperative adjuvant chemotherapy for breast carcinoma. *Cancer, 85,* 640–650.

Servaes, P., Verhagen, C. A., & Bleijenberg, G. (2002). Relations between fatigue, neuropsychological functioning, and physical activity after treatment for breast carcinoma. *Cancer, 95,* 2017–2026.

Smets, E., Garssen, B., Bonke, B., & deHaes, J. C. (1995). The multidimensional fatigue inventory: psychometric qualities of an instrument to assess fatigue. *Journal of Psychosomatic Research, 39,* 315–329.

Stein, K. D., Martin, S. C., Hann, D. M., & Jacobsen, P. B. (1998). A multidimensional measure of fatigue for use with cancer patients. *Cancer Practice, 6,* 143–152.

Tuxen, M. K., & Hansen, S. W. (1994) Neurotoxicity secondary to antineoplastic drugs. *Cancer Treatment Reviews, 20,* 191–214.

van Dam, F. S., Schagen, S. B., Muller, M. J., et al. (1998). Impairment of cognitive function in women receiving adjuvant treatment for high-risk breast cancer: high-dose versus standard-dose chemotherapy. *Journal of the National Cancer Institute, 90,* 210–218.

Vercoulen, J. H., Swanink, C. M., Fennis, J. F., Galama, J. M., Van-der-Meer, J. W., & Bleijenberg, G. (1994). Dimensional assessment of chronic fatigue syndrome. *Journal of Psychosomatic Research, 38,* 383–392.

Weitzner, M. A., Moncello, J., Jacobsen, P. B., & Minton, S. (2002). A pilot trial of paroxetine for the treatment of hot flashes and associated symptoms in women with breast cancer. *Journal of Pain and Symptom Management, 23,* 337–345.

Wessely, S., Hotopf, M., & Sharpe, M. (1998). *Chronic Fatigue and Its Syndromes.* New York: Oxford University Press.

Winer, E. P., Lindley, C., Hardee, M., et al. (1999). Quality of life in patients surviving at least 12 months following high dose chemotherapy with autologous bone marrow support. *Psycho-Oncology, 8,* 167–176.

Winningham, M. L., Nail, L. M., Burke, M. B., et. al. (1994). Fatigue and the cancer experience: the state of the knowledge. *Oncology Nursing Forum, 21,* 23–36.

17   Psychoneuroimmunology and Fatigue

Nancy G. Klimas, Mary Ann Fletcher, Kevin Maher, and Rasha Lawrence

The aim of this chapter is to review the psychoneuroimmunology of fatigue. Much of psychoneuroimmunology research has focused on the response of the brain and the immune system to emotional or physical stressors and the interrelationship of soluble mediators including hormones, neuropeptides, and cytokines. We review the impact of changes in the equilibrium of these soluble mediators on the brain and end organs, as they relate to fatigue, and explore the hypothesis that chronic immune activation mediates chronic fatigue. Finally, the chapter reviews the impact of brain–immune interactions on the quality of restorative sleep.

Psychoneuroimmunology

Psychoneuroimmunology, one of the newer fields of research, explores how the immune system and brain may interact to influence health. In 1964, George Solomon published the first article on the subject, entitled "Emotions, Immunity and Disease: A Speculative Theoretical Integration" (Solomon & Moos, 1964). Since that time, it has been increasingly accepted that stress influences health; data show increased risk of sickness and death during times of extreme stress, such as bereavement, and increased risk of illness during times of lesser stress, including short-term stress such as exam week or chronic stress such as work burnout. Research focusing on the biological explanation for these health consequences has resulted in an ever-increasing understanding of how the brain and the immune system function and interact. Research shows that a wide range of stresses can deplete immune resources, causing B and T cell levels and function to decrease, inflammatory cytokines to elevate, natural killer cells to become less responsive, and fewer immunoglobulin A (IgA) antibodies to be secreted in the saliva or IgG antibodies to be produced in response to vaccine challenge (reviewed by Kiecolt-Glaser et al., 2002).

Another way to approach the study of brain and immune-mediated health consequences of stress is to evaluate the influence of stress on health outcomes in chronic illnesses. Studies of chronic viral illness, such as human immunodeficiency virus

(HIV), have shown clinically important decrements in immune function as a result of a physiologic stress response, which can be mediated by behavioral management interventions (Antoni et al., 1997; 2000; 2002). In posttraumatic stress disorder and chronic fatigue syndrome, patient's inflammatory cytokine release has been seen as a consequence of a sudden severe environmental stressor, such as a hurricane (Ironson, Wynings, Schneiderman et al., 1997; Lutgendorf, Antoni, Ironson, Fletcher, Penedo, VanRiel, Baum, Schneiderman, & Klimas, 1995a).

The response of the immune system to stress can be explained by the biological links between the immune system and the central nervous system that exist at several levels. The autonomic nervous system links directly to the immune system, with "hard wiring" of the sympathetic nervous system to organs such as the spleen and lymph nodes (Cano et al., 2001). Nerve fiber networks have been found that connect to the thymus gland, spleen, lymph nodes, and bone marrow. Micrographs even demonstrate lymphocyte–synaptic junctions (Ackerman et al., 1991). Moreover, experiments show that immune function can be altered by chemical sympathectomy (Callahan & Moynihan, 2002).

Lymphocytes have receptors for a number of neuropeptides (hormonelike chemicals released from nerve cells), and macrophages, T cells, and NK cells encode and release neuropeptides in addition to the cytokines known to be the messengers of the immune system such as interferons and interleukins. These cytokines can, in turn, transmit information to the nervous system. Hormones produced by the thymus gland, also act on cells in the brain (Glaser & Kiecolt-Glaser, 1994).

One well-known pathway involves the hypothalamic-pituitary-adrenal axis (HPA axis), which, in response to stress messages from the brain, causes the release of corticosteroid hormones from the adrenal glands into the blood. In addition to helping a person respond to emergencies by mobilizing the body's energy reserves to fight or flight, these "stress hormones" decrease antibody production and reduce lymphocytes in both number and function. As an acute stress response, these responses would be adaptive. But they become maladaptive in chronic stress models, exhausting resources and leaving the individual more susceptible to the consequences of reduced immune function, such as infection and cancer, as well as more prone to the consequence of long-term immune activation and immune-mediated illness such as autoimmune diseases or allergy. There is also a direct link to the symptom of fatigue, as chronic glucocorticoid elevation results in metabolic imbalance and muscle atrophy (Glaser & Kiecolt-Glaser, 1994). The concept of chronic stress and the cumulative impact of stress on health are of great interest. McEwen developed the concept of "allostatic load" to describe the cumulative long-term effects of physiological responses to stress, mediated primarily by the HPA axis and the autonomic nervous system (ANS) (McEwen, 1998). Laboratory studies of acute stress models demonstrate immune, autonomic, and HPA axis change. Chronic stress has an impact on immune function as well, such as the chronic elevations of cortisol seen in caregivers of Alzheimer's patients, resulting in lymphocyte insensitivity to glucocorticoids (Bauer et al., 2000).

The image that is emerging is of closely interlocked systems facilitating a two-way flow of information, through the language of hormones, neuropeptides, and cytokines. Immune cells, it has been suggested, may function in a sensory capacity, detecting the arrival of foreign invaders and relaying chemical signals to alert the brain. The brain, for its part, may send signals that direct the traffic of cells through the lymphoid organs. The influence of stress, particularly chronic stress, on this system may result in maladaptive physiological response and a state of chronic immune activation. This state is characterized by elevation of lymphocyte activation markers, a blunting of essential immune functions such as proliferation and cytotoxicity, and the oversecretion of inflammatory cytokines. These cytokines, in turn, interact with the brain and the neuroendocrine system, influence health, and result in the perception of fatigue.

Fatigue, Sickness Behavior, and the Immune System

Hickie and colleagues (2001) carried out an investigation of the etiology of prolonged fatigue and immune activation in 124 pairs of twins (79 monozygotic and 45 dizygotic). For fatigue, the monozygotic correlation was more than double the dizygotic correlation (0.49 versus 0.16), indicating a strong genetic association. In contrast, for in vitro immune activation measures correlations for identical and fraternal twins were similar (0.49–0.69 versus 0.42–0.53) indicating an etiologic role for environment factors. Suggested environmental factors included physical agents such as infection and psychological stress.

Following acute infection, animals and humans display "sickness behavior," consisting of fatigue, malaise, poor motivation to eat, and changes in physical, social, and sleep patterns (Kelley et al., 2003). For example, circulating tumor necrosis factor alpha (TNF-α) and interferon-gamma (IFN-γ) are detectable during acute and convalescent parvovirus B19 infection and associated with prolonged and chronic fatigue (Kerr et al., 2001). In chronic inflammatory illness, including chronic active infections and active autoimmune disorders, sickness behaviors become chronic, and both animal and human subjects display lassitude, exaggerated responses to pain, and poor concentration. In clinical practice, despite this complex symptomatology, fatigue is almost always the chief complaint. The illness behavior is frequently adaptive, facilitating the recovery from an acute illness. Exaggerated symptoms of illness behavior, such as cachexia in oncology patients, can be maladaptive and life-threatening to the individual. Increasingly data implicate the immune system as the prime mediator of these behaviors, with proinflammatory cytokines playing a central role (Kiecolt-Glaser et al., 2002).

Many studies demonstrate the impact of proinflammatory cytokines on both human and animal wellness and behavior. The infusion of TNF-α or interleukin-1 (IL-1) results in disruption of the sleep cycle, enhancing nonrapid eye movement sleep (NREMS) (Krueger et al., 2001). The hypothesis that expression of proinflammatory cytokines within the central nervous system (CNS) plays a role in the pathogenesis of immuno-logically mediated fatigue is underscored by the study by Sheng and colleagues (1996). Using two strains of mice with differential patterns of cytokine expression in response to an injection challenge with *Corynebacterium parvum*, they demonstrated that elevated IL-1 and TNF cytokine mRNA expression in the CNS corresponded to de-velopment of fatigue. Injection of antibodies specific to either IL-1 or TNF-α into the peripheral circulation did not alter immunologically induced fatigue, suggesting that these cytokines were not involved in fatigue induction outside of the CNS. Thus, in this model system, these proinflamatory cytokines must act within the CNS to produce fatigue. Katafuchi and colleagues (2003) have demonstrated an inverse relationship between the amount of brain IFN-α mRNA and spontaneous running wheel activity in rats. This confirms an earlier study by Davis and associates (1998) revealing that IFN-α/β is at least partially responsible for the early fatigue induced by poly I:C (an interferon-α/β induction therapy) during prolonged treadmill running in mice.

In human clinical trials, cytokine therapies also show the direct and indirect effects of cytokines on health and fatigue. Fatigue is a common side effect of IFN therapy, reported in 70 to 100 percent of patients treated with this drug (Malik et al., 2001). The etiology of IFN-mediated fatigue (IMF) is multifactorial, with endocrine failure, neuropsychiatric disturbance, autoimmunity, and cytokine dysregulation as potential contributors. Although the direct cause of IFN-α-induced fatigue is unknown, there are probably both central and peripheral effects, including neuromuscular fatigue, similar to the fatigue observed in patients with postpolio syndrome. The induction of proinflammatory cytokines observed in patients treated with IFN-α is consistent with a possible mechanism of neuromuscular pathology that could manifest as fatigue.

Thyroid dysfunction, associated with the development of autoantibodies, is seen in 8 to 20 percent of patients receiving IFN-α. According to Jones and colleagues (1998), administration of exogenous IFN-γ can be associated with upregulation of class II major histocompatibility antigens in the thyroid and development of thyroiditis. Interferon-α also stimulates the production of IL-6. Jones and colleagues (1998) suggest that IFN-α can initiates a cytokine cascade affecting the hypothalamic-pituitary-adrenal and hypothalamic-pituitary-gonadal axes, and thus the regulation of gluco-corticoid and sex steroid hormone secretion as shown in Figure 17.1.

In addition, IFN-α therapy leads to depression and cognitive slowing, and depressed patients are predisposed to develop fatigue. Clinical management of IMF is challeng-ing because the syndrome is variable in onset and severity and its pathophysiology is poorly understood (Malik et al., 2001). Other cytokines that have been used in ther-

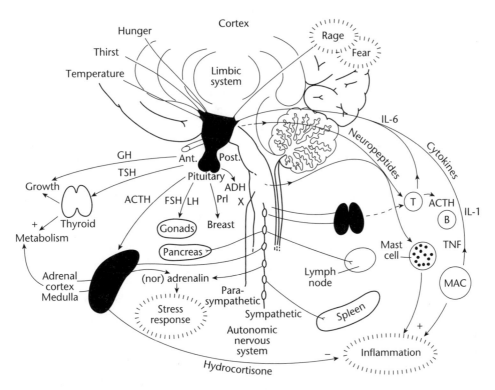

Figure 17.1

Neuroendocrine and immune pathways—soluble mediators from these interactive systems lead to symptoms termed "sickness behavior."

apeutic settings also rate fatigue as the most common limiting side effect, sometimes as a direct effect and sometimes as a result of other cytokines induced by the treatment. Symptoms of depression and fatigue in cancer patients follow elevated plasma levels of IL-6, IL-1, TNFα, and cytokines induced by IL-2 immunotherapy (Neveu et al., 2000).

Cytokine-Mediated Illness and Fatigue

Elevated serum IL-6 levels have been repeatedly shown to correlate with the symptoms of fatigue, wasting, and physical decline in the elderly. In addition to the effects of IL-6 on the CNS, this cytokine is also known to have a negative effect on skeletal muscle and hematopoesis. Leng and associates (2002) recently published a study showing an association between IL-6 levels and lower hematocrit in a geriatric population who met the criteria for the geriatric syndrome of frailty. The inflammatory cytokines may decrease red blood cell formation at two levels: by suppressing bone marrow response to the triggering hormone, erythropoetin, and by suppressing the production of erythropoetin at the renal site of production.

Fatigue is prominent in cancer patients and probably multifactorial in origin (Stasi et al., 2003). Factors contributing to fatigue include anemia, weight loss, fever, pain, medication, and infection. Many of these factors are influenced in cancer patients by a frequently disrupted balance between endogenous cytokine levels and their natural antagonists. Indeed, cancer cells and the immune system appear to overexpress a range of cytokines in patients with malignancies. Some of these cytokines act as autocrine or paracrine growth factors for the neoplastic tissue while simultaneously causing secondary symptoms related to fatigue. For instance, cancer-associated anemia may be due to a blunted erythropoietin response and cytokines (IL-1, IL-6, TNF-α) that suppress erythropoiesis. Cachexia, a wasting syndrome and hallmark of cancer, can be attributed to loss of appetite or enhanced energy expenditure. Several interleukins as well as TNF-α, INF-γ, and leukemia inhibitory factor act as cachectins in animal models. Bower and colleagues (2002) examined whether 20 fatigued breast cancer survivors would experience elevated in proinflammatory cytokines and markers of cytokine activity compared with 20 nonfatigued survivors. Both groups were studied an average of 5 years after diagnosis. The fatigued breast cancer survivors had significantly higher serum levels of several markers associated with immune activation than nonfatigued survivors, including interleukin-1 receptor antagonist (IL-1ra), soluble tumor necrosis factor receptor type II (sTNF-RII), and neopterin. The fatigued survivors had significantly lower serum levels of cortisol than the nonfatigued group. Recently, molecules that function as cytokine antagonists have been identified and are being tested as potential treatments of cancer-related fatigue (Kurzrock, 2001). For more on cancer and fatigue, see chapter 16.

Multiple sclerosis is a chronic illness characterized by profound fatigue. Although peripheral mechanisms have some role in the pathogenesis of fatigue, in MS there are clear indications that "central" abnormalities play a more important role. Neurophysiological studies show that fatigue does not depend on involvement of the pyramidal tracts and implicate impaired volitional drive of the descending motor pathways as a physiopathological mechanism. Metabolic abnormalities of the frontal cortex and basal ganglia revealed by positron emission tomography and correlations between fatigue and magnetic resonance imaging lesion burden support this hypothesis. Some recent studies also suggest that proinflammatory cytokines contribute to the sense of tiredness (Comi et al., 2000). For more on MS and fatigue, see chapter 4.

Persistent postinfection fatigue is another example of immune-mediated fatigue. Studies of cytokine production by stimulated peripheral blood mononuclear cells from patients with post-Q-fever fatigue syndrome (QFS; inappropriate fatigue, myalgia and arthralgia, night sweats, and mood and sleep pattern changes follow about 20 percent of laboratory-proven, acute primary Q-fever cases) showed an accentuated release of IL-6 significantly in excess of medians for all four control groups (resolving QFS, acute primary Q-fever without subsequent QFS, healthy Q-fever vaccines, and healthy controls). Levels of induced IL-6 significantly correlated with total symptom scores and scores for other key symptoms (Penttila et al., 1998). Bennett and associates (1998) reported on the relationship between fatigue and psychological and immunological variables in serologically proven acute infectious illnesses due to Epstein-Barr virus (EBV), Ross River virus (RRV), or Q fever. During the acute phase, profound fatigue and malaise were the most common symptoms. Initially, 46 percent of cases had no delayed-type hypersensitivity skin response (DTH) indicative of impaired cellular immunity. Over a 4-week period, both somatic and psychological symptoms improved markedly, although fatigue remained a prominent feature in 63 percent of subjects. Reduction in reported fatigue was correlated with improvement in the DTH skin response ($p = 0.001$).

Another illness associated with prolonged fatigue, that most frequently follows acute viral syndrome, is chronic fatigue syndrome (CFS) (Kerr & Tyrrell, 2003). The types of soluble immune mediator dysfunctions in CFS patients reported by some investigators certainly may be regarded as potentially important in the syndrome's pathophysiology. One model of CFS pathophysiology proposes chronic lymphocyte activation with cytokine dysregulation characterized by episodic increased proinflammatory cytokines in plasma and a shift in the ratio of type 1 to type 2 cytokines produced by in vitro stimulated lymphocytes. Our model for the subsequent chronicity of this disorder holds that the interaction of psychological factors (distress associated with either CFS-related symptoms or other stressful life events) and immunologic dysfunction contribute to (a) both direct and indirect (HPA and autonomic) mediated symptoms (e.g., perception of fatigue and cognitive difficulties, fever, muscle and joint pain) and increases in illness burden and (b) impaired immune surveillance associated with cytotoxic lymphocytes, with resulting activation of latent herpes viruses (Patarca et al., 1995a; Patarca-Montero, 2001).

The signs and symptoms of CFS including fatigue, myalgia, and cognitive dysfunction are similar to those experienced by patients infused with cytokines such as IL-1. Elevated serum levels of IL-6 found in a significant number of CFS patients could underlie several of the clinical symptoms. The levels of spontaneously produced IL-6 by both adherent monocytes and nonadherent lymphocytes were significantly increased in CFS patients compared to controls (Gupta et al., 1997). The abnormality of IL-6 was also observed at mRNA level. Buchwald and coworkers (1997) found that circulating IL-6 levels were elevated in febrile CFS patients compared to those without CFS and therefore considered it an epiphenomenon possibly secondary to infection. Chao and coworkers (Chao et al., 1990, 1991) also found elevated plasma IL-6 levels in CFS patients, but other groups found no difference (Buchwald et al., 1997; Linde et al., 1992; Patarca et al., 1994; Peakman et al., 1997). CFS patients have higher levels of sIL-6R (Patarca et al., 1995b), and sIL-6R enhances the effects of IL-6. Some of the differences between groups are likely due to the remit/relapse course seen in many CFS patients as well as heterogeneity in the defined population. Efforts to classify the illness by pathphysiologic subtype, including studies of potential immune biomarkers, are underway.

The association between CFS physical symptoms, illness burden, and lymphocyte activation markers in a sample of 27 CFS patients was also reported by our group (Wagner et al., 1999). Increased activated cytotoxic/suppressor cells (CD38 + HLA − DR + CD8+) were associated with greater severity of tender lymph nodes ($r = 0.45$), fatigue ($r = 0.34$), and sleep problems ($r = 0.34$). Elevations in T-helper/inducer cells were associated with a greater frequency and severity of tender lymph nodes, greater severity of memory and concentration difficulties, and headaches ($r = 0.35$ to 0.46). Greater numbers of activated T cells (CD2 + CD3 + CD26+) were associated with a greater frequency of tender lymph nodes ($r = 0.52$) and cognitive difficulties ($r = 0.34$). Conversely, lower percentage of regulatory cells such as CD3 + CD8 cells were associated with a greater number of cognitive difficulties ($r = -0.61$), greater SIP-Total ($r = -0.47$), SIP Physical Impairment ($r = -0.39$), and increased frequency ($r = -0.43$) and severity of memory problems ($r = -0.43$), increased frequency of headaches ($r = -0.70$), and increased severity of fatigue ($r = -0.39$). A multiple regression equation predicted 29 percent of the variance in fatigue severity from higher CD38 + HLADR + CD8+ cells (+ 0.41) and lower CD3 + CD8+ cells (= −0.41). Thus, among CFS patients the degree of cellular immune activation is associated with the severity of CFS-related physical symptoms, cognitive complaints, perceived illness burden, and fatigue.

A maladaptive stress response in illnesses mediated by inflammatory cytokines may contribute to both their severity and chronicity in immune-mediated illnesses. In studies of CFS, data in our lab showing that distress levels in response to the stressor Hurricane Andrew were positively correlated with alterations in natured killer (NK) cells and elevated (compared to prestorm values) circulating levels of the cytokines, exacerbation in CFS symptoms, including fatigue severity, and increases in SIP-based illness burden scores among 49 CFS patients (Lutgendorf et al., 1995a). We found that CFS patients living in a hurricane exposure area (Dade County) had significantly more severe CFS symptom relapses (using clinician-rated fatigue levels and ability to engage in work-related activities) and significantly greater increases in illness burden than age- and gender-matched CFS patients from the same clinical practice living in an adjacent geographical region not in the storm's path (Broward/Palm Beach counties). We also found that pre-post hurricane NKCC changes were associated with pre-post storm symptom severity changes including patient-reported cognitive symptoms ($r = -0.54$, $p < 0.01$), muscle weakness ($r = -0.61$, $p < 0.01$), and muscle pain ($r = -0.43$, $p < 0.05$).

These data suggested that stressor-induced decrements in NKCC were associated with greater increases in the severity of perceived cognitive difficulties, muscle weakness, and pain symptoms. A final regression analysis on NKCC indicated that appraisals of greater storm impact and low social support predicted the greatest pre-post storm decrements in NKCC (total $R^2 = 0.35$, $p < 0.01$). Avoidance coping predicted higher levels of IL-6. Higher degrees of negative emotions conveyed through essays predicted greater SIP total, physical, and psychosocial symptoms and displayed a trend toward higher IL-6 levels.

For more on CFS, see chapter 9.

Cytokine/Endocrine Interactions and Fatigue

Knowledge is accumulating on cytokine–nervous system interactions that may be mediated by endocrine mechanisms (Berkenbosch et al., 1987; Besedovsky et al., 1986; Uehara et al., 1987; Demitrack & Dale, 1991; Kamilaris et al., 1987; Lowy et al., 1988). For example, the proinflammatory cytokine IL-1 interacts with corticotropin-releasing hormone (CRH) at the hypothalamus, and subsequent HPA activation is hypothesized to follow (Besedovsky et al., 1986). This interaction between cytokines and the HPA axis may act to downregulate inflammatory processes and limit the clonal expansion of antigen-specific lymphoid cells. Conversely, states characterized by dysregulation of the HPA axis and hypocortisolemia may be associated with sustained elevations in cytokines and subsequent physical symptoms (e.g., fatigue) related to pyrogenic and proinflammatory agents (Sternberg, 1993). Glucocorticoid insufficiency is associated with extreme fatigue and its onset is precipitated by stressors, myalgias, exacerbation of allergic responses, and sleep disturbances (Demitrack & Crofford, 1998; Moldovsky, 1995). Persistent cytokine elevations may also contribute to HPA axis dysregulation, and subsequent endocrine abnormalities may relate to some of the physical symptoms of CFS. Of course, the picture is complicated by the possibility that HPA abnormalities may also be impacted by coexisting affective disturbance or distress responses in CFS patients, which in turn interact with the physical symptoms (Scott & Dinan, 1998; Scott et al., 1998; Visser et al., 1998).

In CFS, elevated serum levels of IL-1α could underlie several clinical symptoms. IL-1 has direct effects on the pituitary; it has been shown to augment release of prolactin and growth hormone and inhibit release of thyrotropin and luteinizing hormone (Bernton, Beach, Holaday, Smallridge, & Fein, 1987; Rettori, Gimeno, Karara, Gonzalez, & McCann, 1991). It has been hypothesized that the growth hormone deficiency state associated with CFS may be a reflection of the defect in hypothalamic feedback loop that renders it inadequately responsive to IL-1 (Allain et al., 1997; Buskila, 1999).

Cytokines and the Autonomic Nervous System and the Central Nervous System

The relationship between immune, autonomic neuroendocrine, and central neuro-transmitter processes is multidirectional. Systemic immune challenges have been shown to involve the prefrontal cortex, nucleus accumbens, and amygdyla, which are also responsible for mood and fatigue symptoms (Anisman & Merali, 1999). Immune system activation affects the CNS through stimulation of the afferent vagal fibers (Herman & Cullnan, 1997; Dantzer et al., 1996; Maier & Watkins, 1998).

Various models have been used to study autonomic–immune interactions and their impact on sickness behavior. The influence of cytokines autonomic function has been studied. For instance, IL-1β increases norepinephrine turnover within areas of the central nervous system, particularly the locus coeruleus. TNF-α increases use of nor-epinephrine (NE) and 5-hydroxytriptamine (5-HT) within the hypothalamus, partic-ularly the paraventricular nuclei (PNV), and it increases the turnover of NE within the central amygdyla and locus coeruleus (Hayley et al., 2001; Brebner, 2001). Beyond their acute effects on the brain and autonomic system, repeated cytokine exposure may have long-term consequence. Studies of physiologic levels of cytokine challenge demonstrate sensitization of receptors so that subsequent exposures greatly augment the CNS/autonomic effect, particularly of proinflammatory cytokines TNF-α and IL-1β, elevating HPA activity and NE, sensitization in the areas of the brain controlling sickness behavior such as fatigue and mood, in animal models, sickness behavior increases with continually lower levels of cytokine exposure (Hayley et al., 1999; 2001). This time-dependent sensitization in animal models allows one to hypothesize that earlier cytokine exposures may leave individuals vulnerable to fatigue and other sickness behavior symptoms with lesser intermittent or chronic cytokines exposures, such as those seen in infectious illness or stress responses.

Cytokines and Sleep

Sleep is an important component of mammalian homeostasis, and is vital for survival. Sleep disorders are common in the general population, associated with significant medical, psychological, and social disturbances. Abnormalities of sleep physiology present as fatigue, daytime sleepiness, and cognitive dysfunction and can contribute to the severity of comorbid conditions. Sleep, in particular deep sleep, has an inhibitory influence on the HPA axis, whereas activation of the HPA axis or adminis-tration of glucocorticoids can lead to arousal and sleeplessness. Insomnia, the most common sleep disorder, is associated with a 24-hour increase of adrenocorticotropic hormone and cortisol secretion, consistent with CNS hyperarousal. Sleepiness and fatigue are very prevalent in the general population, and recent studies have demon-strated that the proinflammatory cytokines IL-6 and TNF-α are elevated in disorders associated with excessive daytime sleepiness, such as sleep apnea, narcolepsy, and idiopathic hypersomnia. Sleep deprivation leads to sleepiness and daytime hypersecretion of IL-6. Combined, these observations suggest that the HPA axis stimulates arousal, while IL-6 and TNF-α are possible mediators of excessive daytime sleepiness in humans (Vgontzas et al., 1999).

Animal models using physiological ranges of cytokine infusion into the brain showed that IL-1 and TNF-α provoke slow-wave sleep when placed in the lateral ventricles of experimental animals (Shoham et al., 1987). Different doses of highly purified endotoxin to induce a short-lived inflammatory response under human lab conditions shed additional light on this complex area. Dose-dependent studies demonstrated that doses capable of causing a 1.5°C increase in temperature, as well as an increase in cortisol and inflammatory cytokine levels, produced an increase in slow-wave sleep. Most interesting, a dosage that did not raise the temperature produced no increase in cortisol but a significant increase in circulating inflammatory cytokines and had a marked effect on slow-wave sleep (Mullington et al., 2000). Studies of sleep in humans following infusion of IL-6 and granulocyte colony-stimulating factor demonstrate decreases in REM sleep and a shift of slow-wave sleep to later in the sleep cycle. Similar findings were seen after administration of clozapine, a CNS active antipsychotic agent known to have immunomodulatory properties (Schuld et al., 1999; Spath-Schwaldbe, 1998; Mullington, 2001). See chapter 13 for more on sleep and fatigue.

Conclusion

Increasing evidence shows that the soluble mediators of the immune system interact with the CNS, ANS, and neuroendocrine system resulting in sickness behavior. Proinflammatory cytokines induce a constellation of behavioral changes, with fatigue as the most prominent symptom. Animal studies of CNS responses to infused cytokines reveal the intriguing observation of sensitization of the CNS, and its autonomic and HPA axis, to additional doses of minute amounts of cytokine, augmenting the autonomic and central responses. Extending this observation to the human condition may reframe current concepts of chronic illnesses characterized by fatigue. Activation of the inflammatory response system with subsequent cytokine synthesis and release can provoke neuroendocrine and brain neurotransmitter changes that the brain interprets as stressors. Furthermore, these effects are subject to sensitization so that a history of stressful experiences or cytokine activation augments the response to later challenges (Anisman & Merali, 2003). Fatigue-mediating cytokine interaction with tissues such as muscle and CNS centers that control cognition, alertness, and restorative sleep may play key roles in illnesses characterized by chronic immune activation.

Activation of the primary host defense system may lead to increased or decreased slow-wave sleep and sleep quality, depending on the degree of immune activation. Modest elevations of certain inflammatory cytokines are found during experimental sleep loss in humans and, in addition, relatively small elevations of cytokines are seen after immunomodulatory pharmacological treatments are started. Cytokines such as TNF-α, its soluble receptors, and IL-6 in the periphery and CNS link peripheral immune stimulation and CNS-mediated behaviors and experiences such as sleep, sleepiness, and fatigue. The debilitating fatigue experienced in illnesses with known chronic immune activation such as chronic fatigue syndrome, multiple sclerosis, and some oncologic disorders may also be related to diminished levels of restorative sleep.

References

Ackerman, K. D., Bellinger, D. L., Felton, S. Y., & Felton, D. L. (1991). Ontogeny and the senescence of noradrenergic innervation of the rodent thymus and spleen. In R. Adler, D. L., Felten, & N. Cohen, eds. *Psychoneuroimmunology*, 2nd ed. Pp. 72–114. San Diego: Academic Press.

Allain, T. J., Bearn, J. A., Coskeran, P., Jones, J., Checkley, A., Butler, J., Wessely, S., & Miell, J. P. (1997). Changes in growth hormone, insulin, insulin-like growth factors, and IGF-binding protein-1 in chronic fatigue syndrome. *Biological Psychiatry*, *41*, 567–573.

Arnason, B. G. W. (1991). Nervous system–immune system communication. *Reviews in Infectious Diseases*, *13(1)*, S134–S137.

Anisman, H., & Merali, Z. (1999). Anhedonic and anxiogenic effects of cytokine exposure. *Advances in Experimental Biology*, *461*, 199–233.

Anisman, H., & Merali, Z. (2003). Cytokines, stress and depressive illness: brain-immune interactions. *Annals of Medicine*, *35(1)*, 2–11.

Antoni, M. H. (1997). Cognitive-behavioral intervention for persons with HIV. In J. R. Spira, ed. *Group Therapy for Medically Ill Patients*. Pp. 55–91. New York: Guilford Press.

Antoni, M. H., Cruess, D. G., Cruess, S., Lutgendorf, S., Kumar, M., Ironson, G., Klimas, N., Fletcher, M. A., & Schneiderman, N. (2000). Cognitive-behavioral stress management intervention effects on anxiety, 24-hr urinary norepinephrine output, and T-cytotoxic/suppressor cells over time among symptomatic HIV-infected gay men. *Journal of Consulting Clinical Psychology*, *68(1)*, 31–45.

Antoni, M. H., Cruess, D. G., Klimas, N., Maher, K., Cruess, S., Kumar, M., Lutgendorf, S., Ironson, G., Schneiderman, N., & Fletcher, M. A. (2002). Stress management and immune system reconstitution in symptomatic HIV-infected gay men over time: effects on transitional naive T cells (CD4(+)CD45RA(+)CD29(+)). *American Journal of Psychiatry*, *159(1)*, 143–145.

Bauer, M. E., Vedhara, K., Perks, P., Wilcock, G. K., Lightman, S. L., & Shanks, N. (2000). Chronic stress in caregivers of dementia patients is associated with reduced lymphocyte sensitivity to glucocorticoids. *Journal of Neuroimmunology*, *103*, 84–92.

Bennett, B. K., Hickie, I. B., Vollmer-Conna, U. S., Quigley, B., Brennan, C. M., Wakefield, D., Douglas, M. P., Hansen, G. R., Tahmindjis, A. J., & Lloyd, A. R. (1998). The relationship between fatigue, psychological and immunological variables in acute infectious illness. *Australia and New Zealand Journal of Psychiatry, 32(2)*, 180–186.

Berkenbosch, F., VanOers, J., del Rey, A., Tilders, F., & Besedovsky, H. (1987). Corticotropin-releasing factor-producing neurons in the rat activated by interleukin-1. *Science, 238*, 524–526.

Bernton, E. W., Beach, J., Holaday, J. W., Smallridge, R. C., & Fein, H. G. (1987). Release of multiple hormones by a direct action of interleukin-1 on pituitary cells. *Science, 238*, 519–521.

Besedovsky, H., del Ray, A., Sorkin, E., & Dinarello, C. A. (1986). Immunoregulatory feedback between interleukin-1 and glucocorticoid hormones. *Science, 233*, 652–654.

Bower, J. E., Ganz, P. A., & Fahey, J. L. (2002). Fatigue and proinflammatory cytokine activity in breast cancer survivors. *Psychosomatic Medicine, 64*, 604–611.

Brebner, K., Hayley, S., Merali, Z., & Anisman, H. (2000). Synergistic effects of IL-1beta, IL-6, and TNF-alpha. Central monamine, corticosterone and behavioral variations. *Neuropsychopharmacology, 22*, 566–580.

Buchwald, D., Wener, M. H., Pearlman, T., & Kith, P. (1997). Markers of inflammation and immune activation in chronic fatigue and chronic fatigue syndrome. *Journal of Rheumatology, 24(2)*, 372–376

Buskila, D. (1999). Fibromyalgia, chronic fatigue syndrome and myofacial pain syndrome. *Current Opinion in Rheumatology, 11*, 119–126.

Callahan, T. A., & Moynihan, J. A. (2002). Contrasting pattern of cytokines in antigen- versus mitogen-stimulated splenocyte cultures from chemically denervated mice. *Brain Behavioral Immunology, 16(6)*, 764–773.

Cano, G., Sved, A. F., Rinaman, L., Rabin, B. S., & Card, J. P. (2001). Characterization of the central nervous system innervation of the rat spleen using viral transneuronal tracing. *Journal Computational Neurology, 8;439(1)*, 1–18.

Chao, C. C., Gallagher, M., Phair, J., & Peterson, P. K. (1990). Serum neopterin and interleukin-6 levels in chronic fatigue syndrome. *Journal of Infectious Diseases, 162*, 1412–1413.

Chao, C. C., Janoff, E. N., Hu, S., Thomas, K., Gallagher, M., Tsang, M., & Peterson, P. K. (1991). Altered cytokine release in peripheral blood mononuclear cell cultures from patients with the chronic fatigue syndrome. *Cytokine, 3*, 292–298.

Cohen, S., Tyrrell, D. A., & Smith, A. P. (1991). Psychological stress and susceptibility to the common cold. *New England Journal of Medicine, 325(9)*, 606–612.

Comi, G., Leocani, L., Rossi, P., & Colombo, B. (2000). Physiopathology and treatment of fatigue in multiple sclerosis. *Journal of Neurology, 248(3)*, 174–179.

Dantzer, R. (2000). Cytokine-induced sickness behavior. *Brain, Behavior & Immunity, 14*, 88–89.

Dantzer, R., Bluthe, R. M., Aubert, A., et al. (1996). Cytokine action on behavior. In N. J. Rothwell, ed. *Cytokines and the Nervous System.* Pp. 117–44. London: Landes.

Davis, J. M., Weaver, J. A., Kohut, M. L., Colbert, L. H., Ghaffar, A., & Mayer, E. P. (1998). Immune system activation and fatigue during treadmill running: role of interferon. *Medicine and Science in Sports and Exercise, 30(6)*, 863–868.

Dejana, E., Brenario, F., Erroi, A., et al. (1987). Modulation of endothelial cell function by different molecular species of interleukin-1. *Blood, 69*, 635–699.

Demitrack, M., & Crofford, L. (1998). Evidence for and pathophysiologic implications of hypothalamic-pituitary-adrenal axis dysregulation in fibromyalgia and chronic fatigue syndrome. *Annals of the New York Academy of Sciences, 840*, 684–697.

Demitrack, M., & Dale, J. (1991). Evidence for impaired activation of the hypothalamic-pituitary-adrenal axis in patients with chronic fatigue syndrome. *Journal of Clinical Endocrinology and Metabolism, 73*, 1224–1234.

Dinarello, C. A. (1991). Interleukin-1 and interleukin-1 antagonism. *Blood, 77(8)*, 1627–1652.

Dinarello, C. A. (1992). Interleukin-1 and tumor necrosis factor: effector cytokines in auto-immune diseases. *Seminars in Immunology, 4(3)*, 133–145.

Dreisbach, A. W., Hendrickson, T., Beezhold, D., Riesenberg, L. A., & Sklar, A. H. (1998). Elevated levels of tumor necrosis factor alpha in postdialysis fatigue. *International Journal of Artificial Organs, 21(2)*, 83–86.

Glaser, R., & Kiecolt-Glaser, J. K., eds. (1994). *Handbook of Human Stress and Immunity*. San Diego: Academic Press.

Gupta, S., Aggarwal, S., See, D., & Starr, A. (1997). Cytokine production by adherent and non-adherent mononuclear cells in chronic fatigue syndrome. *Journal of Psychiatric Research 31(1)*, 149–156.

Hayley, S., Brebner, K., Lacosta, S., Merali, Z., & Anisman, H. (1999). Sensitization to the effects of TNF-alpha: neuroendocrine, central monoamine and behavioral variations. *Journal of Neuroscience, 19*, 5654–5665.

Hayley, S., Staines, W. M., Merali, Z., & Anisman, H. (2001). Time dependent sensitization of corticotropin releasing hormone, arginine vasopressin and c-fos immunoreactivity within the mouse brain in response to TNF-alpha. *Neuroscience, 106*, 137–148.

Herman, J. P., & Cullnan, W. E. (1997). Neurocircuitry of stress: central control of HPA axis. *Trends in Neuroscience, 20*, 78–84

Hickie, I. B., Bansal, A. S., Kirk, K. M., Lloyd, A. R., & Martin, N. G. (2001). A twin study of the etiology of prolonged fatigue and immune activation. *Twin Research, 4(2)*, 94–102.

Ironson, G., Wynings, C., Schneiderman, N., et al. (1997). Posttraumatic stress symptoms, intrusive thoughts, loss and immune function after Hurricane Andrew. *Psychosomatic Medicine, 59*, 128–141.

Jones, T. H., Wadler, S., & Hupart, K. H. (1998). Endocrine-mediated mechanisms of fatigue during treatment with interferon-alpha. *Seminars in Oncology, 25(1 Suppl 1)*, 54–63.

Kamilaris, T., Debold, C. R., Pavlous, S. N., Island, D. P., Hoursanidis, A., & Orth, D. N. (1987). Effect of altered thyroid hormone levels on hypothalamic-pituitary-adrenal function. *Journal of Clinical Endocrinology and Metabolism, 65*, 994–999.

Katafuchi, T., Kondo, T., Yasaka, T., Kubo, K., Take, S., & Yoshimura, M. (2003). Prolonged effects of polyriboinosinic:polyribocytidylic acid on spontaneous running wheel activity and brain interferon-alpha mRNA in rats: a model for immunologically induced fatigue. *Neuroscience, 120(3)*, 837–845.

Kelley, K. W., Bluthe, R. M., Dantzer, R., Zhou, J. H., Shen, W. H., Johnson, R. W., & Broussard, S. R. (2003). Cytokine-induced sickness behavior. *SR. Brain Behavioral in Immunology, 17(Suppl 1)*, S112–S118.

Kerr, J. R., Barah, F., Mattey, D. L., Laing, I., Hopkins, S. J., Hutchinson, I. V., & Tyrrell, D. A. (2001). Circulating tumour necrosis factor-alpha and interferon-gamma are detectable during acute and convalescent parvovirus B19 infection and are associated with prolonged and chronic fatigue. *Journal of General Virology, 82(Pt 12)*, 3011–3019.

Kerr, J. R., & Tyrrell, D. A. (2003). Cytokines in parvovirus B19 infection as an aid to understanding chronic fatigue syndrome. *Current Pain Headache Report, 7(5)*, 333–341.

Kiecolt-Glaser, J., McGuire, L., Robles, T. F., & Glaser, R. (2002). Psychoneuroimmunology: psychological influences on immune function and health. *Journal of Consulting and Clinical Psychology, 70;3*, 537–547.

Klimas, N. G., & Fletcher, M. A. (1999). Alteration of type 1/type 2 cytokine pattern following adoptive immunotherapy of patients with chronic fatigue syndrome (CFS) using autologous ex vivo expanded lymph node cells. Presented 2nd International Conference on Chronic Fatigue Syndrome, Brussels.

Klimas, N., Patarca, R., & Fletcher, M. A. (1992). Psychoneuroimmunology and chronic fatigue syndrome. In N. Schneiderman & A. Baum, eds. *Perspectives in Behavioral Medicine Hillsdale*, NJ: Erlbaum.

Krueger, J. M., Obal, F. J., Fang, J., Kubota, T., & Taishi, P. (2001). The role of cytokines in physiological sleep regulation. *Annals of the New York Academy of Science, 933*, 211–221.

Kurzrock, R. (2001). The role of cytokines in cancer-related fatigue. *Cancer, 15;92(6 Suppl)*, 1684–1688.

Leng, S., Chavos, P., Koenig, K., & Walston, J. (2002). Serum IL-6 and hemoglobin as physiologic correlates in the geriatric syndrome of frailty: a pilot study. *Journal of American Geriatric Society, 50*, 1268–1271.

Linde, A., Soderstrom, R., Smith, C. I., Sallberg, M., Dahl, H., Grubb, R., Bjorkander, J., & Hammenstrom, L. (1992). Herpes virus serology, aberrant specific immunoglobulins G2 and G3 subclass patterns and GM also types in individuals with low levels of I, 63. *Clinical and Experimental Immunology, 90*, 199–203.

Lowy, M. T., Reder, A. T., Gormley, G. J., & Meltzer, H. Y. (1988). Comparison of in vivo and in vitro glucocorticoid sensitivity in depression: relationship to the dexamthanone suppression test. *Biological Psychiatry*, 24, 619–630.

Lutgendorf, S., Antoni, M. H., Ironson, G., Fletcher, M. A., Penedo, F., VanRiel, F., Baum, A., Schneiderman, N., & Klimas, N. (1995a). Physical symptoms of chronic fatigue syndrome are exacerbated by the stress of Hurricane Andrew. *Psychosomatic Medicine*, 57, 310–323.

Lutgendorf, S., Klimas, N., Antoni, M. H., Brickman, A., & Fletcher, M. A. (1995b). Relationships of cognitive difficulties to immune measures, depression and illness burden in chronic fatigue syndrome. *Journal of Chronic Fatigue Syndrome*, 1(2), 23–41.

Maier, S. F., & Watkins, L. R. (1998). Cytokines for psychologists: implications of bidirectional immune-to-brain communication for understanding behavior, mood, and cognition. *Psychology Review*, 105, 83–107.

Malik, U. R., Makower, D. F., Wadler, S. (2001). Interferon-mediated fatigue. *Cancer*, 15:92(6 Suppl), 1664–1668.

McEwen, B. S. (1998). Stress adaptation and disease. Allostasis and allostatic load. *Annals of the New York Academy Science*, 840, 33–44.

Moldovsky, H. (1989). Nonrestorative sleep and symptoms after a febrile illness in patients with fibrosis and chronic fatigue syndrome. *Journal of Rheumatology*, 16(19), 150–153.

Moldovsky, H. (1995). Sleep, neuroimmune and neuroendocrine functions in fibromyalgia and chronic fatigue syndrome. *Advances in Neuroimmunology*, 5, 39–56.

Morag, A., Tobi, M., Ravid, Z., Ravel, M., & Schattner, A. (1982). Increased (2′-5′)-oligo-a synthetase activity in patients with prolonged illness associated with serological evidence of persistent Epstein-barr virus infection. *Lancet*, 1, 744.

Mullington, J. M., Hinze-Selch, D., & Pollmacher, T. (2001). Mediators of inflammation and their interaction with sleep: relevance for chronic fatigue syndrome and related conditions. *Annals of the New York Academy of Science*, 933, 201–210.

Mullington, J. M., Korth, C., & Hermann, D. (2000). Dose dependent effects of a stimulating factor on a nights sleep in humans. *American of Journal of Physiology*, 278, R947–R955.

Neveu, P. J., Capuron, L., Ravaud, A., Gualde, N., Bosmans, E., Dantzer, R., & Maes, M. (2000). Early depressive symptoms correlated with an increased cytokine production in cancer patients treated with interleukin-2. *Brain, Behavior and Immunity*, 14, 118–119.

Patarca, R., Klimas, N. G., Garcia, M. N., Pons, H., & Fletcher, M. A. (1995b). Dysregulated expression of soluble immune mediator receptors in a subset of patients with chronic fatigue syndrome: categorization of patients by immune status. *Journal of Chronic Fatigue Syndrome*, 1(1), 79–94.

Patarca, R., Klimas, N. G., Sandler, D., Garcia, M. N., & Fletcher, M. A. (1995c). Interindividual immune status variation patterns in patients with chronic fatigue syndrome: association with the tumor necrosis factor system and gender. *Journal of Chronic Fatigue Syndrome*, 2(1), 13–19.

Patarca, R., Sandler, D., Walling, J., Klimas, N. G., & Fletcher, M. A. (1995a). Assessment of immune mediator expression levels in biological fluids and cells: a critical appraisal. *Critical Reviews in Oncogenesis, 6(2)*, 117–149.

Patarca-Montero, R., Antoni, M., Fletcher, M. A., & Klimas, N. G. (2001). Cytokine and other immunologic markers in chronic fatigue syndrome and their relation to neuropsychological factors. *Applied Neuropsychology, 8(1)*, 51–64.

Peakman, M., Deale, A., Field, R., Mahalingam, M., & Wessely, S. (1997). Clinical improvement in chronic fatigue syndrome is not associated with lymphocyte subsets of function or activation. *Clinical Immunology and Immunopathology, 82(1)*, 83–91.

Penttila, I. A., Harris, R. J., Storm, P., Haynes, D., Worswick, D. A., & Marmion, B. P. (1998). Cytokine dysregulation in the post-Q-fever syndrome. *Quarterly Journal of Medicine, 91(8)*, 549–560.

Quan, N., & Herkenham, M. (2002). Connecting cytokines and brain: a review of current issues. *Histology of Histopathology, 17(1)*, 273–288.

Rettori, V., Gimeno, M. F., Karara, A., Gonzalez, M. C., & McCann, S. M. (1991). Interleukin 1 alpha inhibits protaglandin E2 release to suppress pulsatile release of luteinizing hormone but not follicle-stimulating hormone. *Proceedings of the National Academy of Science USA, 88*, 2763–2767.

Rook, G. A., & Zumla, A. (1997). Gulf War syndrome: Is it due to a systemic shift in cytokine balance towards a Th2 profile? *Lancet, 349(9068)*, 1831–1833.

Sapolsky, R., Rivier, C., Yamamoto, G., Plotsky, P., & Vale, W. (1987). Interleukin-1 stimulates the secretion of hypothalamic corticotropin-releasing factor. *Science, 238*, 522–524.

Schuld, A., Mullington, J., Herman, D., et al. (1999). Effects of granulocyte colony stimulating factor on night sleep in humans. *American Journal of Physiology, 276*, R1149–R1155.

Scott, L., & Dinan,T. (1998). Urinary free cortisol excretion in chronic fatigue syndrome, major depression and in healthy volunteers. *Journal of Affective Disorders, 47*, 49–54.

Scott, L., Medbak, S., & Dinan, T. (1998). Blunted adrenocorticotropin and cortisol responses to corticotropin-releasing hormone stimulation in chronic fatigue syndrome. *Acta Psychologica Scandinavia, 97*, 450–457.

Sheng, W. S., Hu, S., Lamkin, A., Peterson, P. K., & Chao, C. C. (1996). Susceptibility to immunologically mediated fatigue in C57BL/6 versus Balb/c mice. *Clinical Immunology & Immunopathology, 81(2)*, 161–167.

Shoham, S., Davenne, D., Cady, A. B., Dinarello, C. A., & Krueger, J. M. (1987). Recombinant tumor necrosis factor and interleukin 1 enhance slow-wave sleep. *American Journal of Physiology, 253*, R142–R149.

Solomon, G. F., & Moos, R. H. (1964). Emotions, immunity and health: a speculative theoretical integration. *Archives of General Psychiatry, II*, 657–674.

Spath-Schwalbe, E., Hansen, K., Schmidt, F., et al. (1998). Acute effects of recombinent IL-6 on endocrine and central nervous system sleep functions in healthy men. *Journal of Clinical Endocrinology and Metabolism, 83,* 1573–1579.

Sternberg, E. (1993). Hypoimmune fatigue syndromes: Disease of the stress response? *Journal of Rheumatology, 20,* 418–421.

Stasi, R., Abriani, L., Beccaglia, P., Terzoli, E., & Amadori, S. (2003). Cancer-related fatigue: evolving concepts in evaluation and treatment. *Cancer, 1;98(9),* 1786–1801.

Uehara, A., Gottschall, P., Dahl, R., & Arimura, A. (1987). Interleukin-1 stimulates ACTH release by an indirect action which requires endogenous corticotropin releasing factor. *Endocrinology, 121,* 1580–1582.

Van Snick, J. (1989). Interleukin-6: an overview. *Annual Review of Immunology, 8,* 253–278.

Vgontzas, A. N., Papanicolalao, D. A., & Bixler, E. O. (1999). Circadian IL-6 secretion and depth of sleep. *Journal of Clinical Endocrinology and Metabolism, 84,* 2603–2607.

Visser, J., Blauw, B., Hinloopen, B., Broomer, E., de Kloet, R., Kluft, C., & Nagelkerken, L. (1998). CD4 T lymphocytes from patients with chronic fatigue syndrome have decreased interferon-γ production and increased sensitivity to dexamathasone. *Journal of Infectious Diseases, 177,* 451–454.

Vojdani, A., Ghoneum, M., Choppa, P. C., Magtoto, L., & Lapp, C. W. (1997). Elevated apoptotic cell population in patients with chronic fatigue syndrome: the pivotal role of protein kinase RNA. *Journal of Internal Medicine, 242(6),* 465–478.

Vojdani, A., & Lapp, C. W. (1999). Interferon-induced proteins are elevated in blood samples of patients with chemically or virally induced chronic fatigue syndrome. *Immunopharmacology and Immunotoxicology, 21(2),* 175–202.

Vollmer-Conna, U., Lloyd, A., Hickie, I., & Wakefield, D. (1998). Chronic fatigue syndrome: an immunological perspective. *Australian New Zealand Journal of Psychology, 32(4),* 523–527.

Wagner, S., Helder, L., Klimas, N., Antoni, M., & Keller, R. (1999). Immunological status correlates with severity of physical symptoms in chronic fatigue syndrome patients. *Journal of Chronic Fatigue Syndrome 5,* 132–133.

V Treatment of Fatigue

18 Rehabilitation and Treatment of Fatigue

Gudrun Lange, Dane B. Cook, and Benjamin H. Natelson

Fatigue, or "a feeling of tiredness or weariness" (Thomas, 1993), is one of the most common complaints reported to primary care physicians (Walker, Katon, & Jemelka, 1993; Kroenke, 2003). About 27 percent of patients in primary care settings (Bates et al., 1993) experience frequent and prolonged tiredness that interferes with their everyday life (David, Wessely, & Pelosi, 1988; Fuhrer & Wessely, 1995; Pawlikowska et al., 1994). Treatment for unusual fatigue, tiredness, or sleepiness in the primary care setting often consists of the recommendation to "get more rest." Because the complaint of frequent tiredness/fatigue is very common, primary care physicians rarely invest much time or effort in evaluating and determining the underlying causes of fatigue. Thus, attempts at identifying the severity of fatigue and appropriately managing fatigue have been rather poor in the primary care setting (Katon & Walker, 1998; Ridsdale et al., 1994; Ruffin & Cohen, 1994), prompting individuals suffering from unusual, prolonged fatigue to use healthcare services more frequently in their search for symptom relief (Walker et al., 1993; Kroenke, 2003).

Fatigue is a multidimensional somatic construct encompassing physical, physiological, and psychological dimensions that vary with the underlying cause of the reported fatigue. As already discussed in previous chapters, fatigue often accompanies chronic medical, neurological, or psychiatric illnesses, but it can also be a symptom of an actual sleep disorder, transient stress at home or the workplace, or just poor sleep hygiene. Thus, effective treatment needs to be tailored to each individual reporting persistent fatigue to his or her primary care physician and often consists of a combination of behavioral, pharmacological, and physical interventions. The goal of this chapter is to acquaint the reader with some of the most common and effective treatment modalities used to manage fatigue. Following is a brief overview of the prominent treatment modalities used across a variety of disorders associated with prolonged fatigue.

Behavioral Treatment and Fatigue

Cognitive behavior therapy (CBT) is a behavioral intervention that has received much attention in the primary and secondary care settings (Akagi, Klimes, & Bass, 2001; Deale, Chalder, Marks, & Wessely, 1997; Kroenke & Swindle, 2000; Looper & Kirmayer, 2002; Sharpe, 1997; Edinger, Wohlgemuth, Radtke, Marsh, & Quillian, 2001a; 2001b). Like many other treatment modalities, CBT is practiced in a variety of ways, thus making it difficult to compare clinical trials using this intervention to help individuals cope with the effects of persistent fatigue on functional status and quality of life. Briefly, some practitioners focus on the *behavioral* aspects of CBT, also known as behavior modification (Bandura, 1977; Wolpe, 1973). This approach uses principles of learning theory that focus on altering and substituting overt behavior that is considered maladaptive by (1) identifying the nature and frequency of the maladaptive behavior, (2) using classical or operant conditioning, counterconditioning, and modeling techniques to reeducate the client and change the behavior, and (3) assessing the effectiveness of the intervention. For example, this treatment approach would be useful in individuals who are fatigued secondary to poor sleep hygiene. Once a physician has determined that an individual suffers from disordered sleep, he or she needs to evaluate the person's sleep needs and ideal sleep duration, provide information about the consequences of sleeping less than needed, and institute a protocol to increase the individual's sleep hygiene (see chapter 13).

Other CBT practitioners bring a *cognitive* orientation to treatment. In general, this approach focuses on the belief that individuals attach faulty and irrational labels to certain situations that, in turn, causes them to respond maladaptively. Once clients learn to appraise situations logically and rationally, cognitive restructuring of the faulty, irrational thinking patterns occurs and the maladaptive behavior disappears (Beck, 1976; Ellis, 1970; Meichenbaum, 1977). For example, persistent fatigue, whether it is associated with a chronic medically explained or unexplained illness or transient stressful life event, may be cognitively appraised as a significant threat to a person's ability to function appropriately in everyday life. This perception may be supported and exaggerated by social circumstances, such as the tendency of solicitous family members or coworkers to cater to the fatigued individual, fostering increased illness behavior and often leading to functional disability and greater healthcare utilization. Cognitive restructuring leads the client to modify his or her cognitive appraisal of the significance and personal saliency of fatigue as a symptom, eventually increasing the client's ability to cope and manage fatigue.

Much of the research establishing the efficacy of CBT for persistent fatigue has been done in secondary or tertiary care settings. Reductions in the effect of fatigue on functional ability and quality of life have been found for many medically explained and unexplained conditions associated with fatigue, including major depression and bipolar disorders (Deckersbach, Gershuny, & Otto, 2000; Patelis-Siotis, 2001; Reinecke, Ryan, & DuBois, 1998; Thase et al., 2000), anxiety disorders (Borkovec & Ruscio, 2001), rheumatoid arthritis (Evers, Kraaimaat, van Riel, & de Jong, 2002; Keefe & Caldwell, 1997; Sharpe et al., 2001), multiple sclerosis (MS) (Mohr, Boudewyn, Goodkin, Bostrom, & Epstein, 2001), HIV/AIDS (Adinolfi, 2001a; Adinolfi, 2001b; Evans, Fishman, Spielman, & Haley, 2003), cancer (Cella, Peterman, Passik, Jacobsen, & Breitbart, 1998; Liossi & Hatira, 1999; Lovejoy, Tabor, Matteis, & Lillis, 2000), coronary artery disease (Writing Committee for the ENRICHD Investigators, 2003), and chronic fatigue syndrome (CFS) (Kroenke & Swindle, 2000; Prins et al., 2001).

In contrast, the applicability of CBT for the primary care setting is equivocal. Raine and colleagues (Raine et al., 2002) undertook a systematic literature review of randomized, controlled CBT trials to determine the efficacy of CBT in three medically unexplained disorders associated with prolonged fatigue including CFS, irritable bowel syndrome, and chronic low back pain in primary and secondary care settings. Since most investigators do not specify the CBT protocols used, Raine and colleagues' review made no distinction between trials that were labeled cognitive behavioural or just behavioural; they identified 20 studies conducted in a primary care setting and 41 studies in a secondary care setting, concluding that the data available were insufficient "to draw conclusions about treatment effectiveness in primary care for behavior therapy in patients with CFS and irritable bowel syndrome." Akagi and associates (Akagi et al., 2001) partially support this impression based on their study conducted in a general hospital setting with 94 individuals diagnosed with CFS. Of the 58 individuals who completed treatment (median of six sessions over a median 6-month period), 32 (55%) were considered moderately improved or recovered by their therapist as reflected in significantly improved functional and social impairment scores as well as reduced healthcare utilization. Although the authors state that CBT "is an acceptable and useful treatment which can be used in a general hospital outpatient setting," they caution that "a proportion of the patients do not benefit and remain significantly disabled by the condition." Likewise, Ridsdale and colleagues (Ridsdale et al., 2001) report that CBT in a sample of 160 primary care patients, all of whom fulfilled Chalder's criteria for fatigue, resulted in 47 percent of these patients no longer meeting fatigue criteria 6 months post treatment. However, CBT was just as efficacious as supportive counseling. In general, primary care patients most benefit from CBT or counseling if they are optimistic, entertain the notion that their fatigue may have a psychological explanation, and are socially well adjusted (Chalder, Godfrey, Ridsdale, King, & Wessely, 2003).

Overall, CBT can significantly improve fatigue and its consequences; however, effectiveness may depend on a variety of individual variables.

Pharmacological Interventions for Fatigue

When the physician has ruled out medical causes of fatigue with a careful medical history and a series of bloodwork analyses, the patient has medically unexplained fatigue. Over-the-counter medications offer a first line of therapeutic possibilities. For instance, if caffeine does not make the person too "jumpy," increasing caffeine intake either through coffee or over-the-counter products such as NO DOZ may be beneficial. Phenylephrine, a common ingredient in cough syrup, is also a mild generalized stimulant. Stronger medications require a physician's prescription. Amantidine, a medicine developed to treat flu, has been reported to reduce fatigue in patients using this drug. A double-blind, placebo-controlled trial showed that it reduced fatigue in persons with multiple sclerosis (MS) (Krupp et al., 1995). Although it is probably always worthwhile to try amantidine, it is not clear whether it is effective in persons with long lasting or chronic fatigue other than those with MS. Chronically fatigued patients usually need a trial with a stimulant such as amphetamine, methylphenidate, or pemoline. These stimulants are thought to work by stimulating arousal areas in the raphe nucleus of the brainstem, increasing alertness while decreasing fatigue. The disadvantage of a generalized stimulant is that it activates many bodily systems, often producing anxiety, fast heart rate, and an uncomfortable feeling of restlessness. Nonetheless, some studies have indicated this class of drugs may be effective in treating fatigue (Olson, Ambrogetti, & Sutherland, 2003).

One major problem with all of these prescription-based medications is that they can be quite addicting. In contrast, a new arousal agent, modafinil, has limited addictive potential and far less generalized arousal effects. The drug was initially approved by the FDA for treatment of sleepiness due to narcolepsy. But once a drug is available in drugstores, physicians often try to use it for other conditions. These so-called nonlabel uses often provide the drug company feedback for clinical trials on the drugs efficacy in other illnesses. For instance, Rammohan and colleagues (2002) conducted a clinical trial on the efficacy and safety of modafinil for fatigue in persons with MS. They reported significant improvement after 2 weeks of treatment with 200 mg/day in self-reported fatigue among persons with MS who were fatigued, with no serious side effects. Based on such reports of modafinil's efficacy in MS-related fatigue and sleepiness due to sleep apnea, the drug company recently asked for FDA approval of the drug for abnormal sleepiness. Initial approval was given, and although full approval has not yet been received, it is anticipated in the near future.

In the meantime, one of the authors (Natelson) has designed a double-blind, placebos-controlled trial of modafinil in patients with CFS from five physician practices. No significant effect in reducing fatigue was found, but further analysis showed this lack of effect was due to a robust placebo effect in the two sites that had recruited the most patients. When a further analysis was done site by site, a therapeutic effect seemed to emerge in some sites. The presence of placebo responders in one site but not in other sites suggests that physicians diagnose CFS differently from site to site. Regardless of the drug's efficacy in CFS, modafinil may have a role in treating substantive fatigue. The U.S. military was involved in its discovery and uses it (with amphetamines) for troops experiencing fatigue.

As part of the medical history, the physician should ask the patient about stress-related symptoms other than fatigue. These include nervousness, dry mouth, upset stomach, and the sensation of tachycardia. The physician can consider whether use of an anxiolytic can reduce the anxiety and related symptoms. For short-term use, a benzodiazepine such as alprazolam is a reasonable choice. If therapy will last more than a few weeks, however, a drug such as buspirone, which lacks the habituating properties of benzodiazepines, is preferable. Depressed mood and loss of interest in things that used to interest the individual are major manifestations of depression. Fatigue is a common somatic complaint of depression, and so a treatment trial with an antidepressant is worth considering. Because "atypical" depression is characterized less by mood problems and more by fatigue and a desire to eat and sleep more than usual, a trial of antidepressant medication in patients with relatively new-onset depression makes sense when fatigue is a prominent complaint.

When fatigue becomes so severe that it reduces daily activity, however, antidepressants are rarely helpful unless the patient also has a mood disturbance. In fact, studies of antidepressants in severe fatigue associated with CFS indicate no efficacy, although some evidence shows these medicines can improve health-related quality of life (Vercoulen et al., 1996; Wearden et al., 1998). Based on our clinical experience, we prescribe selective serotonin reuptake inhibitors (SSRIs) for patients with these medical complaints as well as an obvious mood disorder. In general, antidepressants improve mood but not somatic symptoms including fatigue; however, improving mood often improves patients' abilities to cope with such medical symptoms including fatigue.

We begin with a 20-mg daily dose of either fluoxetine or paroxetine. If symptoms are unchanged 4 weeks later and there are no significant side effects, the dose is doubled for another month. If patients still have significant amounts of mood disturbance at these SSRI doses, they should be referred to a psychopharmacologist for more sophisticated management. The major issue with antidepressants is to find the one that produces the least problem with side effects. The major side effects are weight gain and sexual dysfunction; SSRIs tend to be more problematic while buproprion is less problematic, at least in terms of sexual dysfunction.

Medication management of fatigue is in its infancy, and few medicines target the symptom of fatigue alone. The success of modafinil, a drug with relatively low toxicity and efficacy in improving fatigue, suggests that other agents will be in the drug armamentarium in the future. In the meantime, treatments directed at reducing depression and anxiety which can exacerbate fatigue are often the primary drug treatments used.

Exercise Training and Fatigue

Fatigue is a common and debilitating symptom of a host of diseases including cardiovascular (i.e., coronary heart disease, heart failure, chronic obstructive pulmonary disease), neuromuscular and central nervous system (i.e., postpolio syndrome, multiple sclerosis), cancer (i.e., both treatment and disease), rheumatic (i.e., rheumatoid arthritis, systemic lupus erythematosus), immune (i.e., human immunodeficiency virus, acquired immunodeficiency syndrome), psychiatric (i.e., major depression), and musculoskeletal (i.e., chronic fatigue and fibromyalgia syndromes) disorders (Afari & Buchwald, 2003; Breslin et al., 1998; Fukuda et al., 1994; Jubelt & Drucker, 1993; Portenoy, 2000; Quittan, Sturm, Wiesinger, Pacher, & Fialka-Moser, 1999; Rakel, 1999; Smets, Garssen, Schuster-Uitterhoeve, & de Haes, 1993; Sullivan & Dworkin, 2003; Sutherland & Andersen, 2001; Tavio, Milan, & Tirelli, 2002; Tench, McCurdie, White, & D'Cruz, 2000; Wolfe et al., 1990; Wolfe, Hawley, & Wilson, 1996). In fact, as several other chapters in this book document, fatigue is reported as the most disabling symptom in many diseases by affecting the patient's physical, psychological, and social wellbeing (al Majid & McCarthy, 2001; Fukuda et al., 1994; Guymer & Clauw, 2002; Portenoy, 2000; Portenoy & Itri, 1999).

For many fatiguing illnesses, early standards of care called for patients to rest and avoid physical activities that could potentially exacerbate symptoms associated with the disease, or in some cases increase the rate of disease progression (Afari & Buchwald, 2003; Agre, 1995; McCully, Sisto, & Natelson, 1996; Petajan & White, 1999). In MS, exercise was initially avoided for fear of elevating core body temperature, exacerbating symptoms of fatigue and potentially leading to neurological impairments (Petajan & Whik, 1999). In CFS, physical activity is often avoided for fear of postexertional malaise that is commonly reported by patients (Afari & Buchwald, 2003). Moreover, reports of exaggerated perception of effort in some cases of CFS (Cook et al., 2003a), but not in others (Cook et al., 2003b), combined with limited cardiorespiratory tolerance (Nagelkirk et al., 2003) have made exercise prescription a special challenge for the physician.

In HIV, physical activity is avoided to protect against further immune system compromise (Rigsby, Dishman, Jackson, Maclean, & Raven, 1992). Prolonged rest induces skeletal muscle catabolism, however, and can perpetuate fatigue. This is particularly true for diseases in which avoidance of physical activity is common because of functional limitations (e.g., neuromuscular diseases). In contrast to all this, it is now recognized that a physically inactive treatment approach leads to a vicious cycle of cardiovascular and musculoskeletal deconditioning that exacerbates symptoms of fatigue, increases the risk for morbidity, and has a negative impact on quality of life

Table 18.1

Select studies demonstrating the efficacy of exercise in treating fatigue among several chronic conditions

Disease	Reference
Cancer	Dimeo et al., 1998; Dimeo et al., 1999; Dimeo, 2001; Oldervoll et al., 2003
Chronic fatigue syndrome (CFS)	Fulcher & White, 1997; Peters et al., 2002; Powell et al., 2001
Chronic heart failure (CHF)	Quittan et al., 1999
Chronic obstructive pulmonary disease (COPD)	Boueri et al., 2001; Lacasse et al., 2002
Fibromyalgia (FM)	Busch et al., 2002; Peters et al., 2002
Heart disease	McCartney, 1998
Human immunodeficiency virus (HIV)	Smith et al., 2001
Multiple sclerosis (MS)	Petajan et al., 1996; Petajan et al., 1999; Sutherland & Andersen, 2003
Neuromuscular diseases	Consensus Conference Summary, 2002
Postpolio syndrome	Agre, 1995
Rheumatoid arthritis (RA)	Neuberger et al., 1997
Systemic lupus erythematosus (SLE)	Tench et al., 2003

(QOL). Thus, exercise training and recommendations to increase physical activity are becoming more commonplace. The primary goal of most exercise programs is to stop the decline in physical function and improve cardiovascular and muscular conditioning, thus improving the patients' QOL.

A review of the literature indicates that exercise training has beneficial effects on fatigue for virtually all of the diseases discussed in this chapter (see table 18.1). In fact, decreases in self-reported fatigue and increases in self-reported energy, along with numerous additional symptom improvements, have been consistently demonstrated following aerobic exercise training (Afari & Buchwald, 2003; Agre, 1995; Boueri, Bucher-Bartelson, Glenn, & Make, 2001; Busch, Schachter, Peloso, & Bombardier, 2002; Dimeo, 2001; Dimeo, Stieglitz, Novelli-Fischer, Fetscher, & Keul, 1999; Lacasse et al., 2002; McCartney, 1998; McCully et al., 1996; Neuberger et al., 1997; Petajan & White, 1999; Quittan et al., 1999; Singh, Clements, & Fiatarone, 1997; Smart, Fang, & Marwick, 2003; Smith et al., 2001; Sutherland & Andersen, 2001; Tench, McCarthy, McCurdie, White, & D'Cruz, 2003). In MS, for example, 15 weeks (3 days per week) of cycling exercise for 30 minutes at 60 percent of aerobic capacity resulted in decreases in self-reported fatigue, anger, and depression and improved self-reports of physical function and social interaction (Petajan et al., 1996). In persons with rheumatoid arthritis, 2 weeks (3 hours/week) of low-impact aerobic exercise resulted in decreases in pain and fatigue with no detrimental effects on disease status in terms of joint count and sedimentation rate (Neuberger et al., 1997). In persons with COPD, a review of 23 random controlled trials of exercise showed that exercise training resulted in large and clinically meaningful effects on fatigue and sense of control, with modest improvements in aerobic capacity (Lacasse et al., 2002). Finally, in persons with CFS and FM, exercise training has been consistently associated with improvements in self-reported fatigue, physical functional status, and overall QOL (Afari & Buchwald, 2003; Busch et al., 2002; Fulcher & White, 1997; Guymer & Clauw, 2002; McCully et al., 1996; Powell, Bentall, Nye, & Edwards, 2001).

The mechanisms for improved feelings of fatigue with exercise training are unknown and undoubtedly vary with the specific disease. However, improvements in exercise performance appear to resemble those seen in studies of healthy individuals. These include objective improvements in physiological measures of fatigue such as aerobic fitness, muscular strength, physical function, and exercise endurance. For example, Rigsby and colleagues (Rigsby et al., 1992) reported that men seropositive for HIV-1 experienced improved strength and aerobic fitness following a 12-week exercise-training regimen prescribed in accordance with American College of Sports Medicine Guidelines, and including both aerobic cycling exercise and strength and flexibility training resulted in improved strength and aerobic fitness in men seropositive for HIV-1. Importantly, these changes occurred without changes in the patients' clinical status in terms of total leukocyte, lymphocyte, CD4+ count, CD8+ count, and CD4+/CD8+ ratio.

The physiological adaptations that change one's exercise capacity are likely to contribute to reduced feelings of fatigue. These adaptations include increases in cardiac output and distribution to muscle, oxygen transport and utilization, fat utilization, oxidative enzyme activity and capacity, and lean body mass; decreases in heart rate, fat mass, and lactate production; and improved blood lipid profiles (McArdle et al., 1991). Moreover, resistance exercise can reduce the loss of lean body mass common in several fatiguing diseases. Depending on the disease, compromise of these systems can contribute to fatigue. For example, chemotherapy-related fatigue can result from several factors related to oxygen transport to blood and skeletal muscle. Since oxygen transport is critical for energy production, the body must work harder to supply active tissue, and the system can become quickly compromised. There are no known pharmacological treatments for impaired cellular energy production (Dimeo, 2001). Therefore, exercise training that results in improved oxygen transport and delivery, and thus improved cardiovascular and muscular function, may be a critical factor in cancer-related fatigue. This is supported by research showing improved aerobic tolerance and endurance to exercise training in cancer patients that corresponds with improvements in self-reported fatigue (Dimeo, Rumberger, & Keul, 1998; Dimeo, 2001; Dimeo et al., 1999; Oldervoll, Kaasa, Knobel, & Loge, 2003). Exercise training therefore results in both objective (improved oxygen consumption and endurance) and subjective (improved self reports) improvements in fatigue.

In heart failure, several studies have shown that exercise training results in improved autonomic function in the form of decreased cardiac oxygen demand, improved endothelial function, and improved blood supply to exercising muscle (You & Marwick, 2003). These changes help reduce feelings of fatigue during routine activities of daily living. Thus, improvements in exercise capacity can have numerous beneficial effects on treatment and rehabilitation in most chronic diseases characterized by decreased functional capacity and fatigue symptoms. Exercise training or a physically active lifestyle may also have protective effects, and greater initial fitness may result in lower levels of fatigue initially as well as in response to drugs and chemotherapy.

The effects of exercise training are not limited to better cardiovascular or muscular fitness. Improved physical function may also be accompanied by enhanced feelings of mood, independence, and self-esteem (Busch et al., 2002; Dimeo, 2001; Lacasse et al., 2002; Petajan et al., 1996; Quittan et al., 1999). This can result in improved social interactions, reduced anxiety, and increased adherence to rehabilitation. Exercise may also decrease the need for medications used to treat fatigue. Peters and colleagues (Peters et al., 2002) examined the effect of group aerobic exercise training (at 60 to 65 percent of predicted maximal heart rate) and stretching on sedentary primary care patients presenting with a multitude of unexplained physical symptoms (e.g., pain and fatigue). Results indicated that both healthcare utilization, as documented by the general practitioner (GP), and self-reported measures of symptoms and QOL were improved by exercise training. Specifically, patients who adhered to the program had fewer symptoms, had fewer GP consultations, were prescribed less medication, and were less likely to contact secondary care sources. Self-reported pain, fatigue, anxiety, depression, and social interaction all improved following exercise training.

Exercise gives patients an active role in their treatment and promoting their own health. This can help foster-feelings of control and reduce feelings of fear. It is important to note that exercise or increased physical activity does not necessarily alter the disease course, and it certainly is not an alternative to or replacement for other forms of treatment. However, maintaining physical activity or performing exercise training can have beneficial effects on treatment responses and disease management, as well as on the patients' ability to cope with demanding treatment regimens and the side effects of drug therapies. Exercise training and physical activity thus can have both physiological and psychological benefits in the forms of improved physical and mental health.

In summary, emerging evidence supports aerobic exercise training as a safe and effective treatment for a host of diseases in which fatigue is a dominant symptom. Exercise training results in improved physical performance, increased fitness, decreased ratings of fatigue, increased ratings of energy (vigor), and an overall improvement in QOL. The primary goal of exercise is to avoid the spiral of deconditioning that is common in most fatiguing diseases. It is important to recognize that fatigue is not solely a result of disease processes, but can occur as an indirect consequence of decreased physical activity. Thus, increasing physical activity can decrease symptoms of fatigue and help with managing diseases in which fatigue interferes with recovery and negatively affects the patients' physical function and QOL.

Conclusion

In general, treatment for fatigue typically involves three forms of intervention: psychological (e.g., CBT), pharmacological, and exercise. Which of these are indicated and in what combination should be tailored to each patient's individual needs. While no treatment modalities have proved to be overwhelmingly successful, many studies suggest that a tailored approach to fatigue treatment can potentially reduce fatigue intensity and improve QOL.

CBT may be more efficacious in tertiary care settings with patients who have low self-efficacy of their ability to begin an exercise program or where worries of symptom exacerbation persist. In cases of prolonged fatigue, it is important not to become trapped in a vicious cycle of sedentary behavior, and preventing physical inactivity should be a primary concern for the physician. Although not a mainstream concept in primary care, pharmacological treatment of fatigue should be reserved for severe cases, to get the patient up and about, or when the patient's fatigue is resistant to both CBT and exercise treatment. The idea of promoting rest and avoiding physical activity is, in fact, an antiquated concept. Promotion of an exercise program has consistently resulted in decreased self-reported fatigue and improved QOL.

References

Adinolfi, A. (2001a). Assessment and treatment of HIV-related fatigue. *Journal of the Association of Nurses AIDS Care, 12(Suppl)*, 29–34.

Adinolfi, A. (2001b). The need for national guidelines to manage fatigue in HIV-positive patients. *Journal of the Association of Nurses AIDS Care, 12(Suppl)*, 39–42.

Afari, N., & Buchwald, D. (2003). Chronic fatigue syndrome: a review. *American Journal of Psychiatry, 160*, 221–236.

Agre, J. C. (1995). The role of exercise in the patient with post-polio syndrome. *Annals of New York Academy of Science, 753*, 321–334.

Akagi, H., Klimes, I., & Bass, C. (2001). Cognitive behavioral therapy for chronic fatigue syndrome in a general hospital—feasible and effective. *General Hospital Psychiatry, 23*, 254–260.

Al Majid, S., & McCarthy, D. O. (2001). Cancer-induced fatigue and skeletal muscle wasting: the role of exercise. *Biological Research Nursing, 2*, 186–197.

Bandura, A. (1977). *Social Learning Theory.* Englewood Cliffs, NJ: Prentice-Hall.

Bates, D. W., Schmitt, W., Buchwald, D., Ware, N. C., Lee, J., Thoyer, E., Kornish, R. J., & Komaroff, A. L. (1993). Prevalence of fatigue and chronic fatigue syndrome in a primary care practice. *Archives of Internal Medicine, 153*, 2759–2765.

Beck, A. T. (1976). *Cognitive therapy and Emotional Disorders.* New York: International Universities Press.

Borkovec, T. D., & Ruscio, A. M. (2001). Psychotherapy for generalized anxiety disorder. *Journal of Clinical Psychiatry, 62(Suppl 11)*, 37–42.

Boueri, F. M., Bucher-Bartelson, B. L., Glenn, K. A., & Make, B. J. (2001). Quality of life measured with a generic instrument (Short Form-36) improves following pulmonary rehabilitation in patients with COPD. *Chest, 119*, 77–84.

Breslin, E., van der, S. C., Breukink, S., Meek, P., Mercer, K., Volz, W., & Louie, S. (1998). Perception of fatigue and quality of life in patients with COPD. *Chest, 114*, 958–964.

Busch, A., Schachter, C. L., Peloso, P. M., & Bombardier, C. (2002). Exercise for treating fibromyalgia syndrome. *Cochrane Database System Review*, CD003786.

Cella, D., Peterman, A., Passik, S., Jacobsen, P., & Breitbart, W. (1998). Progress toward guidelines for the management of fatigue. *Oncology (Huntingt), 12*, 369–377.

Chalder, T., Godfrey, E., Ridsdale, L., King, M., & Wessely, S. (2003). Predictors of outcome in a fatigued population in primary care following a randomized controlled trial. *Psychological Medicine, 33*, 283–287.

Consensus conference: Role of Physical Activity and Exercise Training in Neuromuscular Diseases. (2002). San Diego, California. September 30–October 3, 2001. *American Journal of Physical Medicine and Rehabilitation, 81*, S1–195.

Cook, D. B., Nagelkirk, P. R., Peckerman, A., Poluri, A., Lamanca, J. J., & Natelson, B. H. (2003a). Perceived exertion in fatiguing illness: civilians with chronic fatigue syndrome. *Medical Science of Sports and Exercise, 35*, 563–568.

Cook, D. B., Nagelkirk, P. R., Peckerman, A., Poluri, A., Lamanca, J. J., & Natelson, B. H. (2003b). Perceived exertion in fatiguing illness: Gulf War veterans with chronic fatigue syndrome. *Medical Science of Sports and Exercise, 35*, 569–574.

David, A. S., Wessely, S., & Pelosi, A. J. (1988). Postviral fatigue syndrome: time for a new approach. *British Medical Journal (Clinical Research Edition), 296*, 696–699.

Deale, A., Chalder, T., Marks, I., & Wessely, S. (1997). Cognitive behavior therapy for chronic fatigue syndrome: a randomized controlled trial. *American Journal of Psychiatry, 154*, 408–414.

Deckersbach, T., Gershuny, B. S., & Otto, M. W. (2000). Cognitive-behavioral therapy for depression. Applications and outcome. *Psychiatric Clinics of North America, 23,* 795–809, VII.

Dimeo, F., Rumberger, B. G., & Keul, J. (1998). Aerobic exercise as therapy for cancer fatigue. *Medical Science of Sports and Exercise, 30,* 475–478.

Dimeo, F. C. (2001). Effects of exercise on cancer-related fatigue. *Cancer, 92,* 1689–1693.

Dimeo, F. C., Stieglitz, R. D., Novelli-Fischer, U., Fetscher, S., & Keul, J. (1999). Effects of physical activity on the fatigue and psychologic status of cancer patients during chemotherapy. *Cancer, 85,* 2273–2277.

Edinger, J. D., Wohlgemuth, W. K., Radtke, R. A., Marsh, G. R., & Quillian, R. E. (2001a). Cognitive behavioral therapy for treatment of chronic primary insomnia: a randomized controlled trial. *Journal of the American Medical Association, 285,* 1856–1864.

Edinger, J. D., Wohlgemuth, W. K., Radtke, R. A., Marsh, G. R., & Quillian, R. E. (2001b). Does cognitive-behavioral insomnia therapy alter dysfunctional beliefs about sleep? *Sleep, 24,* 591–599.

Ellis, A. (1970). *The Essence of Rational Psychotherapy: A Comprehensive Approach to Treatment.* New York: Institute for Rational Living.

Enhancement of Energy Capacity (1991). In W. D. McArdle, F. I. Katch, & V. L. Katch, eds. *Exercise physiology: Energy, nutrition and human performance,* 3rd ed. pp. 423–451. Philadelphia: Lea & Febiger.

Evans, S., Fishman, B., Spielman, L., & Haley, A. (2003). Randomized trial of cognitive behavior therapy versus supportive psychotherapy for HIV-related peripheral neuropathic pain. *Psychosomatics, 44,* 44–50.

Evers, A. W., Kraaimaat, F. W., van Riel, P. L., & de Jong, A. J. (2002). Tailored cognitive-behavioral therapy in early rheumatoid arthritis for patients at risk: a randomized controlled trial. *Pain, 100,* 141–153.

Fuhrer, R., & Wessely, S. (1995). The epidemiology of fatigue and depression: a French primary-care study. *Psychological Medicine, 25,* 895–905.

Fukuda, K., Straus, S. E., Hickie, I., Sharpe, M. C., Dobbins, J. G., & Komaroff, A. (1994). The chronic fatigue syndrome: a comprehensive approach to its definition and study. International Chronic Fatigue Syndrome Study Group. *Annals of Internal Medicine, 121,* 953–959.

Fulcher, K. Y., & White, P. D. (1997). Randomised controlled trial of graded exercise in patients with the chronic fatigue syndrome. *British Medical Journal, 314,* 1647–1652.

Guymer, E. K., & Clauw, D. J. (2002). Treatment of fatigue in fibromyalgia. *Rheumatic Disease Clinics of North America, 28,* 367–378.

Jubelt, B., & Drucker, J. (1993). Post-polio syndrome: an update. *Seminars in Neurology, 13,* 283–290.

Katon, W. J., & Walker, E. A. (1998). Medically unexplained symptoms in primary care. *Journal of Clinical Psychiatry, 59(Suppl 20)*, 15–21.

Keefe, F. J., & Caldwell, D. S. (1997). Cognitive behavioral control of arthritis pain. *Medical Clinics of North America, 81*, 277–290.

Kroenke, K. (2003). Patients presenting with somatic complaints: epidemiology, psychiatric comorbidity and management. *International Journal of Methods in Psychiatric Research, 12*, 34–43.

Kroenke, K., & Swindle, R. (2000). Cognitive-behavioral therapy for somatization and symptom syndromes: a critical review of controlled clinical trials. *Psychotherapy Psychosomatic, 69*, 205–215.

Krupp, L. B., Coyle, P. K., Doscher, C., et al. (1995). Fatigue therapy in multiple sclerosis: results of a double-blind, randomized, parallel trial of amantidine, pemoline, and placebo. *Neurology, 45*, 1956–1961.

Lacasse, Y., Brosseau, L., Milne, S., Martin, S., Wong, E., Guyatt, G. H., & Goldstein, R. S. (2002). Pulmonary rehabilitation for chronic obstructive pulmonary disease. (Cochrane review). In: The Cochrane Library, Issue 3, 2004.

Liossi, C., & Hatira, P. (1999). Clinical hypnosis versus cognitive behavioral training for pain management with pediatric cancer patients undergoing bone marrow aspirations. *International Journal of Clinical Experimental Hypnosis, 47*, 104–116.

Looper, K. J., & Kirmayer, L. J. (2002). Behavioral medicine approaches to somatoform disorders. *Journal of Consulting Clinical Psychology, 70*, 810–827.

Lovejoy, N. C., Tabor, D., Matteis, M., & Lillis, P. (2000). Cancer-related depression: Part I— Neurologic alterations and cognitive-behavioral therapy. *Oncology Nursing Forum, 27*, 667–678.

McCartney, N. (1998). Role of resistance training in heart disease. *Medical Science of Sports and Exercrcise, 30*, S396–S402.

McCully, K. K., Sisto, S. A., & Natelson, B. H. (1996). Use of exercise for treatment of chronic fatigue syndrome. *Sports Medicine, 21*, 35–48.

Meichenbaum, D. (1977). *Cognitive Behavior Modification.* New York: Plenum Press.

Mohr, D. C., Boudewyn, A. C., Goodkin, D. E., Bostrom, A., & Epstein, L. (2001). Comparative outcomes for individual cognitive-behavior therapy, supportive-expressive group psychotherapy, and sertraline for the treatment of depression in multiple sclerosis. *Journal of Consulting Clinical Psychology, 69*, 942–949.

Nagelkirk, P. R., Cook, D. B., Peckerman, A., Kesil, W., Sakowski, T., Natelson, B. H., & Lamanca, J. J. (2003). Aerobic capacity of Gulf War veterans with chronic fatigue syndrome. *Military Medicine, 168*, 750–755.

Neuberger, G. B., Press, A. N., Lindsley, H. B., Hinton, R., Cagle, P. E., Carlson, K., Scott, S., Dahl, J., & Kramer, B. (1997). Effects of exercise on fatigue, aerobic fitness, and disease activity measures in persons with rheumatoid arthritis. *Research in Nursing Health, 20*, 195–204.

Oldervoll, L. M., Kaasa, S., Knobel, H., & Loge, J. H. (2003). Exercise reduces fatigue in chronic fatigued Hodgkins disease survivors—results from a pilot study. *European Journal of Cancer, 39,* 57–63.

Olson, L. G., Ambrogetti, A., & Sutherland, D. C. (2003). A pilot randomized controlled train of dexamphetamine in patients with chronic fatigue syndrome. *Psychosomatics, 44,* 38–43.

Patelis-Siotis, I. (2001). Cognitive-behavioral therapy: applications for the management of bipolar disorder. *Bipolar Disorders, 3,* 1–10.

Pawlikowska, T., Chalder, T., Hirsch, S. R., Wallace, P., Wright, D. J., & Wessely, S. C. (1994). Population based study of fatigue and psychological distress. *British Medical Journal, 308,* 763–766.

Petajan, J. H., Gappmaier, E., White, A. T., Spencer, M. K., Mino, L., & Hicks, R. W. (1996). Impact of aerobic training on fitness and quality of life in multiple sclerosis. *Annals of Neurology, 39,* 432–441.

Petajan, J. H., & White, A. T. (1999). Recommendations for physical activity in patients with multiple sclerosis. *Sports Medicine, 27,* 179–191.

Peters, S., Stanley, I., Rose, M., Kaney, S., & Salmon, P. (2002). A randomized controlled trial of group aerobic exercise in primary care patients with persistent, unexplained physical symptoms. *Family Practice, 19,* 665–674.

Portenoy, R. K. (2000). Cancer-related fatigue: an immense problem. *Oncologist, 5,* 350–352.

Portenoy, R. K., & Itri, L. M. (1999). Cancer-related fatigue: guidelines for evaluation and management. *Oncologist, 4,* 1–10.

Powell, P., Bentall, R. P., Nye, F. J., & Edwards, R. H. (2001). Randomised controlled trial of patient education to encourage graded exercise in chronic fatigue syndrome. *British Medical Journal, 322,* 387–390.

Prins, J. B., Bleijenberg, G., Bazelmans, E., Elving, L. D., de Boo, T. M., Severens, J. L., van der Wilt, G. J., Spinhoven, P., & Van der Meer, J. W. (2001). Cognitive behaviour therapy for chronic fatigue syndrome: a multicentre randomised controlled trial. *Lancet, 357,* 841–847.

Quittan, M., Sturm, B., Wiesinger, G. F., Pacher, R., & Fialka-Moser, V. (1999). Quality of life in patients with chronic heart failure: a randomized controlled trial of changes induced by a regular exercise program. *Scandinavian Journal of Rehabilitation Medicine, 31,* 223–228.

Raine, R., Haines, A., Sensky, T., Hutchings, A., Larkin, K., & Black, N. (2002). Systematic review of mental health interventions for patients with common somatic symptoms: can research evidence from secondary care be extrapolated to primary care? *British Medical Journal, 325,* 1082.

Rakel, R. E. (1999). Depression. *Primary Care, 26,* 211–224.

Rammohan, K. W., Rosenberg, J. H., Lynn, D. J., Blumenfeld, A. M., Pollak, C. P., & Nagaraja, H. N. (2002). Efficacy and safety of modafinil (Provigil) for the treatment of fatigue in multiple sclerosis: a two centre phase 2 study. *Journal of Neurology, Neurosurgery, Psychiatry, 72,* 179–183.

Reinecke, M. A., Ryan, N. E., & DuBois, D. L. (1998). Cognitive-behavioral therapy of depression and depressive symptoms during adolescence: a review and meta-analysis. *Journal of the American Academy of Child and Adolescent Psychiatry, 37*, 26–34.

Ridsdale, L., Evans, A., Jerrett, W., Mandalia, S., Osler, K., & Vora, H. (1994). Patients who consult with tiredness: frequency of consultation, perceived causes of tiredness and its association with psychological distress. *British Journal of General Practice, 44*, 413–416.

Ridsdale, L., Godfrey, E., Chalder, T., Seed, P., King, M., Wallace, P., & Wessely, S. (2001). Chronic fatigue in general practice: is counselling as good as cognitive behaviour therapy? A UK randomised trial. *British Journal of General Practice, 51*, 19–24.

Rigsby, L. W., Dishman, R. K., Jackson, A. W., Maclean, G. S., & Raven, P. B. (1992). Effects of exercise training on men seropositive for the human immunodeficiency virus-1. *Medical Science of Sports and Exercercise, 24*, 6–12.

Ruffin, M. T., & Cohen, M. (1994). Evaluation and management of fatigue. *American Family Physician, 50*, 625–634.

Sharpe, L., Sensky, T., Timberlake, N., Ryan, B., Brewin, C. R., & Allard, S. (2001). A blind, randomized, controlled trial of cognitive-behavioural intervention for patients with recent onset rheumatoid arthritis: preventing psychological and physical morbidity. *Pain, 89*, 275–283.

Sharpe, M. (1997). Cognitive behavior therapy for functional somatic complaints. The example of chronic fatigue syndrome. *Psychosomatics, 38*, 356–362.

Singh, N. A., Clements, K. M., & Fiatarone, M. A. (1997). A randomized controlled trial of progressive resistance training in depressed elders. *Journal of Gerontology A Biological Science and Medical Science, 52*, M27–M35.

Smart, N., Fang, Z. Y., & Marwick, T. H. (2003). A practical guide to exercise training for heart failure patients. *Journal of Cardiac Failure, 9*, 49–58.

Smets, E. M., Garssen, B., Schuster-Uitterhoeve, A. L., & de Haes, J. C. (1993). Fatigue in cancer patients. *British Journal of Cancer, 68*, 220–224.

Smith, B. A., Neidig, J. L., Nickel, J. T., Mitchell, G. L., Para, M. F., & Fass, R. J. (2001). Aerobic exercise: effects on parameters related to fatigue, dyspnea, weight and body composition in HIV-infected adults. *AIDS, 15*, 693–701.

Sullivan, P. S., & Dworkin, M. S. (2003). Prevalence and correlates of fatigue among persons with HIV infection. *Journal of Pain Symptomatology Management, 25*, 329–333.

Sutherland, G., & Andersen, M. B. (2001). Exercise and multiple sclerosis: physiological, psychological, and quality of life issues. *Journal of Sports Medicine and Physical Fitness, 41*, 421–432.

Tavio, M., Milan, I., & Tirelli, U. (2002). Cancer-related fatigue (review). *International Journal of Oncology, 21*, 1093–1099.

Tench, C. M., McCarthy, J., McCurdie, I., White, P. D., & D'Cruz, D. P. (2003). Fatigue in systemic lupus erythematosus: a randomized controlled trial of exercise. *Rheumatology, 42*, 1050–1054.

Tench, C. M., McCurdie, I., White, P. D., & D'Cruz, D. P. (2000). The prevalence and associations of fatigue in systemic lupus erythematosus. *Rheumatology (Oxford), 39*, 1249–1254.

Thase, M. E., Friedman, E. S., Berman, S. R., Fasiczka, A. L., Lis, J. A., Howland, R. H., & Simons, A. D. (2000). Is cognitive behavior therapy just a 'nonspecific' intervention for depression? A retrospective comparison of consecutive cohorts treated with cognitive behavior therapy or supportive counseling and pill placebo. *Journal of Affective Disorders, 57*, 63–71.

Thomas, P. K. (1993). The chronic fatigue syndrome: what do we know? *British Medical Journal, 306*, 1557–1558.

Vercoulen, J. H. M. M., Swanink, C. M. A., Zitman, F. G., et al. (1996). Randomised, double-blind, placebo-controlled study of fluoxetine in chronic fatigue syndrome. *Lancet, 347*, 858–861.

Walker, E. A., Katon, W. J., & Jemelka, R. P. (1993). Psychiatric disorders and medical care utilization among people in the general population who report fatigue. *Journal of General Internal Medicine, 8*, 436–440.

Wearden, A. J., Morriss, R. K., Mullis, R., et al. (1998). Randomised, double-blind, placebo-controlled treatment trial of fluoxetine and graded exercise for chronic fatigue syndrome. *British Journal of Psychiatry, 172*, 485–490.

Wolfe, F., Hawley, D. J., & Wilson, K. (1996). The prevalence and meaning of fatigue in rheumatic disease. *Journal of Rheumatology, 23*, 1407–1417.

Wolfe, F., Smythe, H. A., Yunus, M. B., et al. (1990). The American College of Rheumatology 1990 Criteria for the Classification of Fibromyalgia. Report of the Multicenter Criteria Committee. *Arthritis Rheumatism, 33*, 160–172.

Wolpe, J. (1973). *The Practice of Behavior Therapy*. 2nd ed. New York: Pergamon Press.

Writing Committee for the ENRICHD Investigators (2003). Effects of treating depression and low perceived social support on clinical events after myocardial infarction. *Journal of the American Medical Association, 289*, 3106–3116.

You, F. Z., & Marwick, T. H. (2003). Mechanisms of exercise training in patients with heart failure. *American Heart Journal, 145*, 904–911.

VI Conclusions

19 Fatigue: Its Definition, Its Study, and Its Future

John DeLuca

As discussed throughout this book, fatigue is not a unitary concept in terms of its definition or measurement. Over the twentieth century, it became clear that fatigue was viewed as both a symptom and a disease. As a symptom, fatigue has many causes, ranging from physiological states (sleep deprivation) to medical conditions (thyroid abnormalities, infections, cancer, coronary heart disease or CHD), insults to the brain (traumatic brain injury, multiple sclerosis, stroke), psychiatric disorders such as depression, medications (antihistamines), and even unhealthy lifestyles. As a disease, fatigue is often part of a group of "unexplained" illnesses (e.g., neurasthenia, DeCosta syndrome, chronic fatigue syndrome) with little understanding of its causes.

What is it about fatigue that it can be a consequence of so many different factors? Does fatigue have a single mechanism, or is it so multidimensional that each dimension has a different underlying mechanism? While these questions remain elusive, this book has tried to address how the question of fatigue is related to brain function or dysfunction. We cannot definitively answer this question, but by examining fatigue through a variety of disorders and conditions, we may find some commonalities that can serve as testable hypotheses for future research and clinical treatment.

Wessely and colleagues (1998) state that because fatigue is universal, commonly observed among the healthy, and in those with psychiatric and physical medical conditions, it is nonspecific and therefore of little diagnostic interest. There is thus little interest in understanding the mechanism of fatigue. This book takes the opposite view—fatigue is so common that understanding its mechanism and expression is essential for developing effective treatments.

Defining Fatigue

Even after 100 years of scientific inquiry, the definition of fatigue remains elusive. There is no general consensus on a universal definition, even in the broadest sense of

Table 19.1
Components of fatigue

Behavior (effects on performance)
Feeling   (subjective experience)
Mechanism
Physiological
Psychological
Context (e.g., environment, attitudes)

Adapted from Wessley et al., 1998.

the term. This lack of even a consensual definition remains a major obstacle to understanding the scientific and clinical manifestations of fatigue.

Despite its complexity, the following definition of fatigue in the broad sense is offered with the hope of achieving general acceptance: Fatigue is the reduction in performance with either prolonged or unusual exertion. Thus fatigue can be sensory, motor, cognitive, or subjective.

Components of Fatigue

Problems in defining fatigue become apparent when we break it down into more narrow components. In order to truly understand fatigue broadly, one must finally realize that fatigue is a multidimensional construct. Without this simple understanding, research and clinical manifestations of fatigue will remain in the current stagnant recycling of ideas leading endlessly back to the circular notion of its simplicity. Clearly, fatigue comprises at least four components, first identified in the early experimental work of Mosso (1904): behavioral (or performance decrement), feeling state (or subjective experience), mechanism, and context (table 19.1). After a century of theorizing, research, and identifying illness conditions, these four components remain valid metrics for conceptualizing the nature of fatigue (see Wessely et al., 1998, for a more complete discussion).

The "scientific" approach attempts to operationalize fatigue for analysis by focusing primarily on behavioral fatigue. Viewed as performance decrements, fatigue is usually defined as the inability to sustain physical or "mental" activity over time. The easiest measures are associated with physical manifestations (e.g., muscular or cardiovascular) in which changes in performance are fairly easy to document; mental or cognitive fatigue has proven more elusive (see chapter 3).

In contrast, feeling or subjective states of fatigue are central to the medical context of fatigue, as either an illness or a symptom. However, the poor correlation between subjective, behavioral (or objective, performance-based), and physiological fatigue diminishes the validity or credibility of assessment and treatment of subjective fatigue

(Berrios, 1990). It is this lack of correlation between objective measurement and subjective experience that hinders better understanding of the enigma of fatigue. Medicine has opted for using subject states as the main symptom criterion for various illnesses. Clinical definitions of fatigue focus primarily on global assessments, which emphasize the patient's subjective feeling of fatigue. For instance, the Multiple Sclerosis (MS) Council for Clinical Practice Guidelines (1998) published the following definition of fatigue: "A subjective lack of physical and/or mental energy that is perceived by the individual or caregiver to interfere with usual and desired activities." This lack of uniform definition of subjective fatigue has resulted in little advance beyond what was known about fatigue 100 years ago.

Peripheral versus Central Fatigue

The notion of central versus peripheral fatigue dates back at least to before the turn of the twentieth century (Mosso, 1904; Waller, 1891). Although useful, the concept of peripheral fatigue is most meaningful in studying end organs (e.g., muscles). Central fatigue can be defined as "the failure to initiate and/or sustain attentional tasks ('mental fatigue') and physical activities ('physical fatigue') requiring self motivation (as opposed to external stimulation)" (Chaudhuri & Behan, 2000, p. 35). However, even motor fatigue can result from muscle fatigue (i.e., peripheral state) or brain control over the muscle (central state). Behavioral and subjective manifestations of fatigue may also be related to the peripheral–central distinction. For instance, is decreased cognitive performance with sustained cognitive work due to central processes (e.g., requiring more cerebral effort to sustain performance, see chapter 3) or deconditioning (general physical state of the body) or both? These two potential explanations are separable with proper assessment and may be what is required in the future examination of fatigue (see below).

Proposed Brain Mechanisms of Fatigue

Fatigue has been suggested as a general indicator of brain damage (Heesen et al., 2002) and conceptualized as "the final common pathway of impaired neural processing" (see chapter 7). But what do we really know about the neural mechanisms of central fatigue?

Clearly, the study of the neural mechanism of fatigue is still in its infancy. Yet, mechanisms proposed by this book's various authors with expertise in specific areas of fatigue study overlap considerably. Table 19.2 lists the brain mechanisms proposed for each of the clinical entities discussed in this book. Primary fatigue mechanisms listed include the basal ganglia and frontal lobe regions of the brain, the HPA axis, and proinflammatory cytokines affecting neural metabolism.

Table 19.2
Proposed brain involvement for fatigue by clinical disorder reviewed in this book

Clinical Disorder	Proposed Brain Involvement
Stroke	Basal ganglia, HPA, cytokines and the brain
Other neurological disorders	Basal ganglia, frontal lobes, limbic (hypothalamic), NT
Somatization	HPA, sensory hypersensitivity
HIV	HPA, cytokines
CHD	Cytokines and the brain
Cancer	Cytokines and the brain
TBI	HPA
CFS	Basal ganglia, HPA, frontal lobes, NT
Depression	HPA, cytokines and the brain, limbic–frontal abnormalities
Lupus	Cytokines and the brain
MS	Basal ganglia, thalamus, demyelination, HPA, cytokines, NT
Sleep	Basal ganglia, frontal lobes
Immune disorders	Cytokines and the brain, HPA, NT

HPA, hypothalamic-pituitary-adrenal axis; NT, neurotransmitter systems.

Given these data, what can be proposed? Fatigue is likely the consequence of an interaction between environmental factors such as trauma or stress, and complex physiological activity. As such, consider the following model. Environmental factors can result in a flurry of physiological activity, including cytokine release. Proinflamatory cytokines stimulate HPA activation and neurotransmitter activity. It is also well known that the basal ganglia is particularly vulnerable to multiple insults such as hypoxia, alterations in neurotransmitter balance, and proinflammatory cytokines (Chaudhuri & Behan, 2000). Thus, the basal ganglia may be susceptible to acute or chronic endogenous or exogenous activity and is believed to play a key role in central fatigue. Further, frontal lobe involvement in central fatigue may be secondary to the "association or complex loop" of the basal ganglia, which projects to the prefrontal cortex (striatocortical fibers) while involving the thalamus via a striatothalamocortical loop. A reduction in neurotransmitter activity in the pallidothalamocortical loop is hypothesized to suppress frontal lobe activation. This mechanism of action, involving failure of the nonmotor functions of the basal ganglia, is what Chaudhuri and Behan (2000) propose as the genesis of central fatigue.

Does this proposed mechanism of central fatigue explain the subjective fatigue associated with mental or physical work in clinical populations? Perhaps a new paradigm is needed to understand fatigue.

Table 19.3
Potential mechanisms of fatigue

Primary fatigue: Specific biological mechanisms
Disease activity
Hypothalamic-pituitary-adrenal axis abnormalities
Tryptophan and serotonin
Cytokines
Comorbid medical conditions (e.g., anemia, hypo/hyperthyroidism)
Secondary fatigue: General mechanisms
Deconditioning
Psychological factors (depression, anxiety, perception)
Sleep
Pain
Stress

Adapted from Wessley et al., 1998.

Proposed Study of Primary versus Secondary Fatigue

Perhaps in the broadest sense, we have learned that fatigue may be initiated by factors (e.g., systemic disease) different from those that perpetuate or exacerbate it (Wessely et al., 1998). Physical illness such as MS and CHD may cause the initial symptoms of fatigue through specific biological mechanisms; however, the fatigue symptom may be exacerbated by secondary factors such as deconditioning, sleep disturbance, depression, and pain (table 19.3). These secondary mechanisms are likely associated primarily with the *feeling* of fatigue, and it is this nonspecific feeling that is evaluated in scientific and medical studies of fatigue. The use of such a broad and subjective measure is probably the major reason why disease activity, across most illnesses, does not correlate with objective or behavioral measure of fatigue (Wessely et al., 1998). Until more research focuses on identifying specific or primary mechanisms of fatigue and accounting for the effects of secondary factors, our understanding of fatigue will remain vague, broad, and nonspecific. This approach would simply be unacceptable in other areas of medicine, psychology, and science and should not be for the study of fatigue.

In this light, it is proposed that the future research or clinical study of fatigue acknowledge two new constructs: primary fatigue and secondary fatigue. Primary fatigue is fatigue caused by its primary neural mechanisms. Examples of measures of primary fatigue are: decreases in cognitive performance during sustained cognitive challenges (see chapter 3), changes in basal ganglia activation during fatigue-producing activity, HPA-related activity (e.g., prolactin, 5-HT), and cytokine activity.

Secondary fatigue includes factors that exacerbate its effects (e.g., deconditioning, sleep habits, medication). Peripheral and central fatigue are subsets of primary fatigue in this theoretically based schema. It is incumbent on future research studies to clearly identify whether they are assessing primary or secondary fatigue (or both).

Of course, this proposal is not perfect. For instance, subjective ratings of fatigue may actually reflect both primary and secondary mechanisms responsible for fatigue. However, with over 100 years of research consistently demonstrating the lack of a clear relationship between objective and subjective assessments of fatigue, it is time to claim that the evidence is "in" and propose primary versus secondary fatigue as a legitimate construct, for hypothesis testing and scientific scrutiny. How can the construct of primary and secondary fatigue be useful? Consider just one scenario. The relationship between subjective and objective assessments of fatigue can be used as a theoretical basis for identifying primary versus secondary mechanisms of fatigue. The degree to which objective and subjective measurements of fatigue correlate can potentially be a gauge for assessing primary fatigue, with close agreement indicating primary mechanisms of fatigue while the absence of a relationship suggests secondary fatigue is being measured.

The relative utility of the primary versus secondary fatigue concept must await future investigation. However, one thing is certain, the existing measurement method and understanding of fatigue is obsolete. It is time for a paradigm shift, and the current proposal is likely the best available at this time.

Conclusion

The convergence of work in this volume leaves little doubt that the experience of fatigue is a manifestation of functional brain activity. It is time for a renewed effort toward the investigation of fatigue, its specific mechanism, and its treatment. It is hoped that this book will be the first step toward a new science of fatigue.

References

Berrios, G. E. (1990). Feelings of fatigue and psychopathology: a conceptual history. *Comprehensive Psychiatry*, *31(2)*, 140–151.

Chaudhuri, A., & Behan, P. O. (2000). Fatigue and basal ganglia. *Journal of Neurological Sciences*, *179*, 34–42.

Heesen, C., Gold, S. M., Raji, A., Wiedemann, K., & Schulz, K. H. (2002). Cognitive impairment correlates with hypothalamo-pituitary-adrenal axis dysregulation in multiple sclerosis. *Psychoneuroendocrinology*, *27*, 505–517.

Mosso, A. (1904). *Fatigue*. London: Swan Sonnenschein and Co.

Multiple Sclerosis Council for Clinical Practice Guidelines (1998). Fatigue and multiple sclerosis: evidence-based management strategies for fatigue in multiple sclerosis. Paralyzed Veterans of America.

Waller, A. D. (1891). The sense of effort: An objective study. *Brain, 14*, 179–249.

Wessely, S., Hotopf, M., & Sharpe, M. (1998). *Chronic Fatigue and Its Syndromes*. Oxford: Oxford University Press.

Contributors

Lesley A. Allen, PhD Assistant Professor of Psychiatry, University of Medicine and Dentistry of New Jersey–Robert Wood Johnson Medical School, Piscataway, New Jersey

Gijs Bleijenberg, PhD Professor of Psychology, Expert Center for Chronic Fatigue, University Medical Center Nijmegen, Nijmegen, The Netherlands

William Breitbart, MD Professor of Psychiatry and Behavioral Sciences, Memorial Sloan-Kettering Cancer Center, New York, New York

Christopher Christodoulou, PhD Assistant Professor of Neurology, State University of New York at Stony Brook, Stony Brook, New York

Dane B. Cook, PhD Assistant Professor of Radiology, University of Medicine and Dentistry of New Jersey–New Jersey Medical School, Newark, New Jersey, Health Science Specialist, War-Related Illness and Injury Study Center, New Jersey VA Health Care System, East Orange, New Jersey

John DeLuca, PhD Professor of Physical Medicine and Rehabilitation, University of Medicine and Dentistry of New Jersey–New Jersey Medical School, Newark, New Jersey, Director of Neuroscience Research, Kessler Medical Rehabilitation Research and Education Corporation, West Orange, New Jersey

Kristine A. Donovan, PhD Psychologist, Psychosocial and Palliative Care Program, H. Lee Moffitt Cancer Center and Research Institute, Tampa, Florida

Benoit Dubé, MD, FRCPC Instructor of Psychiatry, University of Pennsylvania School of Medicine, Philadelphia, Pennsylvania, Attending Psychiatrist, Immunodeficiency Program, Hospital of the University of Pennsylvania, Philadelphia, Pennsylvania

Natasha Dufour, MD, FRCPC Clinical Fellow, Department of Psychiatry and Behavioral Sciences, Memorial Sloan-Kettering Cancer Center, New York, New York

Stephen P. Duntley, MD Associate Professor of Neurology, Washington University School of Medicine, St. Louis, Missouri

Elie P. Elovic, MD Associate Professor of Physical Medicine and Rehabilitation, University of Medicine and Dentistry of New Jersey–New Jersey Medical School, Newark, New Jersey; Director of Traumatic Brain Injury Research, Kessler Medical Rehabilitation Research and Education Corporation, West Orange, New Jersey

Javier I. Escobar, MD Professor of Psychiatry, University of Medicine and Dentistry of New Jersey–Robert Wood Johnson Medical School, Piscataway, New Jersey

Luciano Fasotti, PhD Research Department, Rehabilitation Center St Maartenskliniek, Nijmegen, The Netherlands

Jonathan L. Fellus, MD Director of Brain Injury Services, Kessler Institute for Rehabilitation, East Orange, New Jersey

Mary Ann Fletcher PhD Professor of Medicine, University of Miami School of Medicine, Miami, Florida

Susan Torres-Harding, PhD Project Director, Center for Community Research, DePaul University, Chicago, Illinois

Paul B. Jacobsen, PhD Program Leader, Psychosocial and Palliative Care Program, H. Lee Moffitt Cancer Center and Research Institute, Tampa, Florida

Leonard A. Jason, PhD Professor of Psychology, Director, Center for Community Research, DePaul University, Chicago, Illinois

Susan K. Johnson, PhD Associate Professor of Psychology, University of North Carolina at Charlotte, Charlotte, North Carolina

Nancy Klimas MD Professor of Medicine, Universityof Miami School of Medicine, Director, AIDS Research Miami VAMC, Miami, Florida

Elizabeth Kozora, PhD Associate Professor of Medicine, Department of Medicine, National Jewish Medical and Research Center, Associate Professor of Psychiatry, University of Colorado Health Sciences Center, Denver, Colorado

Lauren B. Krupp, MD Professor of Neurology, State University of New York at Stony Brook, Stony Brook, New York

Gudrun Lange, PhD Associate Professor of Psychiatry and Radiology, University of Medicine and Dentistry of New Jersey–New Jersey Medical School, Newark, New Jersey, Associate Director of Education, War-Related Illness and Injury Study Center, New Jersey VA Health Care System, East Orange, New Jersey

Rasha Lawrence MD Research Associate, University of Miami School of Medicine, Miami, Florida

Kevin Maher PhD Assistant Professor of Medicine, University of Miami School of Medicine, Miami, Florida

Benjamin H. Natelson, MD Professor of Neuroscience, University of Medicine and Dentistry of New Jersey–New Jersey Medical School, Newark, New Jersey, Director, War-Related Illness and Injury Study Center, New Jersey VA Health Care System, East Orange, New Jersey

Wahid Rashidzada, MD Postdoctoral Fellow, Department of Physical Medicine and Rehabilitation, University of Medicine and Dentistry of New Jersey–New Jersey Medical School, Newark, New Jersey

Scott Siegel, MA   Graduate student, Clinical Health Psychology, University of Miami, Miami, Florida

Neil Schneiderman, PhD   Professor of Psychology, Director, Behavioral Medicine Research Center, University of Miami, Miami, Florida

Harold Schombert, JD   Thought Leaders Communications, Washington, DC

Edward Shorter, PhD, FRSC   Professor of the History of Medicine, University of Toronto, Toronto, Canada

Maja Stulemeijer, MS   Doctoral student, Expert Center for Chronic Fatigue, University Medical Center Nijmegen, Nijmegen, The Netherlands

Simon Wessely, MA, MSc, MRCP., MRC. Psych   Dept of Psychological Medicine, Institute of Psychiatry and King's College London, London, United Kingdom

Index

Page numbers followed by *f* indicate figures; page numbers followed by *t* indicate tables.